AF606296

WITHDRAWN FROM STOCK

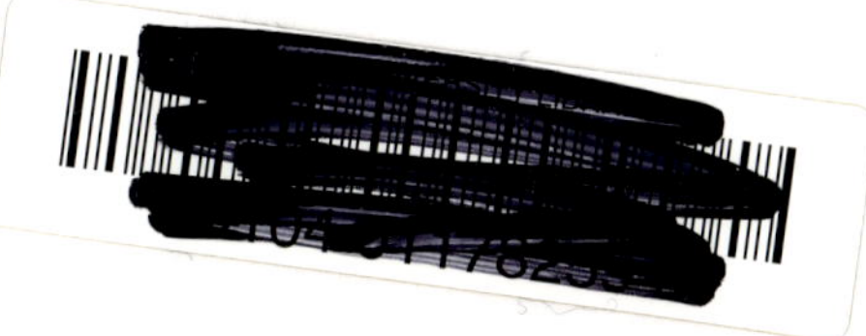

Helicobacter pylori Infection and Immunity

INFECTIOUS AGENTS AND PATHOGENESIS

Series Editors: Mauro Bendinelli, *University of Pisa*
Herman Friedman, *University of South Florida College of Medicine*

Recent volumes in this series:

DNA TUMOR VIRUSES
Oncogenic Mechanisms
Edited by Giuseppe Barbanti-Brodano, Mauro Bendinelli, and Herman Friedman

ENTERIC INFECTIONS AND IMMUNITY
Edited by Lois J. Paradise, Mauro Bendinelli, and Herman Friedman

HELICOBACTER PYLORI INFECTION AND IMMUNITY
Edited by Yoshimasa Yamamoto, Herman Friedman, and Paul S. Hoffman

HERPESVIRUSES AND IMMUNITY
Edited by Peter G. Medveczky, Herman Friedman, and Mauro Bendinelli

HUMAN RETROVIRAL INFECTIONS
Immunological and Therapeutic Control
Edited by Kenneth E. Ugen, Mauro Bendinelli, and Herman Friedman

MICROORGANISMS AND AUTOIMMUNE DISEASES
Edited by Herman Friedman, Noel R. Rose, and Mauro Bendinelli

OPPORTUNISTIC INTRACELLULAR BACTERIA AND IMMUNITY
Edited by Lois J. Paradise, Herman Friedman, and Mauro Bendinelli

PSEUDOMONAS AERUGINOSA AS AN OPPORTUNISTIC PATHOGEN
Edited by Mario Campa, Mauro Bendinelli, and Herman Friedman

PULMONARY INFECTIONS AND IMMUNITY
Edited by Herman Chmel, Mauro Bendinelli, and Herman Friedman

RAPID DETECTION OF INFECTIOUS AGENTS
Edited by Steven Specter, Mauro Bendinelli, and Herman Friedman

RICKETTSIAL INFECTION AND IMMUNITY
Edited by Burt Anderson, Herman Friedman, and Mauro Bendinelli

STAPHYLOCOCCUS AUREUS INFECTION AND DISEASE
Edited by Allen L. Honeyman, Herman Friedman, and Mauro Bendinelli

---

Helicobacter pylori Infection and Immunity

Edited by

Yoshimasa Yamamoto
University of South Florida College of Medicine
Tampa, Florida

Herman Friedman
University of South Florida College of Medicine
Tampa, Florida

and

Paul S. Hoffman
Dalhousie University
Halifax, Nova Scotia, Canada

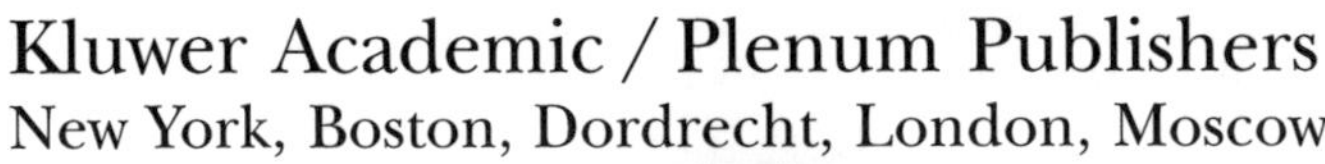

Kluwer Academic / Plenum Publishers
New York, Boston, Dordrecht, London, Moscow

Library of Congress Cataloging-in-Publication Data

Helicobacter pylori infection and immunity/edited by Yoshimasa Yamamoto, Herman Friedman and Paul Hoffman.
p. ; cm. — (Infectious agents and pathogenesis)
Includes bibliographical references and index.
ISBN 0-306-46658-9
1. Helicobacter pylori infections. 2. Helicobacter pylori infections—Immunological aspects. I. Yamamoto, Yoshimasa II. Friedman, Herman, 1931– III. Hoffman, Paul S. IV. Series.
[DNLM: 1. Helicobacter pylori—immunology. 2. Gastritis—parasitology. 3. Helicobacter Infections—drug therapy. 4. Helicobacter Infections—immunology. 5. Helicobacter Infections—pathology. 6. Helicobacter pylori—pathogenicity. QW 154 H4572 2001]
QR201.H44 H463 2002
616′.01423—dc21

2001038408

ISBN: 0-306-46658-9

233 Spring Street, New York, NY 10013

http://www.wkap.nl/

10 9 8 7 6 5 4 3 2 1

A C.I.P. record for this book is available from the Library of Congress

Printed in the United States of America

Contributors

BEN J. APPELMELK • Department of Medical Microbiology, Vrije Universiteit, Amsterdam, The Netherlands

INGRID L. BERGIN • Division of Comparative Medicine, Massachusetts Institute of Technology, Cambridge, MA 02139

THOMAS G. BLANCHARD • Department of Pediatrics, Division of Pediatric Gastroenterology, Case Western Reserve University School of Medicine and Rainbow Babies and Children's Hospital, Cleveland, OH 44106

PELAYO CORREA • Pathology, Louisiana State University Health Sciences Center, New Orleans, LA

JEAN E. CRABTREE • Molecular Medicine Unit, St. James University Hospital, Leeds LS9 7TF, United Kingdom

STEVEN J. CZINN • Department of Pediatrics, Division of Pediatric Gastroenterology, Case Western Reserve University School of Medicine and Rainbow Babies and Children's Hospital, Cleveland, OH 44106

STANLEY FALKOW • Department of Microbiology and Immunology, Stanford University, Stanford, CA

GERHARD FALLER • Department of Pathology, University Erlangen, Erlangen, Germany

JAMES G. FOX • Division of Comparative Medicine, Massachusetts Institute of Technology, Cambridge, MA 02139

YOSHIHIRO FUKUDA • Internal Medicine, Hyogo College of Medicine, Nishinomiya, Hyogo 663-8501, Japan

BENJAMIN D. GOLD • Division of Pediatric Gastroenterology and Nutrition, Department of Pediatrics, Emory University School of Medicine, Children's Healthcare of Atlanta at Egleston Children's Hospital, Foodborne and Diarrheal Disease Branch, Division of Bacterial and Mycotic Diseases, National Center for Infectious Diseases, Centers for Disease Control and Prevention, Atlanta, GA

PAUL S. HOFFMAN • Departments of Microbiology and Immunology and Medicine, Division of Infectious Diseases, Dalhousie University, Halifax, Nova Scotia B3H4H7, Canada

JIA-QING HUANG • Division of Gastroenterology, Department of Medicine, McMaster University Medical Center, Hamilton, Ont., Canada L8N 3Z5

RICHARD H. HUNT • Division of Gastroenterology, Department of Medicine, McMaster University Medical Center, Hamilton, Ont., Canada L8N 3Z5

SHIGERU KAMIYA • Department of Microbiology, Kyorin University School of Medicine, Mitaka, Tokyo 181-8611, Japan

FRANCIS MEGRAUD • Laboratoire de Bacteriologie, Hopital Pellegrin, Bordeaux, France

TAMARA MATYSIAK • INSERM E9925, Faculte Necker—Enfants Malades, Paris, France

STEVEN F. MOSS • Department of Medicine, St. Luke's Roosevelt Hospital Center/Columbia University, New York, NY 10025

KAREN M. OTTERMAN • Department of Biology and Environmental Toxicology, University of California at Santa Cruz, Santa Cruz, CA

TAKASHI SAKAGAMI • Internal Medicine, Hyogo College of Medicine, Nishinomiya, Hyogo 663-8501, Japan

NINA R. SALAMA • Department of Microbiology and Immunology, Stanford University, Stanford, CA

HIROKO SASHIO • Institute Advanced Medical Sciences, Laboratory Hereditary Tumor, Hyogo College of Medicine, Hyogo 663-8501, Japan

YUKIO SAWADA • Internal Medicine, Hyogo College of Medicine, Nishinomiya, Hyogo 663-8501, Japan

PHILIP M. SHERMAN • Division of Pediatric Gastroenterology and Nutrition, The Hospital for Sick Children, Department of Pediatrics, University of Toronto, Toronto, Ont., Canada

TAKASHI SHIMOYAMA • Internal Medicine, Hyogo College of Medicine, Nishinomiya, Hyogo 663-8501, Japan

EMILIA MIA SORDILLO • Department of Pathology and Laboratory Medicine, and Department of Medicine, St. Luke's Roosevelt Hospital Center/Columbia University, New York, NY 10025

KAZUO TAMURA • Institute Advanced Medical Sciences, Laboratory Hereditary Tumor, Hyogo College of Medicine, Hyogo 663-8501, Japan

NORITOSHI TANIDA • Internal Medicine, Hyogo College of Medicine, Nishinomiya, Hyogo 663-8501, Japan

DIANE E. TAYLOR • Department of Medical Microbiology and Immunology, University of Alberta, Edmonton, Alberta, Canada T6G 2H7

CHRISTINA M. J. E. VANDENBROUCKE-GRAULS • Department of Medical Microbiology, Vrije Universiteit, Amsterdam, The Netherlands

GE WANG • Department of Medical Microbiology and Immunology, University of Alberta, Edmonton, Alberta, Canada T6G 2H7

HIROYUKI YAMAGUCHI • Department of Microbiology, Kyorin University School of Medicine, Mitaka, Tokyo 181-8611, Japan

NORIYASU YAMAMOTO • Internal Medicine, Hyogo College of Medicine, Nishinomiya, Hyogo 663-8501, Japan

YOSHIMASA YAMAMOTO • Department of Medical Microbiology and Immunology, University of South Florida College of Medicine, Tampa, FL 33612

Preface to the Series

The mechanisms of disease production by infectious agents are presently the focus of an unprecedented flowering of studies. The field has undoubtedly received impetus from the considerable advances recently made in the understanding of the structure, biochemistry, and biology of viruses, bacteria, fungi, and other parasites. Another contributing factor is our improved knowledge of immune responses and other adaptive or constitutive mechanisms by which hosts react to infection. Furthermore, recombinant DNA technology, monoclonal antibodies, and other newer methodologies have provided the technical tools for examining questions previously considered too complex to be successfully tackled. The most important incentive of all is probably the regenerated idea that infection might be the initiating event in many clinical entities presently classified as idiopathic or of uncertain origin.

Infectious pathogenesis research holds great promise. As more information is uncovered, it is becoming increasingly apparent that our present knowledge of the pathogenic potential of infectious agents is often limited to the most noticeable effects, which sometimes represent only the tip of the iceberg. For example, it is now well appreciated that pathologic processes caused by infectious agents may emerge clinically after an incubation of decades and may result from genetic, immunologic, and other indirect routes more than from the infecting agent in itself. Thus, there is a general expectation that continued investigation will lead to the isolation of new agents of infection, the identification of hitherto unsuspected etiologic correlations, and, eventually, more effective approaches to prevention and therapy.

Studies on the mechanisms of disease caused by infectious agents demand a breadth of understanding across many specialized areas, as well as much cooperation between clinicians and experimentalists. The series *Infectious Agents and Pathogenesis* is intended not only to document the state of the art in this fascinating and challenging field but also to help lay bridges among diverse areas and people.

M. Bendinelli
H. Friedman

Preface

The discovery and concept that *Helicobacter pylori* is associated with gastric disease including gastric cancer which is one of the most common and frequently lethal forms of malignancy, heralded a new and rapidly expanding field recognizing the emergence of many new pathogens and disease syndromes in clinical medicine, as well as basic infectious disease research. There is now an extensive and widely known literature of how *H. pylori* is involved in a wide variety of disease syndromes. As summarized in the introductory chapter of this volume, many major advances have been made in diagnosis, both serologic and endoscopic in time of the involvement of this organism in patients with upper GI ailments as well as its presence in those who are not clinically ill. The Introduction describes the rapid development of understanding the role of this organism in disease.

The basic bacteriology of *H. pylori* is then described in the second chapter. Diagnostic tests for detecting *H. pylori* infection is then highlighted, as well as the role of such infection in gastric cancer. Current knowledge concerning risk factors and peptic ulcer pathology associated with *H. pylori* is then described. Newer information concerning therapy of *H. pylori* infection and colonization is described in a subsequent chapter as well as one concerning the effects of antibiotics on *H. pylori* infection. The extensive literature on natural substances with anti-*H. pylori* activity is then described, followed by a chapter dealing with newer knowledge concerning how this microorganism binds to gastric cells. The involvement of *H. pylori* in autoimmune diseases is then described as well as the pathogenesis of how this organism is related to diseases. The effects of toxins by the organism on host cells as well as development of animal models for *H. pylori* infection studies is described, followed by a review of development of a gerbil model for *H. pylori* infection. New information concerning development of a vaccine against Helicobacter is also presented in the final chapter.

It is anticipated by the editors as well as the authors of the individual chapters, who represent cutting edge laboratories from this country as well as many other countries, that this book will provide useful and valuable information concerning the current status of immunologic, microbiologic, as well as therapeutic prevention studies against the important human pathogen *H. pylori.* The Editors thank Ms. Ilona Friedman for excellent editorial assistance in coordinating and assisting in the preparation of the manuscripts for this volume in this series.

Paul Hoffman
Yoshimasa Yamamoto
Herman Friedman

Contents

7. **Anti-*Helicobacter pylori* Activity of Natural Substances**

YOSHIMASA YAMAMOTO

8. **Adherence of *Helicobacter pylori* to Gastric Cell**

SHIGERU KAMIYA AND HIROYUKI YAMAGUCHI

Introduction and Perspectives

PAUL HOFFMAN

The latter quarter of the 20th century saw the emergence of many new pathogens or disease syndromes, including Legionnaires' disease, toxic shock syndrome, Lyme disease, and AIDS; but perhaps the most surprising finding was that a microbe (*Helicobacter pylori*) was associated with duodenal and gastric ulcers. Prior to the findings of Warren and Marshall in 1983[1] and until general acceptance of the finding by the 90's, most believed that ulcers were due to life style, behavior type, or diet. Interestingly, the spiral-shaped microaerobic bacteria associated with gastric biopsy material had been previously observed at the beginning of the century, but the association with gastric disease was never established. *Helicobacter pylori* became the subject of one of the most intensive investigations in the history of medicine as new knowledge revealed that half or more of all people world-wide are infected by this organism and life long infection is a proven risk-factor in development of gastric cancer, one of the most common and frequently lethal of all cancers. The pharmaceutical industry, once the benefactors of billion dollar ulcer treatment therapeutics (Zantac, Tagamet, Tums and Rolaids to mention a few), now focused on development of new antimicrobials for the potentially worldwide market, while others focused on development of diagnostic tools from endoscopic devices to rapid diagnostic kits for singling out those for eradicative therapy. Pharmaceutical companies provided unprecedented levels of financial support to this area, and were a driving force behind many of the new

PAUL HOFFMAN • Department of Microbiology and Immunology, Dalhousie University, Halifax, Nova Scotia B3H 4H7, CANADA.

Helicobacter pylori Infection and Immunity,
Edited by Yamamoto *et al.*, Kluwer Academic/Plenum Publishers, 2002.

technologies (genomics, bioinformatics and proteomics) that have contributed to characterization of *H. pylori*. Population biology and microbial ecology have also contributed substantially to our understanding of strains and diversity. More recently we have learned that nearly all mammals harbor their own species of *Helicobacter*[2] and some are suggesting now that infection might be benign or even beneficial by protecting against development of esophageal reflux and cancer of the esophagus.[3]

Helicobacter pylori often establishes life long infections of the gastric mucosa, a site generally considered as sterile only a few decades ago, which raises many fundamental questions as to how it persists in this niche, how it survives stomach acid, and why the host immune system, while recognizing the presence of infection, seems incapable of mounting an eradicative immune response. Understanding persistence and host immune response is key to vaccine strategies, be it protective or therapeutic. Physiological studies reveal that *H. pylori* is unremarkable in its resistance to acid,[4] being no more resistant than *Escherichia coli*. The bacteria produce a powerful urease that is regulated in response to acid,[4] so that the ammonia and carbonate produced by this enzyme most likely create a microenvironment that is alkaline, something no other studied pathogen seems capable of doing. Further study shows that the densest colonization by *H. pylori* occurs in the antrum (lower portion of the stomach) where conditions are less acidic. As the infection becomes more pronounced, or under conditions where the antrum becomes more alkaline (e.g., acid suppressive therapeutics like proton pump inhibitors and H2-blockers), the motile bacteria migrate up into the cardia (body) of the stomach. Infection with *H. pylori* bacteria is basically in three dimensions, as these bacteria not only can move north and south in the mucosa in response to acid levels, but they are able to move freely up and down in the mucus layer that coats the gastric mucosa and provides a protective barrier against the diffusion of strong acid onto the epithelium. The notion of being "off shore" and therefore out of reach of the macrophages and cells of host immune defense may also play an important role in survival. Finally, mounting evidence suggests that *H. pylori* may control the immune response through mimicry (LPS displaying Lewis antigens) and selective release of inflammatory factors. The balance between promotion of inflammation and immune suppression are a key to persistence and an area where novel therapeutics, perhaps in combination with vaccine strategies, could be directed.

The discovery of and extreme interest in *Helicobacter*, a relative of *Campylobacter* (bacterial pathogens of the lower GI tract), fortunately coincided with the beginning of the genomics era, and is the beneficiary of two completely sequenced genomes of *H. pylori*.[5,6] The results reveal a small genome (1.67 megabases) containing some 1553 genes encoding around 1,300 proteins. Despite possessing a limited number of genes, *H. pylori* displays auxotropy for only a few amino acids and appears to possess most catabolic and anabolic pathways found in bacteria with larger genomes. Recent studies examining essentiality testing on a genome scale suggested that there are few redundancies and backups in metabolic pathways and thus the percentage of *H. pylori* genes found essential may be greater than expected for organisms with larger genomes, perhaps opening a door for development of *Helicobacter* selective therapeutics.[7] Other caveats from genome gazing is that there are few regulatory genes, particularly two component signal transduction systems, that are so typical of enteric bacteria and many pathogens, perhaps suggesting that other than acid and related stresses, *H. pylori* has little else to worry about in its gastric niche.[8,9,10]

Major interest has focused on genes clustered in a pathogenicity island (PAI) that are associated with strains causing more pathology and gastric manifestations. These CagA positive strains (Cytotoxin associated gene) possess a 40 kilobase region encoding genes with orthologs in the type IV secretion and pathogenesis system of *Agrobacterium* and *Bordetella pertussis* to mention a few.[11] The CagA gene is located at one end of the PAI and serves as a marker for Cag status. Strains lacking the Cag PAI are characterized as less virulent as indicated by colonization at lower microbial densities and producing less inflammation than Cag^+ strains. However, there is still debate over relative association with ulcers and more severe disease. Genes within the Cag PAI promote secretion of a vaculating cytotoxin protein (VacA) whose gene is located outside of the Cag locus. Recently, studies show that the Cag PAI is also responsible for delivery of the CagA protein into mammalian cells and that this protein exhibits tyrosine phosphatase activity.[12] Thus these toxins are considered important in the pathogenesis and severity of disease.

New applications of bioinformatics and proteomics have also contributed to expanded knowledge of protein interactions[13] and assignment of function to many of the *H. pylori* genes whose function is unknown. As more microbial genomes become available and annotated, it is likely that more of the unknown genes will be assigned a biological function. Also anticipated is that selected DNA sequencing from a wide range of strains that are geographically distinct will provide information on genetic diversity of this species. Population biological studies have established genetic differences among European and Asian strains and these warrant further study as the information might be applied to selective therapeutics for strains from a particular region.[14] Other areas of study that will develop in the future will include study of genes common to microaerophiles such as those common between *H. pylori* and *Campylobacter jejuni*, but unique from those of other microbes, might be exploited more generally for therapeutics or vaccines applicable to eliminating these organisms not only from man but from fowl (common reservoir for *Campylobacter*).

Advancements in diagnostics, both serologic, stool antigen test, and invasive (endoscopy) have led to sorting of infected people with upper GI ailments from those who are uninfected. Studies now show that nearly 35% of the world's population suffers from dyspepsia, but only 5 to 20% of these individuals are also infected with *H. pylori.* In western societies, even fewer are infected with more severe CagA strains and in either case, studies have shown that eradication of *H. pylori* infection may not necessarily resolve dyspeptic symptoms.[15] Thus, general practitioners tend not to investigate the basis for dyspepsia and often simply treat the symptoms with anti-acids and or acid secretion blockers. The assumption that *H. pylori* infection is rather benign—particularly in western societies where gastric cancer is rare in the first place (10 on the list of cancers in the US for example)—seems to justify the practice. Where alarm symptoms are noted, referral to a specialist and further investigation by endoscopy is generally pursued. As mentioned earlier, the worry over cure of *H. pylori* and the subsequent development of gastric esophageal reflux disease (GERD) has raised concerns among physicians and the notion that the only good *Helicobacter* is a dead one, has been challenged. It is not clear what the future will bring, but given that 75 to 80% of North Americans are or never were infected with *H. pylori*, needs to be considered in this argument. Are they now at greater risk of developing GERD? Of the remaining 20–23% that are infected in North America, are they more likely upon cure to have a different outcome than those who have never been infected.

Much of the concern associated with whether to treat or not stems from the fact that treatment regimes have variable outcomes. While *H. pylori* is susceptible to a large variety of antimicrobials in vitro, the therapeutic activity in the gastric milieu is often nil and monotherapies have generally demonstrated poor efficacy. The most common practice is to use combinations of drugs, the so called triple or quadruple therapies containing amoxicillin, macrolides like clarithromycin, and or nitroimidazoles like metronidazole in combination with proton pump inhibitors (omeprazole) that reduce acidity and improving therapeutic action of the antimicrobials.[16] Treatments can also contain bismuth salts and tetracycline. The fact that all the current therapeutic agents are old drugs and generally of broad spectrum has alarmed many who do not understand why the pharmaceutical industry has not developed novel therapeutics specifically for treating *Helicobacter* infections. Unfortunately, despite the obvious need, the drug industry market analyses show a rather small market and one that is disappearing—reinfection rates are so low in developed countries that patients would only be treated once and the market would eventually disappear. The need for new therapeutics is still very real for developing countries where resistance to metronidazole and macrolides renders many current therapeutics nearly useless. Unfortunately, the cost of drug development could never be recouped through sales in these markets where need is greatest. In western societies, the educational initiatives associated with efforts to reduce the wide spread practice of prescribing antibiotics have succeeded in that many physicians are reluctant to prescribe first line broad spectrum antibiotics for treatment of non-life threatening infections as *H. pylori* out of fear of contributing to drug resistance.

Animal models of infection, particularly the mouse model and Mongolian gerbil have permitted investigators to follow the course of infection and to examine antimicrobial efficacy and vaccine candidates. The distribution of cytokines and chemokines in the mouse model during infection has yielded much new information on mucosal inflammatory responses. Vaccine strategies using subunits of the urease have shown some promise, but often require toxin adjuvants that will likely never be used in humans. Animal studies with *H. felis*, which produces greater inflammation than *H. pylori* in the mouse model, has yielded much more information on inflammation and development of gastritis.[17] Studies with other species of *Helicobacter* in animals implicate the microbes in other diseases including liver diseases and lower GI diseases such as inflammatory bowel disease. These models my lead to new developments in diseases other than gastritis and stomach ulcers.

The chapters that follow provide state of the art information in many areas of current interest in this exciting field. The authors accurately convey information and where controversies abound, present a balanced view. There are many areas where information is rapidly advancing in diagnostics, genomics and in disease management. There is still much to learn in areas of persistence, vaccine development, and in the basic biology of *Helicobacter* and its activities in the gastric mucosa. It is hoped that readers will be stimulated by historical aspects and as well become motivated by the many existing gaps in knowledge to join the many who are investigating this fascinating microbe.

REFERENCES

1. Warren J. R., and Marshall B., 1983, Unified curved bacilli on gastric epithelium in active chronic gastritis. *Lancet.* **1**:1273–1275.
2. Dewhirst F. E., Fox J. G., and On S. L., 2000, Recommended minimal standards for describing new species of the genus *Helicobacter. Int. J. Syst. Evol. Microbiol.* **6**:2231.
3. Loffeld R. J., Werdmuller B. F., Kusters J. G., Perez-Perez G. I., Blaser M. J., and Kuipers E. J., 2000, Colonization with cagA-positive *Helicobacter pylori* strains inversely associated with reflux esophagitis and Barrett's esophagus. *Digestion.* **62**:95.
4. Scott D. R., Marcus E. A., Weeks D. L., Lee A., Melchers K., and Sachs G., 2000, Expression of the *Helicobacter pylori ureI* gene is required for acidic pH activation of cytoplasmic urease. *Infect. Immun.* **68**:470.
5. Tomb J. F., White O., Kerlavage A. R., Clayton R. A., Sutton G. G., Fleischmann R. D., Ketchum K., Klenk H., Gill S., Dougherty B., Nelson K., Quackenbush J., Zhou L., Kirkness E., Peterson S., Loftus B., Richardson D., Dodson R., Khalak H., Glodek A., McKenney K., Fitzegerald L., Lee N., Adams M., Hickey E., Berg D., Gocayne J., Utterback T., Peterson J., Kelley J., Cotton M., Weidman J., Fujii C., Bowman C., Watthey L., Wallin E., Hayes W., Borodovsky M., Karp P., Smith H., Fraser C., and Venter J., 1997, The complete genome sequence of the gastric pathogen *Helicobacter pylori. Nature* **388**:539–547.
6. Alm R. A., Ling L. S., Moir D. T., King B. L., Brown E. D., Doig P. C., Smith D. R., Noonan B., Guild B. C., deJonge B. L., Carmel G., Tummino P. J., Caruso A., Uria-Nickelsen M., Mills D. M., Ives C., Gibson R., Merberg D., Mills S. D., Jiang Q., Taylor D. E., Vovis G. F., and Trust T. J., 1999, Genomic-sequence comparison of two unrelated isolates of the human gastric pathogen *Helicobacter. pylori. Nature* **397**:176–180.

7. Chalker A. F., Minehart H. W., Hughes N. J., Koretke K. K., Lonetto M. A., Brinkman K. K., Warren P. V., Lupas A., Stanhope M. J., Brown J. R., and Hoffman P. S., 2001, Systematic identification of selective essential genes in *Helicobacter pylori* by genome prioritization and allelic replacement mutagenesis. *J. Bacteriol.* **183**:1259.
8. Berg D. E., Hoffman P. S., Appelmelk B. J., and Kusters J. G., 1997, The *Helicobacter pylori* genome sequence: genetic factors for a long life in the gastric mucosa. *Trends Microbiol.* **13**:468–474.
9. Marais A., Mendz G. L., Hazell S. L., and Megraud F., 1999, Metabolism and genetics of *Helicobacter pylori*: the genome era. *Microbiol. Mol. Biol. Rev.* **63**:642–674.
10. Doig P., De Jonge B. L., Alm R. A., Brown E. D., Uria-Nickelsen M., Noonan B., Mills S. D., Tummino P., Carmel G., Guild B. C., Moir D. T., Vovis G. F., and Trust T. J. 1999, Helicobacter pylori physiology predicted from genomic comparison of two strains. *Microbiol. Mol. Biol. Rev.* **63**:675.
11. Censini S., Lange C., Xiang Z., *et al.*, 1996 *cag*, a pathogenicity island of *Helicobacter pylori*, encodes Type I-specific and disease-associated virulence factors. *Proc. Natl. Acad. Sci., USA* **93**:14648.
12. Odenbreit S., Puls J., Sedlmaier B., Gerland E., Fischer W., and Haas R., 2000, Translocation of *Helicobacter pylori* CagA into gastric epithelial cells by type IV secretion. *Science* **287**:1497.
13. Rain J.-C., Selig L., De Reuse H., Battagila V., Reverdy C., Simon S., Lenzen G., Petel F., Wojcik J., Schachter V., Chemama Y., Labigne A., and Legrain P., 2001, The protein-protein interaction map of *Helicobacter. pylori. Nature* **409**:211.
14. Kersulyte D., Mukhopadhyay A. K., Velapatino B., Su W., Pan Z., Garcia C., Hernandez V., Valdez Y., Mistry R. S., Gilman R. H., Yuan Y., Gao H., Alarcon T., Lopez-Brea M., Balakrish Nair G., Chowdhury A., Datta S., Shirai M., Nakazawa T., Ally R., Segal I., Wong B. C., Lam S. K., Olfat F. O., Boren T., Engstrand L., Torres O., Schneider R., Thomas J. E., Czinn S., and Berg D. E., 2000, Differences in genotypes of *Helicobacter pylori* from different human populations. *J. Bacteriol.* **182**:3210.
15. Talley N. J., Vakil N., Ballard E. D., and Fennerty M. B., 1999, Absence of benefit of eradicating *Helicobacter pylori* in patients with nonulcer dyspepsia. *N. Engl. J. Med.* **341**:1106.
16. de Boer W. A., and Tytgat G. N. J., 2000, Treatment of *Helicobacter pylori* infection. *BMJ.* **320**:31–34.
17. Lee A., O'Rourke J., de Ungria M. C., Robertson B., Daskalopoulos G., and Dixon M. F., 1997, A standardized mouse model of *Helicobacter pylori* infection—introducing the Sydney strain. *Gastroenterology.* **112**:1033.

Helicobacter pylori Infection and Immunity

1

The Bacteriology of *Helicobacter pylori*

PAUL S. HOFFMAN

1. INTRODUCTION

Helicobacter pylori is a gram negative microaerobic bacterium that colonizes the gastric mucosa of some 50% of the world's population, and is one of the most common of human infectious agents.[1] *Helicobacter*-like bacteria have been identified in the stomachs of all mammalian species examined to date, suggesting that these organisms evolved, perhaps with mammalian stomachs, many millions of years ago. It has been suggested that *H. pylori* has undergone a rapid evolution over a 10,000 year period and at one time may have enjoyed an infectivity of nearly 100% of humans.[2] Even today, infectivity in developing countries approaches 100%, while in developed countries the prevalence is between 20 to 40% and decreasing.[3] Until recently, the stomach was considered by the medical community to be refractory to microbial colonization, and while pathologists had seen spiral-shaped bacteria in stomach biopsies from humans and various animals, the connection to disease was never established until Warren and Marshall investigated these organisms in gastric pathologies in the early eighties.[4] At the time of their discovery, the standard therapy for gastritis and ulcers was a life long regime

PAUL S. HOFFMAN • Departments of Microbiology and Immunology and Medicine, Division of Infectious Diseases, Dalhousie University, Rm 7P, Sir Charles Tupper Medical Bldg., Halifax, Nova Scotia B3H 4H7, Canada.

Helicobacter pylori Infection and Immunity,
Edited by Yamamoto *et al.*, Kluwer Academic/Plenum Publishers, 2002.

of drugs that lowered acid secretion (Zantac^R and Tagamet^R), relieving symptoms but not curing infection. Now, antimicrobial intervention together with drugs that decrease acid secretion, leads to eradication of *H. pylori*, resolution of symptoms and in the absence of relapse or re infection, provides a life long cure.

It is not particularly surprising that *Helicobacter pylori* must have evolved several unique biochemical features to enable it to thrive in the seemingly hostile environment of the stomach. Moreover, unlike other mucosal sites, the gastric mucosa harbors no resident flora to be dislodged or organized mucosal immune defense system to circumvent (e.g., Pyers patches), so many virulence associated genes and regulatory mechanisms required by other mucosal pathogens to gain the competitive edge and persist in mucosal tissue, are apparently not required by *H. pylori*. A more complete picture of how *H. pylori*, not only survives, but often persists for the life of the host, are just beginning to emerge. The publication of two complete genomic sequences for *Helicobacter pylori* has greatly facilitated investigations into the physiology, genetics and metabolic capabilities of this organism.[5–7] This information also begins to address adaptation mechanisms, variations in LPS structure and antigenicity, features in other microbial pathogens that enhance chronic infection. This chapter will focus on unique or major features of the organism that enables it to thrive in the gastric mucosa and to thwart efforts by the host immune system to eliminate the infection. For further information, readers are referred to other chapters in this book as well as to the many detailed and specialty reviews that have recently appeared.[1,8–11]

2. TAXONOMY AND EPIDEMIOLOGY

2.1. Human Isolates

When the spiral-shaped bacteria associated with duodenal and gastric ulcers were first cultured by Warren and Marshall, their resemblance to members of the genus *Campylobacter*, a related group of microaerobic bacteria that inhabit the intestines of animals and are the most common cause diarrhea in humans, led to placement in this Genus.[1,12] However, based on ribosomal RNA analysis and other criteria, these gastric campylobacters differed sufficiently to warrant a separate genus, *Helicobacter* and the type species was designated as *pylori*. Genome comparisons between *Helicobacter* and *Campylobacter* reveal a substantial number of specific common genes,[9] suggesting both an early ancestor and that this complement of genes may be required for survival in microaerobic environments. While there are no reservoirs of *H. pylori* in nature, the bacteria have been found in cats and dogs, suggesting one route of transmission to humans. In general, human to human transmission (oral oral or fecal oral), including ingestion of contaminated water are often cited as routes of transmission. While PCR tests show that genomic DNA is present in feces contaminated water, *H. pylori* is rarely isolated from these sources. Several studies show that vomit and diarrhea can spread these organisms, leading to speculation that many of the childhood diseases associated with acute diarrhea may have accounted for the natural spread of *H. pylori* infection among young children. With higher socioeconomic status, clean drinking water, and a reduction of diarrheal diseases in children, the spread of *H. pylori*, at least in western societies, has nearly vanished.

2.2. Related Species of *Helicobacter*

Once methods developed for cultivation of *H. pylori* were applied to cultivation of gastric and other tissue from other animals, it became apparent that nearly all mammals are colonized with *Helicobacter.*[12] A less common species of *Helicobacter* (*H. heilmanii*) is also found in the stomachs of humans.[12] This species is believed to be less virulent, but can be associated with gastritis and ulcer disease. Most diagnostic laboratories do not distinguish between *H. pylori* and *H. heilmanii* species.

The earliest studied non-human strains were *H. mustelae* in ferrets and *H. felis* in cats and dogs.[11] *H. felis* causes inflammation in the stomachs of mice that resembles what is observed in humans infected with *H. pylori* and has been used in the study of pathogenesis and immunity. All of the gastric *Helicobacter* species possess urease activity whereas; most of the non-gastric helicobacters do not.[12] The list of non-gastric helicobacters, including *H. bilus, H. hepaticus* and *H. cinaedi* may be responsible for lower GI manifestations such as inflammatory bowel disease and liver diseases. While most of these sequalae have been studied in animals, the participation of some as yet to be discovered helicobacters, in inflammatory bowl disease (IBD) and extra gastric pathologies is actively being pursued.

3. LIFE IN THE GASTRIC MUCOSA

If one were to design the perfect gastric pathogen, protection from the deleterious effects of hydrochloric acid, which can reach near 100 milimolar concentrations in the lumen of the stomach would be highly desirable. Interestingly, *H. pylori* is not an acidophile, and therefore must cope, perhaps only transiently, with stomach acid during transmission and colonization. An examination of biopsy material reveals that the bacteria are localized to the gastric mucosa and the mucus layer coating the gastric epithelium. The gastric mucus acts as a protective barrier for the underlying epithelial cells by limiting the back diffusion of acid from the lumen. *Helicobacter* can be observed adhering to epithelial cells as well as free swimming in the mucus layer. It has been estimated that 80% of the bacteria are non-adherent, though mutations leading to loss of adherence are associated with decreased infectivity.[13] Both motility and urease activity are critical for colonization and maintenance of infection. These, together with adhesive capabilities provide the bacteria some flexibility and adaptability in response to local acidity or other environmental changes.

4. SURVIVAL IN ACID ENVIRONMENTS

In examining the biology of *H. pylori* in its gastric niche, one must consider how this organism responds to pH changes in the gastric environment. Acidity of the lumen varies, being higher after meals and decreasing in between them. Initially, it was believed that *H. pylori* was an acidophile, based largely on its stomach habitat. Studies of its acid tolerance, however, suggested that the bacteria were in fact neutralophiles and could not grow in vitro in media acidified to below a pH of 5.5. The challenge for acidophiles is to maintain a constant electrochemical gradient across the cytoplasmic membrane of between −75 to −180 mVolts (inside negative), while balancing an internal pH of 6.8 to 7.2 against an external pH as low as 3; the ΔpH alone between 7 and 3 generates a potential of −240 mVolts, which is sufficient to collapse the membrane potential. Acidophiles maintain this balance by compensating for a large ΔpH by concentrating other ions like sodium and potassium (or efflux of chloride or other anions) in the cytoplasm producing a large positive ΔΨ, the other component that determines the electrochemical potential of the cytoplasmic membrane (ΔpH + ΔΨ). A search of the genome sequence reveals no ATP dependent ion transporters (Na/K transporters) typically associated with ion balance. Although several P-type proton pumping ATPases have been identified, which are involved with metal transport, these are unlikely to be associated with ion balance.[5,14] The membrane-spanning proton translocating F_1F_0 ATP synthase takes up protons coupled to phosphorylation of ADP, but this activity is not associated with maintenance of membrane potential. While some of the ATPase subunits have diverged genetically from those in other bacteria, none of these would enable the complex to assume other functions. Taken together, these findings support *H. pylori* as a neutralophile. As will be developed below, *H. pylori* can transiently survive periods of low pH, but there is no evidence that these bacteria can grow under these conditions.

5. ROLE OF UREASE IN PH STASIS

Gastric species of *Helicobacter* produce a powerful urease, whose activity is necessary for colonization. The catalysis of urea by urease produces ammonia that would contribute to localized alkalinity and thereby protect the bacteria from acid. Immuno-electron microscopic localization studies have shown that the urease is found in the cytoplasm, periplasm, and on the bacterial surface. The surface associated urease was initially believed to play a key role in protection from acid, but recent studies by Sachs has demonstrated that the *H. pylori* urease is inhibited by acid.[15] The function of the surface associated urease remains unresolved. Urease genes *ureA* and *ureB* form the functional enzyme while accessory genes, with the exception of *ureI*, are associated with nickel incorporation and include *ureE, ureF, ureG* and *ureH*. Nickel transporting enzymes such as NixA are important in concentrating this essential metal. Other proteins that may be involved in nickel scavenging include HspA, a 10kDa GroES homolog containing a histidine-rich C-terminus capable of binding nickel. This additional function by a heat shock protein is unusual, but given that urease activity is essential for survival in in situ, perhaps *H. pylori* utilizes a variety of nickel binding proteins to ensure an adequate supply of nickel is maintained.

In contrast to other bacterial ureases, the *H. pylori* urease appears to be unregulated in vitro, but there is good clinical evidence that the enzyme may be regulated in vivo. Patients on proton pump inhibitors and infected with *H. pylori* generally are negative by the urea breath test, the standard diagnostic test, suggesting that urease may be inactive under more alkaline conditions. Additionally, constitutive urease activity would also be a liability for *H. pylori*, since the increased alkalinity resulting from ammonia production would render a pH neutral site of colonization too alkaline to support bacterial growth. Interestingly, *Helicobacter pylori* have evolved a novel mechanism to regulate urease activity; rather than regulate enzyme production at a transcriptional level, the bacteria control entry of urea into the cytoplasm through a pH gated transporter. The entry of urea into the bacteria is dependent on pH, and under acidic conditions, the transporter (UreI) permits urea uptake, but once a pH of 6–7 pH is reached, the transporter no longer actively takes up urea.[15,16] Under alkaline conditions, the bacteria produce little ammonia, consistent with the clinical observations with PPIs. Interestingly, loss of function mutations in *ureI* produce a urease negative phenotype,[16] despite their being plenty of enzymatically active urease in the cytoplasm, something demonstrated by permeabilizing the bacterial cells and recovering urease activity. While *ureI* is not essential for in vitro growth, *ureI* mutants are unable to colonize the gastric mucosa in a mouse infection model.[17] It has been speculated that the cytoplasmic urease may be associated with the cytoplasmic sequences of UreI to exchange entering urea with the export of ammonia into the periplasm (see Figure 1). In the absence of numerous two component regulatory systems, alternate sigma factors, or UreR type transcriptional regulators common in other urease positive bacteria, *H. pylori* appears to use pH gating to control uptake of urea and consequently control the microenvironment pH.

6. ACID SHOCK AND OTHER STRESSES

Acid shock also leads to an increase in expression and surface location of heat shock proteins of the Hsp60 and Hsp70 classes.[18,19] The increased surface expression of these proteins has been shown to promote adherence of the bacteria to gastric epithelial cells in an *in vitro* model and presumably, the close association with the epithelial cells in the stomach might provide protection from acid

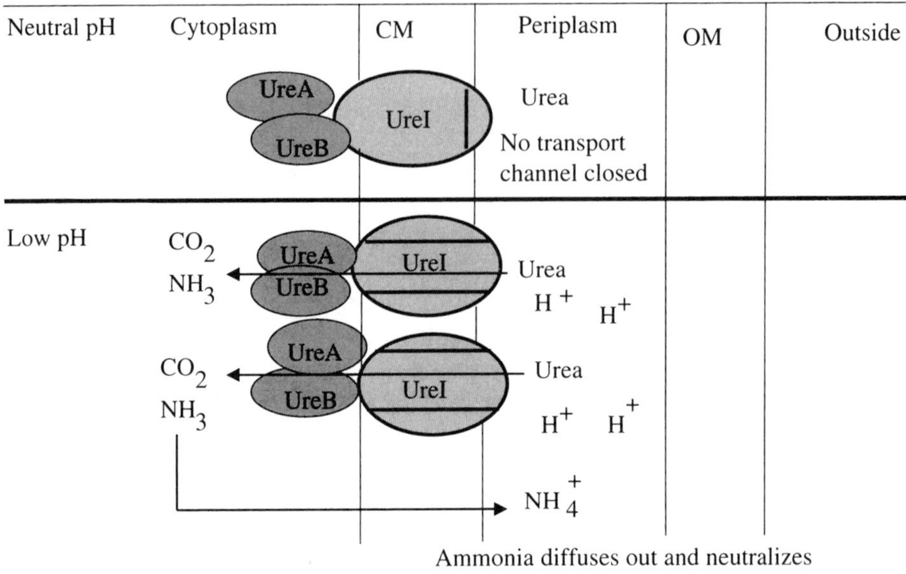

FIGURE 1. pH regulation of Urease Activity. Urease I is a trans-cytoplasmic membrane protein that regulates entry of urea into H. pylori. Under neutral pH, the UreI channel is blocked and no urea enters the bacterial cell. UreA and UreB are the catalytic subunits of urease. Under Low pH conditions, the UreI channel opens and permits entry of urea into the cytoplasm where it is catabolized to ammonia and carbon dioxide. The ammonia diffuses out of the cell as ammonium ions in the periplasmic space.

damage. It follows that under more alkaline conditions Hsp production would decrease and result in the bacteria becoming less adherent, permitting them to swim to more acidic locations. Acid levels, together with where *H. pylori* colonizes in the stomach, have been well studied and it is known that individuals who are hyperchlorhidric tend to have antral *H. pylori* infections; whereas, individuals that are hypochlorhidric have gastric predominant infections. Drug induced changes (proton pump inhibitors) in gastric pH also lead to migration of the bacteria to more acidic areas such as from the antrum up into the body of the stomach. Other adhesins of *H. pylori* that may also contribute to adhesion include babA and Lewis antigens.[20]

Hsp genes are under negative regulation by HspR, an autoregulatory transcription factor that binds to HAIR sequences (HspR-associated inverted repeat) upstream of operons *groELS; cbpA, hspR,* and unknown function *orf;* and *hrcA, grpE* and *dnaK* of *H. pylori.*[21] Knockout mutation in *hspR* leads to over expression of Hsp60, and other Hsps. Measurements of promoter activity revealed that activation of the controlled operons was not affected by heat shock, but was increased by osmotic shock in response to high salt. This study did not determine whether HspR responds to changes in acid levels as might be inferred from the findings of Huesca *et al.*[18,19] It is also possible that HspR might be linked to urease regulation or other cellular activities as part of a coordinated response to acid stress. HrcA, another heat shock negative regulator that binds to CIRCE (controlling inverted repeat of chaperone expression) motif has not been investigated. It is possible that both repressors are associated with control of these Hsp operons.

7. MOTILITY AND CHEMOTAXIS

Motility is also critical for colonization and maintenance of infection. *H. pylori* is highly motile by means of 5 to 7 unipolar flagella, and in biopsy material, bacteria can be readily observed in the mucus associated with the gastric epithelium. The flagella filament of *H. pylori* is composed of two flagellin subunits, FlaA and FlaB, and mutations in these genes lead to nonmotile bacteria that are no longer infectious in the mouse model of infection.[13] The relative abundance of each of these products in the flagella may vary, though the products of these genes are very conserved. The flagella are covered by a sheath, an outgrowth of the outer membrane, composed of double layer of phospholipids that may protect the flagellum from the effects of gastric acid. In general, the genes (approximately 40) associated with flagella assembly and function are similar to counterparts found in other bacteria. Regulation of flagella synthesis may not be as tight as found in other bacteria, where FlgM, a regulator of flagella biosynthesis in other bacteria is absent in *H. pylori*.

As mentioned earlier, *H. pylori* must be able to sense and respond to changes in the environment, including nutrient limitation.[22] A search of the genome has found the bacteria to possess most of the genes associated with chemotactic behavior.[7] Studies show that *H. pylori* is chemo-attracted to urea, so perhaps urea taxis directs the bacteria to the epithelial surface. In addition, *H. pylori* exhibits chemotactic responses to various amino acids such as glutamine, histidine, lysine, and alanine.[8]

8. INFLAMMATION AND NUTRIENT ACQUISITION

Another requirement for gastric colonization and long term survival is nutrient acquisition, something that might not seem so obvious given all the food being digested in the lumen of the stomach. However, most nutrients are not appreciably absorbed by the stomach mucosa, because they poorly pass through the mucus layer. A clue to nutrient acquisition is that all Hp infections produce gastritis, inflammation of the gastric mucosa. Inflammation leads to serum leakage and hence a source of nutrients as well as urea. *Helicobacter pylori,* like most mucosal pathogens has evolved a strategy to produce enough inflammation to gleam nutrients, but not enough to produce sufficient damage to evoke eradication by the host immune system.

An array of surface and secreted proteins together with LPS are most likely to be involved in promoting inflammation by eliciting the production of chemokines like IL-8 and inflammatory cytokines like IL-1β, IL-6, IL-12 and IL-18 by mucosal epithelial cells and infiltrating phagocytic cells. *H. pylori* is typical of many mucosal pathogens, which express highly conserved heat shock proteins of the Hsp60 and Hsp70 classes on the bacterial surface and whose expression appears to be regulated in response to acid.[18,19,23] Other proteins that contribute to inflammation include CagA, produced by *H. pylori* strains containing the Cag locus, a pathogenicity island encoding proteins associated with Type IV secretion and whose function involves insertion of CagA protein into host cells.[24] CagA action on host cells enhances inflammation and is introduced into epithelial cells through a type IV *cag* dependent secretion mechanism (see Chapter for more detail on the pathogenicity island and virulence activities). The VacA cytotoxin is also secreted by the Cag secretion system, and causes vacuoles in host cells. Interestingly, the *vacA* gene is found in all *H. pylori* strains, but in the absence of CagA, the VacA product is not Secreted.[1]

Helicobacter pathogenesis is clearly complex and involves the activities of many genes. The bacteria have evolved mechanisms to cope with acid through a pH regulated urea transporter, to use motility to move to more hospitable regions, surface adhesins to promote adhesion when required, and a strategy to promote inflammation to gain nutrients. With time, many more mechanisms will be added to those outlined herein.

9. METABOLIC CAPABILITIES OF *H. pylori*

An understanding of the biology of *H. pylori* has been greatly aided by the appearance recently of two complete genomic sequences. The reader is referred to Chapter 2 for a more complete discussion of comparative genomes and genetic diversity topics. Despite a relatively small genome (1.67 Megabases), *H. pylori* possesses most of the necessary genes required for central intermediary metabolism, synthesis of vitamins, and most amino acids and nucleic acids. Nutritional studies indicate a requirement for isoleucine, leucine, valine, arginine, histidine, methionine, phenylalanine and some strains require alanine; these requirements are also supported from analysis of the *H. pylori* genomes.[5,6,7]

There is good agreement between genomic and biochemical data in many areas of central metabolism, but there are other areas where differences abound.

The annotation of any genome is dependent on the fidelity of existing databases such that any errors within genomic databases are simply passed along to the new ones. Similarly, enzyme assays, especially those where activities are low, may lack specificity or are attributable to weak activities of different enzymes for substrates used in the particular assay. With time and further studies, these inconsistencies may ultimately be resolved.

Both genomic and biochemical information indicate that other than glucose, sugars are not catabolized by *H. pylori* and while the bacteria possess catabolic glycolysis, pentose cycle, and Entner Doudoroff pathways, there is good agreement that some of these pathways may be incomplete.[7,8,9,25] For example, glycolysis appears to be an anabolic process since two key enzymes considered essential for the catabolic route phosphofructokinase and pyruvate kinase are absent, while the gluconeogenic enzyme counterparts (e.g., fructose 1–6-bisphosphatase and pyruvate dikinase) are present (see Figure 2). While *H. pylori* possesses a glucokinase, the phosphatase counterpart is absent (glucose-6-phosphatase), suggesting that free glucose never accumulates in the cell. The absence of the phosphatase has been pointed out as significant, but should not be that surprising since bacteria generally do not accumulate unphosphorylated sugars. Rather, the phosphorylated glucose would be used in various biosynthetic activities (conversion to NDP-sugars for cell wall and LPS biosynthetic activities). Similarly, one of the key enzymes of the pentose phosphate pathway (6-phosphogluconate dehydrogenase) that reductively decarboxylates 6-phosphogluconate to ribulose-5-phosphate was not found in either of the genome sequences. Activity attributable to this enzyme has been detected in crude extracts of non-sequenced strains, suggesting that the gene for this enzyme may not be present in all strains, has appreciably diverged from its counterparts in other bacteria, or that the particular enzyme assay used lacked specificity. The Entner Doudoroff pathway converts 6-phospho gluconate to pyruvate and glyceraldehyde 3-phosphate, permitting catabolism of glucose directly to pyruvate, thus avoiding the catabolic blocks at phosphofructokinase and pyruvate kinase, while providing 3 carbon phosphates for transaldolase and transketolase interconversions to produce ribulose-5 phosphate for nucleic acid biosynthesis. The pyruvate dikinase is the only gluconeogenic enzyme identified from genome analysis that can move Krebs cycle intermediates up to sugars. While trace activities of PEP carboxylase and pyruvate carboxylase were detected by enzyme assay, it remains to be determined how Krebs cycle intermediates are channeled back into gluconeogenesis. Most studies suggest that the major carbon and energy sources for *H. pylori* are amino acids and organic acids, so with nearly 1/3 of the genome coding for proteins of unknown function, it is reasonable to predict that pathways for Krebs cycle intermediates entering the gluconeogenic path will eventually be elucidated. Further, the observed CO_2 fixation of *H. pylori* also supports a role for novel enzymes in this activity that might involve formation of PEP for gluconeogenesis or in replenishing Krebs cycle intermediates.[26]

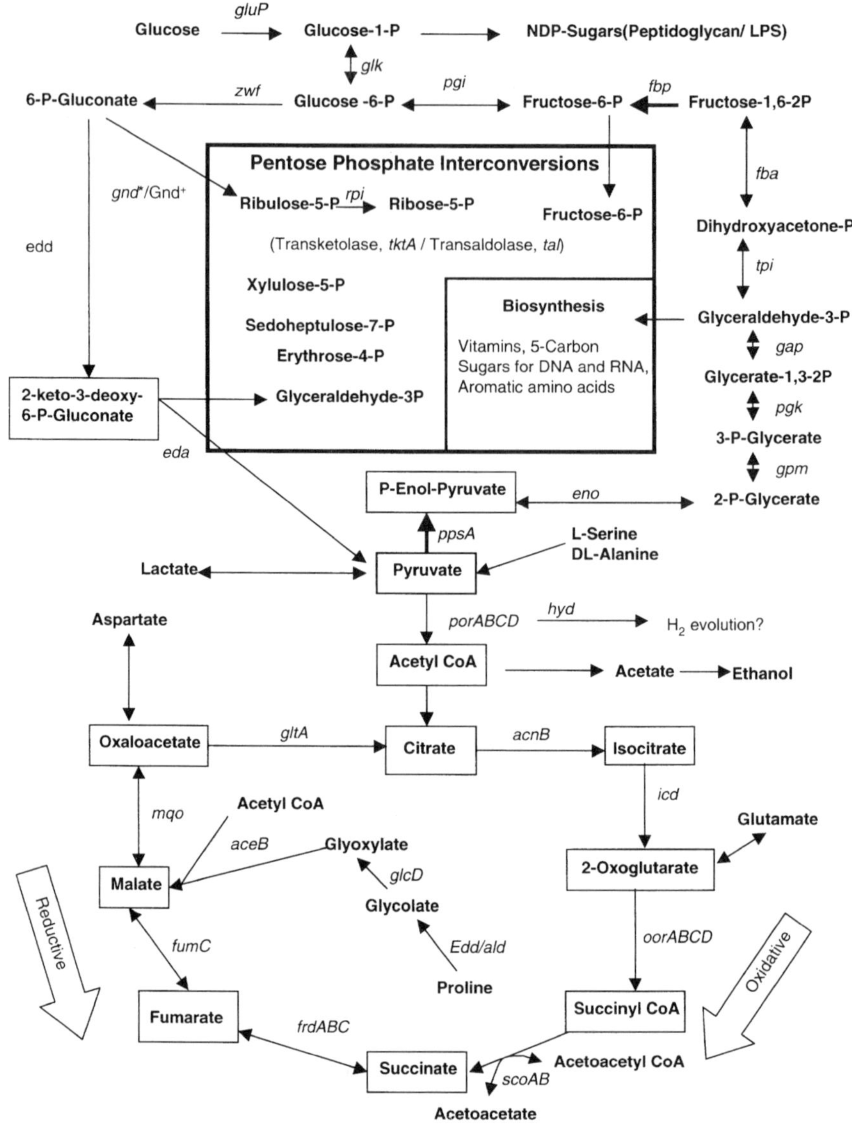

FIGURE 2. Central intermediary metabolism of *H. pylori*. The major pathways of *H. pylori* include glycolysis, Entner Doudoroff, Pentose cycle and the Krebs cycle. Some of the key features include the absence of key enzymatic steps (red arrows) and those where the pathway can go in only the reverse direction (blue arrows). The Krebs cycle operates in both reductive and oxidative directions. The enzymes associated with glycolysis include: glucose transporter (*gluP*), glucokinase (*glk*), phosphoglucoisomerase (*pgi*), fructose-1,6, biphosphatase (*fbp*), fructose biphosphate aldolase (*fba*), triose isomerase (*tpi*), glyceraldehyde-3-P dehydrogenase (*gap*), phosphoglycerate kinase (*pgk*), phosphoglycerate mutase (*gpm*), enolase (*eno*), and pyruvate dikinase (ppsA) and pyruvate oxidoreductase (*porABCD*). The Entner Doudoroff pathway contains the enzymes glucose-6-P dehydrogenase (zwf), 6-P-gluconate dehydratase (*edd*) and the 2-keto-3-deoxy--6-P-gluconate aldolase (*eda*). The Pentose cycle is missing the 6-P-gluconate dehydrogenase (red arrow) but does contain: ribulose-5-P isomerase, transketolase (*tktA*) and transaldolase (*tal*). Enzymes associated with pyruvate catabolism include lactate dehydrogenase, serine and alanine deaminases, and alcohol dehydrogenase. Enzymes of the Krebs cycle include: citrate synthase (*gltA*), aconitate hydratase (*acnB*), isocitrate dehydrogenase (*icd*), 2-oxoglutarate oxidase (*oorABCD*), Succinyl-CoA: acetoacetate-CoA transferase (*scoAB*), fumarate reductase (*frdABC*), fumarase (*fumC*), malate quinone oxidase (*mqo*), glycolate oxidase (*glcD*) and malate synthase (*acdB*, putative). The large arrows indicate that the Krebs cycle may run in both the reductive and oxidative directions.

The Krebs cycle has been extensively studied both enzymatically and through genomic analysis.[5–10,25–28] Several genes/enzymes of this cycle have been identified including citrate synthase, aconitase, isocitrate dehydrogenase and fumarase. *H. pylori* uses a more primitive pyruvate oxidoreductase to oxidize pyruvate to acetyl CoA than the pyruvate dehydrogenase found in many bacteria and eukaryotes. Also, no 2-ketoglutarate dehydrogenase was found in these bacteria, rather, the bacteria produce an oxoglutarate oxidoreductase (OOR) exhibiting an evolutionary relationship with POR.[25–27] While a typical succinate dehydrogenase was not identified in the genome, strong enzymatic activity is readily detected by spectrophotometric assay and with respiring membrane vesicles suggesting that fumarate reductase/succinate dehydrogenase is active in both directions or that one of several putative dehydrogenases of unknown function may perform this oxidation. Interestingly, fumarase activity favors the reverse (fumarate forming) direction suggesting that the left arm of the cycle likely operates in the reductive direction.[27] While weak NAD(P)H malate dehydrogenase activity has been reported, the gene encoding this activity is absent from the genome. However, evidence for a quinone linked malate oxidoreductase has been reported.[10] and recently confirmed experimentally.[29] Malate quinone oxidase is a flavoprotein that interacts directly with quinones and its activity is NAD(P)H independent. The presence of a malate oxidoreductase would certainly be consistent with results from carbon flow studies supporting a role for an enzyme converting oxaloacetate to fumarate.[27] Generally, the deamination of aspartic acid (oxaloacetic acid) would be catabolized via this route. The reason malate is of interest is because several enzymes whose genes have been identified convert substrates to products that in other bacteria would be routed through malate such as glyoxylate from glycolate oxidase (requires malate synthase).[10,25,27] It has been suggested that aspartate catabolism may bypass malate by generating fumarate, though no experimental evidence for this enzyme activity has been presented. Also, weak isocitrate lyase activity has been reported, but no isocitrate lyase gene has been identified in either *H. pylori* genome. As more bacterial genomes are analyzed, we are finding that most bacteria possess incomplete or non mitochondrial-like Krebs cycles.[30] In some cases, the bacteria have compensating pathways to get to key intermediates, but for many, novel genes may be involved. If anything, genomics has changed our understanding of the evolution of intermediary metabolism in bacteria. Also, it suggests that novel enzymes may be associated with critical steps in the cycle, a cry for more research into novel genes. Finally, as mentioned earlier, it cannot be emphasized enough that many of the annotations, particularly those matching at low probability (e^{-10}) may well have a very different function. Similarly, it should be appreciated that all enzymes are able to utilize alternative substrates.[31] Here it is interesting to note that the KDPG aldolase shows similarity to lyases associated with proline metabolism, where splitting of a catabolic intermediate yields glyoxylate and pyruvate. Could this enzyme complex display a dual function? Low specificity might permit splitting isocitrate to glyoxylate and succinate, for example. The only absolute proof for presence of an enzyme activity is purification of the activity, followed by N-terminal sequencing of protein and identification of its gene.

10. RESPIRATION AND ENERGY PRODUCTION

Helicobacter pylori exhibits a strictly respiratory form of metabolism and although fermentation end products are produced from glucose and pyruvate, the bacteria fail to grow in the absence of oxygen. The ability of *H. pylori* to ferment as well as oxidize may be important given that transmission may involve a fecal route where survival under anaerobic conditions may be required. However, at least in the laboratory no one has demonstrated growth of *H. pylori* under anaerobic conditions. Unlike some *Campylobacter* sp. and *Wolenella succinogenes* (close relatives of *Helicobacter*), *Helicobacter* cannot grow anaerobically with alternate electron acceptors such as nitrate, nitrite, nitrous oxide or carry out formate—fumarate or hydrogen—fumarate respiration[32]. Similar to *Campylobacter, H. pylori* contains *b* and *c* type cytochromes and several quinone coupled oxidases. In the gastric mucosa, *H. pylori* most likely scavenges oxygen diffusing from the tissues, and like *C. jejuni*, most likely contains oxidases with high affinity for oxygen. The two microaerophiles share a number of similarities in cytochrome composition and many other genes that may be specific to microaerophiles. The helicobacters are oxidase positive (cytochrome *ccb*3 oxidase) and catalase positive. The catalase is present in the periplasm and may be displayed on the surface, suggesting a role in protection from aspects of the mucosal inflammatory response generated reactive forms of oxygen. These bacteria also express considerable superoxide dismutase, a putative defense mechanism against oxygen toxicity. Thus the aero-intolerance of microaerophiles is not solely due to oxygen toxicity, but could include low respiration rate, diffusion of oxygen into the cells and the oxidation or loss of function of key components of metabolism. At least two Krebs cycle enzymes (aconitate hydratase and fumarase) are oxygen labile and could be damaged by oxygen diffusing into the cells[25]. Another enzyme system Alkyl hydroperoxide reductase (AhpC) is associated with detoxification of alkylhydroperoxides in many bacteria. In enteric bacteria, a second reductase, AhpF provides reducing equivalents for the AhpC reductase, however, in *H. pylori*, like *M. tuberculosis*, there is no AhpF homologue. A search for AhpF homologues identifies some related genes in the thioredoxin reductase family that may function by providing reducing equivalents. Both J99 and 26695 strains of *H. pylori* contain two thioredoxin genes and two thioredoxin reductases. The relative levels of AhpC seem high in *H. pylori*, like *C. jejuni*, suggesting that removal of lipid peroxides may be a necessary task for survival of microaerophiles in aerobic environments.

The NADH dehydrogenase complex from many bacteria is a protein pump, enabling the bacteria to couple proton efflux with ATP synthesis through the ATPase. However, like the related *Campylobacter* sp, the *H. pylori* NADPH dehydrogenase may not be a proton pumping dehydrogenase.[33] This group of microaerophiles probably is energy inefficient with only one proton translocation site likely involving quinone. There are possibly several terminal oxidases though their affinities for oxygen have not been determined. The bacteria also contain hydrogenases, which should enable them to oxidize molecular hydrogen under aerobic conditions. One advantage to hydrogen oxidation is that the hydrogenase is associated with the outside surface of the cytoplasmic membrane enabling protons from hydrogen oxidation to be released in the periplasm, while the reducing equivalents are channeled into the electron transport pathway at the quinone level. Hydrogen was found to be the most energy efficient substrate catabolized by *C. jejuni*. Hydrogenases may also produce molecular hydrogen through proton reduction, a mechanism by which anaerobic bacteria remove reducing equivalents from fermentation. It is possible that hydrogen evolution by *H. pylori* contributes to survival under anaerobic conditions by removing reducing equivalents generated by pyruvate oxidoreductase for example. The *H. pylori* hydrogenase contains four subunits and the enzyme, like urease, requires nickel for activity. Another difference between *H. pylori* and other bacteria is that NADPH, rather than NADH is the major carrier of reducing equivalents in *H. pylori*.[28]

11. IRON AND METAL ACQUISITION

Iron is an essential nutrient for most living organisms and in aerobic environments, most of the iron is in the oxidized form (Fe^{+3}), existing mostly as ferric oxide or rust. Ferric iron is very insoluble in water at neutral pH (~10^{-18} M), so most microorganisms have evolved mechanisms to solubilize iron through chelation via siderophores (iron binding compounds). Ferrous iron (Fe^{+2}) on the other hand is relatively soluble in water under anaerobic conditions. Both forms of iron are soluble in acid, and much of the iron in the lumen of the human stomach would be soluble in stomach acid. It is possible that the mucus layer binds iron, but it is unlikely that iron is concentrated in the gastric mucus, since the acidic lumen would favor accumulation in acid. However, it is known that hog gastric mucin can serve as a source of iron, and so perhaps human gastric mucus also permits accumulation of iron. Alternatively, serum leakage and epithelial cell destruction might provide a source of ferric iron and heme, though most of this iron would be associated with proteins like ferritin or lactoferrin.

Genomic analysis suggests that *H. pylori* does not produce a siderophore, but some of the genes detected are similar to the enterochelin and ferric citrate (*fec* genes) uptake systems of *Campylobacter coli* and *E. coli*, respectively.[7,8] However,

H. pylori is unable to obtain iron from siderophores of the enterochelin or pyrochelin classes. The bacteria also produce outer membrane proteins that bind lactoferrin and heme, enabling the bacteria to scavenge the bound iron. It is interesting that some genes associated with iron acquisition are present while others typically associated with existing genes in *E. coli* are absent. For example, FeoB, a cytoplasmic ferrous iron permease is present, whereas a homolog of FeoA, a small protein that interacts with FeoB in *E. coli* is absent. *H. pylori* produces a cytoplasmic ferritin protein that functions in iron storage. Ordinarily, ferritin proteins serve as a source of stored iron, serving to supply the ferric uptake regulator (Fur) with iron to maintain repression of iron regulated genes. As the ferritin protein becomes depleted of iron, the Fur repressor looses repressor activity. Fur is non-essential for in vitro growth and although Fur binding sequences (Fur boxes) have been found upstream of several genes including the catalase gene, further study will be required to resolve its regulatory role. The complexities of iron acquisition by *H. pylori* suggest that even in seemingly acidic environment of the stomach, iron acquisition requires a concerted effort by the bacterium.

The urease of *H. pylori* requires the metal nickel for activity. Nickel acquisition has been well characterized and a specialized transporter for nickel (NixA) functions in nickel transport.[34] When cloned into *E. coli* containing the *H. pylori* urease operon, NixA expression leads to increased urease activity.[35] Other proteins associated with nickel binding include HspA the Hsp10 GroES homologue. This protein contains histidine-rich sequences in the carboxy region of the protein and it is speculated that HspA participates in assembly and nickel incorporation into the urease enzyme complex. In addition to these proteins, a P-type ATPase has also been found to participate in nickel transport as well as of copper and cobalt.[14] Since nickel acquisition is critical to urease based acid protection, the bacteria likely use a range of metal uptake systems to ensure that an adequate supply of nickel is maintained. The cost of this strategy is the accumulation of toxic heavy metals like copper and zinc. Genes associated with general efflux systems have also been found, but none of these enzymes seems to be associated with drug resistance mechanisms as shown in other bacterial pathogens. Rather, these efflux mechanisms may be involved with removal of toxic heavy metals, other than nickel from the bacteria.

12. CONCLUDING REMARKS

Until the discovery of *H. pylori,* through its association with peptic ulcer disease, microaerophiles were an understudied novelty, essentially out of the mainstream of scientific interest. Thus, the massive and unprecedented international effort to understand this medically significant human pathogen has inadvertently led to a remarkable accumulation of information on the biology of microaerophiles. Gastric colonization by *H. pylori* and the establishment of life long infection has provided new lessons in microbial ecology and the dynamics of the host parasite interaction. With a minimal complement of genes and a paucity of transcriptional regulatory factors, this organism has evolved rather simple strategies for survival in the gastric mucosa, including acid gated urea transport to modulate urease activity; motility, chemotaxis and adherence mechanisms—flexibility in response to host immune activities and local acid changes; and a metabolic capability to scavenge nutrients from the host. With about a third of the genes encoding proteins of unknown function, there is much more to be learned about this unique human pathogen.

REFERENCES

1. Dunn B. E., Cohen H., and Blaser M. J., 1997, *Helicobacter pylori. Clin. Microbiol. Rev.* **10**:720–741.
2. Blaser M. J. 1999, Where does *Helicobacter pylori* come from and why is it going away? *JAMA.* **282**:2260–2262.
3. Taylor D. N., and Parsonnet J., 1995, Epidemiology and natural history of *H. pylori* infections, p. 551–564. In Blaser M. J., Smith P. F., Ravdin J., Greenberg H., and Guerrant R. L. (ed.), *Infections of the gastrointestinal tract.* Raven Press, New York, N. Y.
4. Warren J. R., and Marshall B., 1983. Unified curved bacilli on gastric epithelium in active chronic gastritis. *Lancet.* **I**:1273–1275.
5. Tomb J. F., White O., Kerlavage A. R., Clayton R. A., Sutton G. G., Fleischmann R. D., Ketchum K., Klenk H., Gill S., Dougherty B., Nelson K., Quackenbush J., Zhou L., Kirkness E., Peterson S., Loftus B., Richardson D., Dodson R., Khalak H., Glodek A., McKenney K., Fitzegerald L., Lee N., Adams M., Hickey E., Berg D., Gocayne J., Utterback T., Peterson J., Kelley J., Cotton M., Weidman J., Fujii C., Bowman C., Watthey L., Wallin E., Hayes W., Borodovsky M., Karp P., Smith H., Fraser C., and Venter J., 1997, The complete genome sequence of the gastric pathogen *Helicobacter pylori. Nature.* **388**:539–547.
6. Alm R. A., Ling L. S., Moir D. T., King B. L., Brown E. D., Doig P. C., Smith D. R., Noonan B., Guild B. C., deJonge B. L. Carmel G., Tummino P. J., Caruso A., Uria-Nickelsen M., Mills D. M., Ives C., Gibson R., Merberg D., Mills S. D., Jiang Q., Taylor D. E., Vovis G. F., and Trust T. J., 1999, Genomic-sequence comparison of two unrelated isolates of the human gastric pathogen *Helicobacter pylori. Nature.* **397:**176–180.
7. Berg D. E., Hoffman P. S., Appelmelk B. J., and Kusters J. G., 1997, The *Helicobacter pylori* genome sequence: genetic factors for a long life in the gastric mucosa. *Trends Microbiol.* **13**: 468–474.
8. Marais A., Mendz G. L., Hazell S. L., and Megraud F., 1999, Metabolism and genetics of *Helicobacter pylori*: the genome era. Microbiol. *Mol. Biol. Rev.* **63**:642–674.
9. Doig P., De Jonge B. L., Alm R. A., Brown E. D., Uria-Nickelsen M., Noonan B., Mills S. D., Tummino P., Carmel G., Guild B. C., Moir D. T., Vovis G. F., and Trust T. J., 1999, Helicobacter pylori physiology predicted from genomic comparison of two strains. Microb iol. *Mol. Biol. Rev.* **63**:675–707.
10. Kelly D. J. 1998, The physiology and metabolism of the human gastric pathogen *Helicobacter pylori. Adv. Microb. Physiol.* **40**:138–189.
11. Ge Z., and Taylor D. E., 1999, Contributions of genome sequencing to the understanding of the biology of Helicobacter pylori. *Ann. Rev. Microbiol.* **53**:353–387.

12. Lee A., and Robertson B., 1998, New *Helicobacter* species. p. 3–12. In Hunt R. H., and Tytgat G. N. T., (ed.), Basic mechanisms to clinical cure. Kluwer Academic Publishers Dordrect, The Netherlands.
13. Lee A., and Mitchell H., 1994, Basic bacteriology of *H. pylori* colonization factors, p. 59–72. In Hunt R. H., and Tytgat G. N. T., (ed.), Basic mechanisms to clinical cure. Kluwer Academic Publishers Dordrect, The Netherlands.
14. Melchers K., Hermann L., Mauch F., Bayle D., Heuermann D., Weitzenegger T., Schuhmacher A., Sachs G., Haas R., Bode G., Bensch K., and Schafer K. P., 1998, Properties and function of the P type inon pumps cloned from *Helicobacter pylori. Acta. Physiol. Scand. Suppl.* **643**:123–135.
15 Weeks D. L., Eskandari S., Scott D. R., and Sachs G., 2000, A H+–-gated urea channel: the link between Helicobacter pylori urease and gastric colonization. *Science.* **287**:482–485.
16. Scott D. R., Marcus E. A., Weeks D. L., Lee A., Melchers K., and Sachs G., 2000, Expression of the *Helicobacter pylori ureI* gene is required for acidic pH activation of cytoplasmic urease. *Infect. Immun.* **68**:470–477.
17. Skouloubris S., Thiberge J.-M., Labigne A., and De Reuse H., 1998, The *Helicobacter pylori* UreI protein is not involved in urease activity but is essential for bacterial survival in vivo. *Infect. Immun.* **66**:4517–4521.
18. Huesca M,. Goodwin A., Bhagwansingh A., Hoffman P., and Lingwood C. A., 1998, Characterization of an acidic-pH-inducible stress protein (hsp70), a putative sulfatide binding adhesin, from Helicobacter pylori. *Infect. Immun.* **66**:4061–4067.
19 Huesca M., Borgia S., Hoffman P. S., and Lingwood C. A., 1996, Acidic pH changes receptor binding specificity of *Helicobacter pylori*: a binary adhesion model in which surface heat shock (stress) proteins mediate sulfitide recognition in gastric colonization. *Infect. Immun.* **64**:2643–2648.
20. Guruge J. L., Falk P. G., Lorenz R. G., Dans M., Wirth H. P., Blaser M.J., Berg D. E., and Gordon J. I., 1998, Epithelial attachment alters the outcome of *Helicobacter pylori* infection. *Proc. Natl. Acad. Sci. U. S. A.* **95**:3925–3930.
21. Spohn, G., and Scarlato V., 1999, The autoregulatory HspR repressor protein governs chaperone gene transcription in *Helicobacter pylori. Mol. Microbiol.* **34**:663–674.
22. Yoshiyama, H., Nakamura H., Kimoto M., Okita K., and Nakazawa T., 1999, Chemotaxis and motility of *Helicobacter pylori* in a viscous environment. *J. Gastroenterol. 34, Suppl.* **11**:18–23.
23. Hoffman, P. S., and Garduno R., 1999, Surface-associated heat shock proteins of Legionella pneumophila and Helicobacter pylori: roles in pathogenesis and immunity. *Infect. Dis. Obstetrics and Gynecology* **7**:58–63.
24. Odenbreit S., Puls J., Sedlmaier B., Gerland E., Fischer W., and Haas R., 2000, Translocation of *Helicobacter pylori* CagA into gastric epithelial cells by type IV secretion. *Science.* **287**:1497–1500.
25. Hoffman, P. S., Goodwin A., Johnsen J., Magee K., and Veldhuyzen van Zanten S. J. O., 1996, Metabolic activities of metronidazole-sensitive and -resistant strains of *Helicobacter pylori*: Repression of pyruvate oxidoreductase and expression of isocitrate lyase activity correlate with resistance. *J. Bacteriol.* **178**:4822–4829.
26. Hughes, N. J., Chalk P. A., Clayton C. L., and Kelly D. J., 1995, Identification of carboxylation enzymes and characterization of a novel four-subunit pyruvate:flavodoxin oxidoreductase from *Helicobacter pylori. J. Bacteriol.* **177:**3953–3959.
27. Pitson, S. M., Mendz G. L., Srinivasan S., and Hazell S. L., 1999, The tricarboxylic acid cycle of *Helicobacter pylori. Eur. J. Biochem.* **260**:258–267.
28. Hughes, N. J., Clayton C. L., Chalk P. A., and Kelly D. J. 1998, *Helicobacter pylori* porCDAB and oorDABC genes encode distinct pyruvate:flavodoxin and 2-oxoglutarate:acceptor oxidoreductases which mediate electron transport to NADP. *J. Bacteriol.* **180:**1119–1128.
29. Kather, B., Stingl K., van der Rest M. E., Altendorf K., and Molenaar D., 2000, Another unusual type of citric acid cycle enzyme in *Helicobacter pylori*: the malate:quinone oxidoreductase. *J. Bacteriol.* **182**:3204–3209.

30. Huynen, M. A., Dandekar T., and Bork P., 1999, Variation and evolution of the citric-acid cycle: a genomic perspective. *Trends. Microbiol.* **7**:281–291.
31. 'D'Ari, R., and Casadesus J., 1998, Underground metabolism. *BioEssays.* **20**:181–186.
32. Payne, W. J., Grant M. A., Shapleigh J., and Hoffman P., 1982, Nitrogen oxide reduction in Wolinella succinogenes and *Campylobacter* species. *J. Bacteriol.* **152**:915–918.
33. Hoffman, P. S., and Goodman T. G., 1982, Respiratory physiology and energy conservation efficiency of *Campylobacter jejuni*. *J. Bacteriol.* **150**:319–326.
34. McGee, D. J., and Mobley H. L., 1999, Mechanisms of *Helicobacter pylori* infection: bacterial factors. *Curr. Top. Microbiol. Immunol.* **241**:155–180.
35. Mobley, H. L., Garner R. M., and Bauerfeind P., 1995, *Helicobacter pylori* nickel transport gene nixA: synthesis of catalytically active urease in *Escherichia coli* independent of growth conditions. *Mol. Microbiol.* **16**:97–109.

2

Diagnosis of *Helicobacter pylori* Infection

FRANCIS MÉGRAUD and TAMARA MATYSIAK

1. INTRODUCTION

Several methods are used to diagnose *Helicobacter pylori* infection. They are usually divided into two groups: invasive tests, which are all direct tests for which an endoscopy must be performed; and non-invasive tests, which are indirect tests that do not necessitate an endoscopy. The exception is the newly introduced antigen stool test which is a direct but non-invasive test. Each method has its advantages and disadvantages, and none can be considered to be perfect, i.e., to have a sensitivity and a specificity close to 100%, to be quick, readily available and inexpensive. Other characteristics which may be very useful are: 1) the possibility to detect pathogenic properties of *H. pylori*, 2) the globality of the test, and depending on the technique, 3) the added value of histology due to information gathered on the gastric mucosa status, and 4) for culture, the possibility to perform antimicrobial susceptibility testing.[1] The choice will also depend on the clinical situation, i.e., initial diagnosis or follow-up post-eradication treatment. In this chapter, the tests currently used will be described. Their advantages, disadvantages and optimal applications will be noted.

FRANCIS MÉGRAUD • Laboratoire de Bactériologie, Hôpital Pellegrin, Bordeaux, France.
TAMARA MATYSIAK • INSERM E9925, Faculté Necker—Enfants Malades, Paris, France.

Helicobacter pylori Infection and Immunity,
Edited by Yamamoto *et al.*, Kluwer Academic/Plenum Publishers, 2002.

2. TESTS PERFORMED DIRECTLY BY THE PHYSICIAN

Two tests can be classified in this category: the urease test which is performed by the endoscopist, and serology on whole blood which can be performed by any physician.

2.1. Tests Performed by the Endoscopist

The urease test is performed during endoscopy and does not need the intervention of a medical laboratory. It is based on the production of a large amount of urease by *H. pylori.* This enzyme breaks down urea generating ammonia and carbon dioxide. Commercially available kits consist of a urea solution in agar with a pH indicator on which the biopsy is normally placed. The ammonia generated increases the pH of the medium and the pH indicator changes color. Several kits are now commercially available, the first proposed being the CLOtest®.[2] This test is designed to be read after one hour and 24 hours. Its sensitivity ranges from 70 to 97% and its specificity from 90 to 100%.[3] Its sensitivity is dependent on the number of bacteria present in the biopsy; 10^4 CFU of bacteria are needed to obtain a positive result.[4] Such a quantity may not be present 4 weeks after an eradication treatment, and therefore this test is not recommended to test *H. pylori* eradication.[5] To increase the sensitivity, the use of two biopsies, the incubation of the kit at 37°C, and the use of a weakly buffered medium have been recommended. A membrane-based test (PyloriTek®) has been proposed more recently. It is designed to be read within one hour, but most of the results are obtained after only 20 minutes. Its sensitivity and specificity are high.[6,7]

The urease test is one of the most simple and inexpensive tests currently available. It provides an immediate result and then allows the immediate implementation of *H. pylori* eradication therapy when necessary.

3. TESTS PERFORMED BY ANY PHYSICIAN

The serology on whole blood test can be performed in the doctor's office within a few minutes. It is based on an indirect solid-phase immunoassay. A whole blood drop is mixed with an appropriate test developer solution and added to a pad. By capillary action the specimen and the developer solution move toward the *H. pylori* antigens immobilized as a dot or a band on the test membrane, and mobilize a dye conjugated with anti-human IgG. If specific antibodies are present, the complex consisting of *H. pylori* IgG and the conjugated dye binds to the antigen and a color change occurs within few minutes.

A variety of these so-called "doctor tests" have been proposed. The whole blood serology tests are quite practical and cheap. Despite the fact that their

TABLE 1
Sensitivity and specificity of several whole blood serological tests for *Helicobacter pylori*

Test	Author	n	Reference tests	Sensitivity	Specificity
Helisal	Moayyedi *et al.* (8)	114	H, C, UT, UBT	92	92
BM-test	Enroth *et al.* (9)	144	H, C	96	83
Flesxure	Graham *et al.* (10)	551	UT, S	96	95.1
CLOser	Chen *et al.* (11)	86	H, UT	95.7	72.5
AccuStat	Harrison *et al.* (12)	50	UBT, S	89.5	93.5
Pyloriset Screen	Oksanen *et al.* (13)	207	H, S	95	94

H: histology; C: culture; UT: urease test; UBT: urea breath test; BM: Boehringer Mannheim; S: serology.

sensitivities and specificities have been found satisfactory in published studies (Table 1), it must be emphasized that these studies have involved special settings where the same person systematically performed the tests, whereas they were designed primarily for general practitioners who will only use them from time to time. Nevertheless, we can expect increased accuracy of these tests which will ultimately contribute to the improvement in the diagnosis of *H. pylori* infection.

A rapid test detecting antibodies in urine (Rapirun®) is also being evaluated.

4. TESTS FOR WHICH A LABORATORY IS NEEDED

These tests require an endoscopy and collection of gastric biopsy specimens. As for all *H. pylori* tests except antibody tests, consumption of antibiotics and antisecretory drugs must be stopped at least 2 weeks before biopsy sampling.

It is recommended that biopsies be obtained from both the antrum and the corpus since there are situations when the bacteria can be present in one part or the other of the stomach.

4.1. Standard Bacteriological Tests

Gastric mucus can be obtained and observed either directly by dark-field microscopy to determine the motility of the bacteria, or after fixation and staining by Gram, Giemsa or acridine orange.

This test is a quick, cheap and specific method; its sensitivity is, however, limited and in the range of 80%. Bacteria can be evaluated semi-quantitatively. This method can be used in endoscopic wards if a microscope and expertise are available.

Culture has not been extensively used in routine testing until recently because it was wrongly considered to be a difficult technique. Currently, the emergence of resistant strains has rendered culture necessary, because it is the only method which allows antimicrobial susceptibility testing of the isolates. This information is becoming critical for the administration of the proper treatment, especially after an initial failure.[14]

To succeed in culturing *H. pylori*, special care must be taken during handling and processing of the specimens.[15] Biopsies (two from the antrum, two from the fundus) must be protected from dehydration and air, maintained at a low temperature, and ground with an electric homogenizer. Media with and without antibiotics must be freshly prepared and incubated in a proper atmosphere (5% oxygen) over long periods (10–12 days). In-house media may contain Wilkins Chalgren agar (Oxoid, Basingstoke, UK) supplemented with 10% blood, preferably of human origin, and the Dent selective supplement (Oxoid). The commercially available pylori agar (bioMérieux, Marcy l'Etoile, France) also allows good growth and selectivity.

To obtain an adequate atmosphere, either a special incubator filled with the gas mixtures producing 5% oxygen or anaerobe jars containing either a microaerobic gas generating kits or flushed and filled with the appropriate gas mixture can be used for routine culture.

Colonies of *H. pylori* grow after a minimum of 3 days. They appear as small, round, and smooth colonies. Identification involves microscopic examination and detection of enzymes (urease, catalase, and oxidase).

Under doubtful circumstances, molecular tests can be used. They consist of the identification of genes specific for *H. pylori* such as the urease gene, or the sequencing of the 16S rRNA gene.

By definition, culture has a 100% specificity because once a colony is present, all identification tests can be performed. Theoretically, the sensitivity should also be 100%, since a positive test can be obtained with only one organism. However, the difficulty in assuring both proper transport conditions and specimen handling in the lab usually leads to decreased sensitivity.

Molecular tests performed on colonies by PCR or hybridization allow the detection of genes considered as virulence markers such as *cagA*[16] and *vacA* alleles. In the case of relapse, other molecular tests can be employed: PCR-RFLP, RAPD and other techniques allowing differentiation between recurrence and re-infection.[17]

The drawback of culture is the delay in obtaining the result. At least three to five days are necessary to visualize colonies and an additional three to five days to get the results of the antimicrobial susceptibility tests. This technique is also ranked among the most costly. It can be considered as a reference technique.

Culture can also be performed on gastric juice although with less success. There is a turnover of gastric epithelial cells and *H. pylori* that adhere to these cells can be found in gastric juice. Positive cultures have been obtained by induced vomiting.[18] The detection of *H. pylori* in feces by culture is not a reliable method.

Positive results have only been obtained in cases of spontaneous or induced diarrhea.[18,19] This latter method is still limited to the research domain.

4.2. Histological Detection

The Sydney System recommends obtaining two biopsies each from the antrum and the fundus. In the revised version, biopsies from the angulus were also requested.[20] These biopsies must be fixed in formaldehyde and processed within two weeks. The preparation and staining of histological slides is critical. Spiral bacteria can be observed microscopically at high magnification on the epithelium surface, in the mucus and in the crypts sometimes adhering to the epithelial cells but not intracellularly nor in areas of intestinal metaplasia. These bacteria can be seen after hematein eosin staining but special stains are highly recommended.[21] A small biopsy which has been poorly oriented or inadequately fixed or stained can jeopardize the results of the examination.

The specificity and sensitivity of histology can be decreased when there are few atypical bacteria present. In such cases, immunohistochemistry or molecular methods (*in situ* hybridization or PCR) can be helpful.

Indeed, the results of histology are very much dependent on the experience of the observer. Inter-observer reproducibility is not good.[22] Histology is not a quantitative test but allows a semi-quantitative evaluation. Similar to culture, this test is considered to be relatively costly, but the delay in obtaining results is shorter (two to three days). It also allows a retrospective evaluation since the paraffin blocks are usually kept in the laboratory.

The added value of histology is the possibility to study the gastric mucosa. During the post-eradication follow-up, the disappearance of activity can be considered as a surrogate of *H. pylori* eradication.

4.3. Polymerase Chain Reaction (PCR)

This technique is reputed to be highly sensitive and specific. It consists of amplifying DNA sequences specific for *H. pylori* in gastric biopsies. Bacteria do not have to be viable, so no specific transport conditions are required.

The biopsy is first disrupted to release the bacteria and lysed with a specific buffer in order to make the DNA accessible. Then the PCR *per se* is performed with a special thermostable DNA polymerase (*Taq* polymerase), nucleotides and primers usually derived from the urease gene. The amplified products are then identified according to their size by electrophoresis after staining with ethidium bromide.[23] Another approach is to perform a DNA-enzyme immunoassay. The hybrids are detected by an immunoenzymatic reaction, which consists of applying an anti-double strand DNA antibody, a conjugate, and a chromogenic substrate allowing colorimetric detection.

Theoretically, it is possible to detect a unique copy of bacterial DNA present in the specimen. This is true when a PCR is performed on culture. In contrast, a PCR which is performed directly on biopsy specimens is less sensitive, first, because the nucleic acids must be released and, second, because *Taq* polymerase inhibitors may be present.

PCR specificity can be compromised by cross-contamination between the specimens studied and amplified products from a previous reaction. Therefore, very strict procedures must be followed. To increase the sensitivity, nested PCR has been proposed. This method consists of a second PCR using primers inside the DNA fragment which was first amplified. However, nested PCR is not generally recommended because of the risk of false positive reactions.[24]

Quantitative PCR is also possible using specific thermocyclers. The main advantage of PCR is that it does not require specific transport conditions and the results are obtained within a day. The absence of commercial kits has been a limit to the development of this technique as a standardized procedure for *H. pylori* detection. Its current use is focused on detecting the presence of virulence genes such as *cagA*, the allelic type of *vacA*,[25] or mutations causing macrolide resistance[26] which can be performed directly on biopsy specimens. The point mutations on the 23S rRNA can be detected using a DEIA[27] and even more rapidly by dissociation of the amplicons in the Light Cycler®.[28]

4.4. Tests Performed by any Physician

As for the urease test, this test is based on the great amount of urease produced by *H. pylori*. Urea labeled with a carbon isotope is ingested, and broken down into ammonia and labeled carbon dioxide when *H. pylori* is present in the stomach; the labeled carbon dioxide is absorbed into the blood and eliminated in the expired air. When *H. pylori* is not present, most of the labeled urea is eliminated in the urine.

Two carbon isotopes can be used: one is a radioactive isotope with a very long half life, carbon 14 (^{14}C), which is used as a tracer;[29] the other is a non-radioactive stable isotope, carbon 13 (^{13}C).[30]

Different protocols have been proposed with regard to the use of ^{13}C labeled urea. It is recommended that the patient fast and ingest something to delay gastric emptying. The first protocol to be recommended included a test meal. It was then recognized that ingestion of citric acid had a better effect and was more convenient.[31] More recently, orange juice has also been used, alleviating the need to include citric acid in the kit. It is more pleasant to drink while the effect is slightly inferior. The dose of urea can also vary: 75 mg seems to be sufficient and corresponds to the dose present in certain kits while others contain 100 mg.

The ratio of $^{13}C/^{12}C$ is always determined prior to ingesting the isotope because the amount of ^{13}C present in the expired air (collected by blowing into a tube) may vary according to the patient's diet. A second sample is collected 30 minutes after the ingestion and the difference in the ratios before and after the ingestion is calculated. The cut-off considered for positivity varies between 3.5 and 5 delta per mil.

The analysis is performed using an isotope-ratio mass spectrometer on a small amount of breath air. Another technology, non-dispersive infrared spectrometry, may also be used but a larger amount of breath air is required and must be collected in a bag.[32]

The ^{13}C-UBT is very accurate with both high sensitivity and specificity and is not dependent on special transport conditions (it can be sent by normal mail) nor on the observer, contrary to most other tests.

Other urease positive bacteria can theoretically be present in case of hypochlorhydria and bacterial proliferation can lead to positive results but this situation is very seldom found. False negative results may occur when only a low number of bacteria are present in the stomach, for instance when there is extensive intestinal metaplasia, or consumption of antibiotics or antisecretory drugs. In the latter case, the anti-urease activity of PPIs may also be responsible.

The ^{13}C-UBT can be used as a screening test, as well as a post-treatment follow-up test. It is definitely the most appealing method available for this last purpose.

There are attempts to use UBT as a quantitative test but, in comparison to culture or histology, the results are controversial. When the $^{13}C/^{12}C$ ratio was tested in the blood (serum bicarbonate assay), the overall accuracy was indeed inferior.

A new test measuring the $^{13}C/^{12}C$ ratio on-line by the patient blowing directly into a tube connected to a special apparatus is currently being developed (Oridion, Israel).

The possibility of using an isotope other than ^{13}C, e.g., ^{15}N, has also been explored. For this test, urine samples are assayed for ^{15}N. No clear advantage has been demonstrated to this test.

The cost of UBT is very high in the US while, in most European countries, it is only slightly higher than that of culture and histology.

A special scintillation counter has been developed to measure ^{14}C radioactivity when performing ^{14}C-UBT. The dose absorbed is very low, but this test cannot be used in children and pregnant women. The breath collection normally occurs after 20 minutes.

4.5. Antigen Stool Test

This direct non-invasive test has been recently introduced. It concerns the detection of *H. pylori* antigens in stools, using specific antibodies and an ELISA. The commercially available test is the Premier Platinum Hp SA® (Meridian

TABLE 2
Sensitivity and specificity of the antigen stool test in several studies

Country	Patient No.	Reference tests	Sensitivity	Specificity
Europe (33)	501	C or H + UT	94.1	91.8
Austria (35)	100	UBT – S	89	94.6
Italy (36)	154	UT + H	94	93
France (41)	99	C or H + UT	89	94
Spain	105	RT + UBT	91.8	83.3
Canada	137	C-H-UT – UBT	98	95
Taiwan	59	C or H + UT – UBT	94.4	87
Japan	188	UT + H + UBT	95.5	93.9
Italy	124	UT-H – UBT	97	91
Israel	73	H-UT – S	83	96
Germany	94	UBT	93	95

H: histology; C: culture; UT: urease test; UBT: urea breath test; BM: Boehringer Mannheim; S: serology.

Diagnostics). The plates are coated with *H. pylori* antibodies and a fecal suspension is added to the well followed by a conjugate.

This test is easy to perform and does not require special transport conditions. Its sensitivity and specificity were 94.1% and 91.8%, respectively, in a large European multicenter study published in 1999.[33] The results of other studies presented in Table 2 show comparable good results with two exceptions where the sensitivity in one case, and the specificity in another, were only 83%.

This test can also be used for post-treatment follow-up. In the European multicenter study, sensibility was equivalent but specificity was even higher (90.9%) to the screening test.[34] However, such a good specificity was not confirmed by Makristathis *et al.* (68%)[35] and Trevisiani *et al.* (82%).[36] The limitation can be the difficulty in obtaining stool samples from adult patients in certain countries. However, this test may become a standard for children in the future based on the promising results reported.

4.6. Detection of Specific Antibodies in Serum

Serology is a standard method of indirect diagnosis in infectious diseases, and therefore was one of the first to be applied to *H. pylori.* This bacterium is so different from most bacteria colonizing humans that a specific reaction can be obtained even when using a sonicate of the organism as the antigen. However, because it is a mucosal infection, the antibody titer may not be very high. Despite the general sensitivity of the ELISA, in a good proportion of cases, the values obtained are close to the cut-off.

TABLE 3
Comparative study of sensitivity and specificity of eight kits on the same 59 serums samples and performed in 17 laboratories (adapted from reference 38)

Test	Mean sensitivity (%)	Mean specificity (%)
Hel-p Test (Amrad)	89.4	93.3
Malakit (Biolab)	79.9	98.6
GAP IgG (Bio-Rad)	94.9	91.3
Pyloriset EIA-G (Orion)	95.8	95.5
Helico - G (Porton)	92.3	87.1
H. pylori IgG Kit Radim (Radim)	81.6	90.7
Roche MTP (Roche)	99.3	86.5
Pylori-stat (Whittaker)	92.9	89.4

There is also an important heterogeneity in the response of individuals to *H. pylori*, either due to the diversity of antibody production or to the diversity of antigen expression by the bacteria.[37]

Because of cross-reactions which can theoretically occur with campylobacter flagella, commercial kits have turned to a second generation of antigens consisting of a mixture of purified antigens, some highly immunogenic. There are more than 20 such kits now available. Our experience concerns essentially the Pyloriset IgG EIA (Orion, Espoo, Finland) and the Hp Check EIA (Hoffman La Roche, Basel, Switzerland) which are both excellent. These commercial kits have never all been compared in the same study. However, Feldman *et al.* compared 10 of them on the same sera in 15 laboratories and obtained the best results with Pyloriset IgG EIA (Table 3).[38] A comparison based on all published studies has recently been made.[39]

Serology detecting specific IgG antibodies is a good technique but it suffers from the fact that antibodies persist months and possibly years after *H. pylori* eradication and even then can be the sign of either a current infection or an infection which has already been cured. For this reason, serology cannot be used for post-treatment follow-up, unless it is possible to test the pre-treatment serum and a follow-up serum obtained 6 months after the treatment on the same plate.[40] Some kits detecting *H. pylori* specific IgA antibodies have been proposed but do not seem to be very promising since not all patients raise specific IgA antibodies in serum.

Important developments have been made in the field of serology in recent years: immunoblot (western blot) is now commercially available (Helicoblot 2.0, Genelabs, Singapore). This test is very practical because it is highly specific.[41] It can be used to confirm doubtful ELISA results as done for HIV infection. Furthermore, the specific detection of a 120–130 KD protein band can identify patients harboring *cagA* positive strains.

ELISA to detect the CagA antigen. Specific ELISAs using recombinant CagA antigen have been developed and can also identify patients infected with strains which are suspected to be more pathogenic than others: CagA IgG EIA Well® (Radim, Pomezia, Italy) and Helori-CTX® (Eurospital SPA, Trieste, Italy).

4.7. Detection of Specific Antibodies in Saliva

IgG antibodies can transude from the serum into saliva. Their concentration is much lower than in serum but there are also fewer substances which can interfere in the reaction so it is not necessary to dilute the specimens. Devices to collect either saliva (Omnisal®, Cortex Diagnostics, Clwyd, UK) or saliva plus gingival transudate (OraSure®, Epitope, Beaverton, Oregon, USA) have been designed. Using saliva collected with OraSure® and the Roche ELISA, we obtained specific results but with a lower sensitivity than serum testing.[42] A kit calibrated to be used with OraSure® is being developed (Enteric Products, Stony Brooke, NY, USA). The first results also show a sensitivity inferior to serum testing.

4.8. Detection of Specific Antibodies in Urine

A test detecting *H. pylori* specific IgG antibodies in urine (Urinelisa *H. pylori* antibody®) has recently been proposed (Otsuka, Tokyo, Japan). Only one study has been published but its results are quite promising.[43]

4.9. Detection of *H. pylori* DNA in Stools

This approach has always been faced with the problem of the presence of PCR inhibitors. These PCR inhibitors have been identified as complex polysaccharides of food origin, especially issued from vegetables.[44] Therefore, their quality and quantity may vary according to diet.

There is, at present, no simple and efficient method to eliminate these PCR inhibitors. However, several groups claim to have succeeded. Reliable results were obtained by Makristathis *et al.* using a very complicated purification procedure.[35] Because of its timescale and complexity, this method cannot be used in routine testing.

5. HOW TO USE THE DIFFERENT TESTS?

Few studies have compared all the different tests on the same patients and furthermore the choice of a gold standard is always a problem. Nevertheless, it was possible to show that most of the tests have a sensitivity and a specificity higher than 90% (Table 4). The exception concerns the lower sensitivity of the urease

TABLE 4
Comparison of the sensitivity of different tests for the diagnosis of *Helicobacter pylori* (excluding post-treatment follow-up)

	Monteiro *et al.* n = 104	Lerang *et al.* n = 351	Andersen *et al.* n = 97		Thijs *et al.* n = 105	Soulé *et al.* (multicenter) n = 104	Olson *et al.* (multicenter) n = 845	Cutler *et al.* n = 228	Vandenplas *et al.* n = 95	Logan *et al.* n = 195
^{13}C UBT	93%	95%	87%	77%	100%	94%	91%	90%	96%	98%
Serology	95%	99%	81%	69%	98%	–	–	91%	96%	91%
Immunoblot	–	–	100%	97%	–	–	–	–	–	–
Histology	95%	–	100%	78%	97%	100%	99%	93%	100%	95%
Urease test (24 h)	89%	85%	84%	65%	90%	–	–	89%	100%	92%
Culture	100%	93%		64%	98%	86%	83%	–	–	83%
PCR	93%	–	90%	80%	97%	91%	–	–	–	–
Reference test	Culture + or histology[+] and urease test[+]	association of three tests	culture or histology[+]	association of two tests	association of two tests	association of two tests	association of three tests	Association of four tests	Culture	association of two tests

test, but PyloriTek® was not performed nor the whole blood serology tests, and saliva tests. In addition, some serological kits have a lower specificity.

It must be said, first, that the decision to test implies the decision to treat according to several consensus conferences held in recent years, because it does not seem ethical to tell a patient that he has this infection and not give him an eradication treatment.[45,46]

The method to be used may vary widely according to country. The elements to be taken into consideration are the rate of infection, the rate of gastric cancer, the availability of the tests and their cost.

6. INITIAL DIAGNOSIS

In the US, the rate of infection and of gastric cancer is low and the cost of endoscopy is very high, so it is cost-effective to use a "test and treat" strategy for patients under 50 years of age. For this purpose, any non-invasive test can be used but serology is the least costly. The most convenient would be to use doctor tests but in our opinion their performance is not yet adequate. The same strategy may be useful in other countries where the possibility of endoscopy is limited by the low number of endoscopists such as in the UK.

In other European countries, endoscopy is widely available and relatively cheap so the "test and scope" strategy or the "scope and treat" strategy is more useful, taking into account the reassuring value of a negative endoscopy for the patient. The "test and scope" strategy will also include laboratory serology and the sero-positive patients will be scheduled for endoscopy and treatment.

The "scope and treat" strategy leaves the diagnosis in the hands of the specialist who can use any of the invasive tests. In young adults, performing a urease test may be sufficient especially if the most accurate one (PyloriTek®) is used. Other tests will increase the costs but histology may be important in older patients to evaluate the status of the mucosa, and ideally culture should be performed to test macrolide resistance before prescribing clarithromycin. At this stage, the unavailability of PCR kits renders this method impractical for routine *H. pylori* diagnosis.

However, PCR may be routinely used in the future to detect clarithromycin resistance directly from a biopsy specimen using the new real-time PCR apparatus LightCycler®. In children, the tendency is to avoid endoscopy as often as possible. In this context, non-invasive tests have to be considered. However, they have not been properly validated in this population, except the UBT in children older than 5 years of age. It is possible that false positives occur in younger children. The antibody response may be weak in children, so the cut-off value needs to be adapted to this population. Furthermore, it must be noted that antibodies may appear a few weeks after the onset of the infection leading to the possibility of false negatives using serology. The antigen stool test may indeed be the most accurate method according to the first studies performed. A large European study is currently being conducted to answer these questions. But once endoscopy is performed, the same tests used in adults can be performed.

In patients older than 50 years, endoscopy becomes mandatory because of the increased risk of gastric cancer at this age. Histology will also be systematically performed to gain information on the mucosa.

The detection of *H. pylori* becomes more difficult in patients older than 70 years due to the prevalence of atrophy and intestinal metaplasia, as well as the common use of antisecretory drugs and antibiotics (up to 40% in our experience). Considering patients who had not taken medication, UBT and culture had the highest sensitivity, and histology the lowest (Montaudon). The antigen stool test has not yet been evaluated in this age group.

7. POST-TREATMENT FOLLOW-UP

While post-treatment follow-up concerns the detection of the same bacterium, the accuracy of the tests may be different than before treatment, because the bacterial load tends to be lower and its distribution in the stomach may be different with less bacteria in the antrum. The consequence is that when using biopsy based tests, it is mandatory to obtain biopsies both from the antrum and the corpus. The least sensitive test (urease test) is not recommended in this context. Since a positive biopsy result means failure of the previous treatment, it may be advised to use culture which allows susceptibility testing in view of a second line treatment. However, non-invasive tests are favored, especially the UBT.

In a comparative study, the UBT performed favorably in comparison to culture and histology (Table 5). The first results obtained with the antigen stool test are also very promising.

TABLE 5
Comparison of the sensitivity of three tests for post-treatment follow-up in three multicentrer studies

	French multicenter study Soulé *et al.* (n = 104)	International multicenter study Olson *et al.* (n = 634)	European multicenter study Mégraud *et al.* (n = 97)
^{13}C UBT	97%	89% Europe 95% / USA 83%	87.5%
Histology	95%	97% Europe 96% / USA 99%	95%
Culture	76%	81% Europe 75% / USA 86%	90%

8. CONCLUSION

In conclusion, biopsy-based tests remain the reference tests but, now that the spectrum of diseases related to *Helicobacter pylori* infection is expanding, there is a trend to obtain more rapid results using convenient and inexpensive tests. For this purpose, non-invasive tests are the most suitable and several have been developed. The urea breath tests remain the most accurate, but progress in antigen stool tests and antibody tests may challenge this leadership in the future.

REFERENCES

1. Mégraud F., 1996, Advantages and disadvantages of *Helicobacter pylori* diagnostic tests for the detection of *Helicobacter pylori. Scand. J. of Gastroenterol.* **31**(suppl 215):57–62.
2. Marshall B. J., Warren J. R., Francis G. J., Langton S. R., Goodwin C. S., and Blincow E. D., 1987, Rapid urease test in the management of *Campylobacter pyloridis*—associated gastritis. *Am. J. Gastroenterol.* **82**:200–210.
3. Lee N., Lee T. T., and Fang K. M., 1994, Assessment of four rapid urease test systems for detection of *Helicobacter pylori* in gastric biopsy specimens. *Diagn. Microbiol. Infect Dis.* **18**:69–74.
4. Laine L., Chun D., Stein C., Le-Beblawi I., Sharma V., and Chandrasoma P., 1996, The influence of size or number of biopsies on rapid urease test results: a prospective evaluation. *Gastrointest. Endosc.* **43**:49–53.
5. Louw J. A., Zak J., Jaskiewicz K., Lastovica A. J., Kotze T. J., Lucke W., Le Roux E., and Marks I. N., 1992, Omeprazole may clear but does not eradicate *H. pylori. Eur. J. Gastroenterol. Hepatol.* **4**:481–485.
6. Rogge J. D., Wagner D. R., Carrico R. J., Glowinski E. A., Mahoney S. J., Boguslawski R. C., and Genta R. M., 1995, Evaluation of a new urease reagent strip for detection of *Helicobacter pylori* in gastric specimens. *Am. J. Gastroenterol.* **90**:1965–1969.
7. Yousfi M. M., El-Zimaity H. M. T., Genta R. M., and Graham D. Y., 1996, Evaluation of a new reagent strip rapid urease test for detection of *Helicobacter pylori* infection. *Gastrointest. Endosc.* **44**:519–522.
8. Moayyedi P., Carter A. M., Herppell R. M., *et al.*, 1997, Validation of a rapid whole blood test for the diagnosing of *Helicobacter pylori* infection. *BMJ* **314**:7074–7119.
9. Nilson I., Ljungh A., Aleljung P., *et al.*, 1997, Immunoblot assay for serodiagnosis of *Helicobacter pylori* infections. *J. Clin. Microbiol.* **35**:427–432.
10. Enroth H., Rigo R., Hulten K., *et al.*, 1997, Diagnostic accuracy of a rapid whole blood test for detection of *Helicobacter pylori. J. Clin. Microbiol.* **35**:2695–2697.
11. Sörberg M., Engstrand L., Ström M., *et al.*, 1996, The diagnosis value of enzyme immunoassay and immunoblot in monitoring eradication of *Helicobacter pylori. Scand. J. Infect Dis.* **6**:579–583.
12. Graham D. Y., Evans D. J. Jr, Peacock J., *et al.*, 1996, Comparison of rapid serological tests (FexSure and QuickVue) with conventional ELISA for detection of *Helicobacter pylori* infection. *Am. J. Gastroenterol. Hepatol.* **91**:942–948.
13. Thijs J. C., van Zwet A. A., Meyer B. C., *et al.*, 1997, Serology to monitor the efficacy of anti-*Helicobacter pylori* treatment. *Eur. J. Gastroenterol. Hepatol.* **6**:184–186.
14. Mégraud F., 1998, Epidemiology and mechanism of antibiotic resistance in *Helicobacter pylori. Gastroenterology* **115**:1278–1282.
15. Mégraud F., 1998, A growing demand for *Helicobacter pylori* culture in the near future? *Ital. J. Gastroenterol. Hepatol.* **29**:574–576.

16. Jenks P. J., Mégraud F., and Labigne A., 1998, Clinical outcome after infection with *Helicobacter pylori* does not appear to be reliably predicted by the presence of any of the genes of the *cag* pathogencity island. *Gut* **43**(6):752–758.
17. Hua J., Birac C., and Mégraud F., 1996, PCR-based RAPD (random amplified polymorphic DNA) "fingerprinting" of clinical isolates of *Helicobacter pylori*. *In*: *Helicobacter pylori*: techniques for clinical diagnosis & basic research. A. Lee and F. Mégraud (Eds.). W.B. Saunders Company Ltd: London 121–127.
18. Parsonnet J., Shmuely H., and Haggerty T., 1999, Fecal and oral shedding of *Helicobacter pylori* from healthy infected adults. *JAMA* **282**:2240–2245.
19. Thomas J. E., Gibson G. R., Darboe M. K., Dale A., and Weaver L. T., 1992, Isolation of *Helicobacter pylori* from human faeces. *Lancet* **340**:1194–1195.
20. Dixon M. F., Genta R. M., Yardley J. H., Correa P., and the participants in the International Workshop on the Histopathology of Gastritis, Houston 1994, 1996, Classification and grading of gastritis. The updated Sydney System. *Am. J. Surg. Pathol.* **20**:1161–1181.
21. Price A. B., 1995, The histological recognition of *Helicobacter pylori*. *In*: *Helicobacter pylori*. Techniques for clinical diagnosis and basic research. A. Lee and F. Mégraud (Eds.). W.B. Saunders Company Ltd, London, 33–49.
22. Kolts B. E., Joseph B., Achem S. R., Bianchi T., and Monteiro C., 1993, *Helicobacter pylori* detection: a quality and cost analysis. *Am. J. Gastroenterol.* **88**:650–655.
23. Monteiro L., Birac C., and Mégraud F., 1995, Detection of *Helicobacter pylori* in gastric biopsy by polymerase chain reaction. *In: Helicobacter pylori*. Techniques for clinical diagnosis and basic research. A. Lee and F. Mégraud (Eds.). W.B. Saunders Company Ltd, London, 112–120.
24. European *Helicobacter pylori* Study Group, 1997, Guidelines for clinical trials in *Helicobacter pylori* infection. *Gut* **41**(suppl 2).
25. van Doorn L. J., Figueiredo C., Mégraud F., *et al.*, 1999, Geographic distribution of *vac*A allelic types of *Helicobacter pylori*. *Gastroenterology* **116**:823–830.
26. Occhialini A., Urdaci M., Doucet-Populaire F., Bébéar C. M., Lamouliatte H., and Mégraud F., 1997, Macrolide resistance in *Helicobacter pylori*: rapid detection of point mutations and assays of macrolide binding to ribosomes. *Antimicrob. Agents Chemother.* **41**:2724–2728.
27. Marais A., Monteiro L., Occhialini A., Pina M., Lamouliatte H., and Mégraud F., 1999, Direct detection of *Helicobacter pylori* resistance to macrolides by a polymerase chain reaction/DNA enzyme immunoaasay in gastric biopsy specimens. *Gut* **44**.
28. Gibson J. R., Saunders N. A., Burke B., and Owen R. J., 1999, Novel method for rapid determination on clarithromycin sensitivity in *Helicobacter pylori*. *J. Clin. Microbiol.* **37**:3746–3748.
29. Marshall B. J., and Surveyor I., 1988, Carbon-14 urea breath test for the diagnosis of *Campylobacter pylori* associated gastritis. *J. Nucl. Med.* **29**:11–16.
30. Graham D. Y., Klein P. D., Evans D. J., *et al.*, 1987, *Campylobacter pylori* detected non-invasively by the ^{13}C-urea breath test. *Lancet* **ii**:1174–1177.
31. Dominguez-Muñoz J. E., Leodolter A., Sauerbruch T., and Malfertheiner P., 1997, A citric acid solution is an optimal test drink in the ^{13}C-urea breath test for the diagnosis of *Helicobacter pylori* infection. *Gut* **40**:459–462.
32. Koletzko S., Haisch M., Seeboth I., Braden B., Hengels K., Loketzko B., and Hering P., 1995, Isotope-selective non-dispersive infrared spectrometry for detection of *Helicobacter pylori* infection with ^{13}C-urea breath test. *Lancet* **345**:961–962.
33. Vaira D., Malfertheiner P., Mégraud F., Axon A. T. R., Deltenre M., Hirschl A. M., Gasbarrini G., O'Morain C., Pajares Garcia J. M., Quina M., Tytgat G. N. J., and the HpSA European, 1999, Diagnosis of *Helicobacter pylori* infection with a new non-invasive antigen-based assay. *Lancet* **354**:30–33.
34. Vaira D., Malfertheiner P., Mégraud F., Axon A. T. R., Deltenre M., Gasbarrini G., O'Morain C., Pajares Garcia J. M., Quina M., and Tytgat G. N. J., 2000, Non-invasive antigen based assay

for assessing *Helicobacter pylori* eradication. A european multicenter study. *Am. J. Gatsroenterol.* (in press).

35. Makristhatis A., Pasching E., Schutze K., Wimmer M., Rotter M. L., and Hirschl A. M., 1998, Detection of *Helicobacter pylori* in stool specimens by PCR and antigen enzyme immunoassay. *J. Clin. Microbiol.* **36**:2772–2774.
36. Trevisani L., Sartoni S., Galvani F., Rossi M. R., Ruina M., Chiamenti C., and Caselli M., 1999, Evaluation of a new enzyme immunoassay for detecting *Helicobacter pylori* in faeces: a prospective pilot study. *Am. J. Gastroenterol.* **94**:1830–1833.
37. Mayo K., Pretolani S., Gasbarrini G., Ghironzi G., and Mégraud F., 1998, Heterogeneity of IgG response to *Helicobacter pylori* measured by The Unweighted Pair Group method with Averages. *Clin. Drap. Lab. Immunol.* **5**:70–73.
38. Feldman R. A., Deeks J. J., and Evans J. J. W., 1995, The *Helicobacter pylori* serology study group. Multi laboratory comparison of eight commercially available *Helicobacter pylori* serology kits. *Eur. J. Clin. Microbiol. Inf. Dis.* **14**:428–433.
39. Laheij R. J. F., Straatman H., Jansen J. B. M. J., and Verbeek A. L. M., 1998, Evaluation of commercially available *Helicobacter pylori* serology kits: a review. *J. Clin. Microbiol.* **36**:2803–2809.
40. Kosunen T. U., Seppalä K., Sarna S., and Sipponen P., 1992, Diagnostic value of decreasing IgG, IgA and IgM antibody titers after eradication of *Helicobacter pylori*. *Lancet* **339**:893–895.
41. Monteiro L., de Mascarel A., Sarasqueta A. M., Bergey B., Barberis C., Talby P., Roux D., Shouler L., Goldfain D., Lamouliatte H., and Mégraud F., 2000, Diagnosis of *Helicobacter pylori* infection: non-invasive methods compared to invasive methods and evaluation of the antigen stool test. *Am. J. Gastroenterol.* (submitted for publication).
42. Mégraud F., Bouchard S., and Manier C., 1994, Detection of IgG in gingival transudate using a special collection device. *Gastroenterology* **106**:135.
43. Katsuragi K., Noda A., Tachikawa T., *et al.*, 1998, Highly sensitive urine-based enzyme-linked immunosorbent assay for detection of antibody to *Helicobacter pylori*. *Helicobacter* **3**:289–295.
44. Monteiro L., Bonnemaison D., Vekris A., *et al.*, 1997, Complex polysaccharides as PCR inhibitors in feces. *Helicobacter pylori* model. *J. Clin. Microbiol.* **35**:995–998.
45. Current European concepts in the management of *Helicobacter pylori* infection, 1997, The Maastricht Consensus Report. *Gut* **41**:8–13.
46. The Report of the Digestive Health Initiative international Update Conference on *Helicobacter pylori*, 1997, *Gastroenterology* **113**(suppl):S4–S8.
47. Salles-Montaudon N., Monteiro L., Gras N., de Mascarel A., Rainfray M., Emerian J. P., and Mégraud F., 2000, Résultats préliminaires d'une étude prospective. *Gastroenterol. Clin. Biol.* (in press).

3

Helicobacter pylori Infection and Gastric Cancer

PELAYO CORREA

1. INTRODUCTION

Although histopathologists described the bacterium we now call *Helicobacter pylori* more than 100 years ago,[1,2] recognition of its importance as a human pathogen dates back only to 1983, when Warren and Marshall reported their finding of "unidentified curved bacilli" in the stomachs of Australian patients with gastritis, peptic ulceration and gastric cancer.[3,4] The role of the bacterium as a cause of chronic gastritis and peptic ulceration has been documented.[5,6] Its role as a human carcinogen has been considered controversial by some investigators. The weight of the epidemiologic evidence, however, led the International Agency for Research on Cancer to declare the infection with the bacterium as a human carcinogen.[7]

This chapter will discuss the evidence to support the carcinogenic role of the bacterium, its involvement in the precancerous process and the hypothetical mechanisms leading to neoplastic events, as well as the cancer prevention potential.

PELAYO CORREA • Pathology, Louisiana State University Health Sciences Center, New Orleans, Louisiana

Helicobacter pylori Infection and Immunity,
Edited by Yamamoto *et al.*, Kluwer Academic/Plenum Publishers, 2002.

2. EPIDEMIOLOGY

The proposition that *H. pylori* infection may "have a part to play" in gastric cancer was mentioned by Marshall in his original report in 1983. It has since been methodically addressed by the scientific community utilizing classical epidemiologic techniques: correlation studies, retrospective case-control studies and prospective cohort studies. Epidemiologic techniques have also been utilized to investigate how the bacterium is transmitted, which may be relevant to the outcome of the infection.

Correlation (also called "ecologic") studies examine the association in diverse populations of 2 separate events: in this case the prevalence of *H. pylori* infection and gastric cancer rates. Such studies have been recently summarized.[8,9] Six such studies have shown a positive association between infection and gastric cancer; in 3 of them the difference was statistically significant. In 46 rural counties of China, gastric cancer rates were matched with results of serologic testing for *H. pylori* in each population. A significantly high correlation between the 2 events (46%) was reported.[10] Significant associations were also reported in a serologic study of 17 different populations,[11] chosen to reflect the global range of gastric cancer incidence. Correlation studies only provide weak evidence of association, but are useful as indicators of the need for more sophisticated studies to test the causality of the association.

At least 17 retrospective case-control studies examining the association between *H. pylori* infection and gastric cancer have been reported and recently summarized.[8,9,12] Most of the studies that were conducted in low or intermediate cancer risk countries showed an increased risk of gastric cancer in *H. pylori* infected subjects; however, that was not always the case in several studies in high risk countries. The divergent findings have been in large part clarified by a consideration of the issue of temporality. In retrospective case-control studies disease and exposure status are documented at the same time: in this case the presence of gastric cancer and the infection with *H. pylori*. Infection is usually acquired in childhood and may disappear in older individuals, especially if atrophic gastritis or intestinal metaplasia progress to the point of rendering the gastric microenvironment hostile to *H. pylori* colonization. The infection, however, may have triggered events which influence the initiation and/or progression of the precancerous process. Several reports indicate that this might have been the case: in Swedish and Japanese[13,14] studies, the relative risk of cancer in infected subjects decreases as the age increases. The same phenomenon is reported in meta-analysis of case-control studies, as seen in Table 1.[12] The same general message is found in the Japanese study by Fukuda *et al.*: higher risk in early or small cancers, in which the precancerous atrophic and metaplastic lesions are expected to be less advanced.[14] In summary, retrospective case-control studies may yield conflicting or negative results only if the temporality issue is not addressed.

TABLE 1
Meta-Analysis of *H. pylori*-Gastric Cancer Case-Control Studies

20–29	9.29
30–39	7.27
40–49	3.65
50–59	1.86
60–69	1.46
>70	1.05

Prospective (cohort) studies may provide stronger test of causality. In such studies exposure is determined prior to the onset of clinical disease, thereby avoiding the temporality issue and recall biases. In the case of the *H. pylori*-gastric cancer association, they are particularly helpful because the infection is documented long before the cancer event, implicating that the precancerous lesions of atrophy and metaplasia were not advanced. In the case of *H. pylori* infection, the original event was documented by examining samples of serum which were kept frozen for many years. Although the testing for *H. pylori* antibodies was performed at the time that the presence of cancer (cases) or its absence (controls) was documented, the serum sample represented the infection status many years before. This type of design is usually called: "nested case-control." Findings from cohort studies were key to the classification of the *H. pylori* infection as carcinogenic to humans by the International Agency for Research on Cancer in 1994. At that time 3 independent cohorts studies were reported: Japanese-Americans in Hawaii,[15] Kaiser Permanente subscribers in California[16] and Union workers in the United Kingdom.[17] All reported an elevated risk of gastric cancer in patients whose serum obtained years before were positive for *H. pylori* antibody. A combined analysis showed that the risk increased with the time between serum sample collection and the cancer diagnosis. The relative risk was 2.1 when the time interval was less than 5 years and 8.7 when it was 15 years or greater.[18] This provides a strong argument for causality: the longer the exposure (dose), the greater the cancer risk (effect). More recent studies of similar design have supported the findings of the 3 original cohort reports.[9]

It has been estimated that approximately 50% of the world's population are infected with *H. pylori*, and only a very small minority develops cancer. It is therefore of great interest to examine the factors which lead to a neoplastic outcome in *H. pylori* infected individuals. One factor that has been proposed as a determinant of risk is the age at first infection. The earlier the age at infection, the greater the risk. Some indicators of early infection, such as larger sibship size and higher birth order, are associated with higher risk of infection.[19] In Colombian children with very high prevalence of infection, the risk of infection increases with the

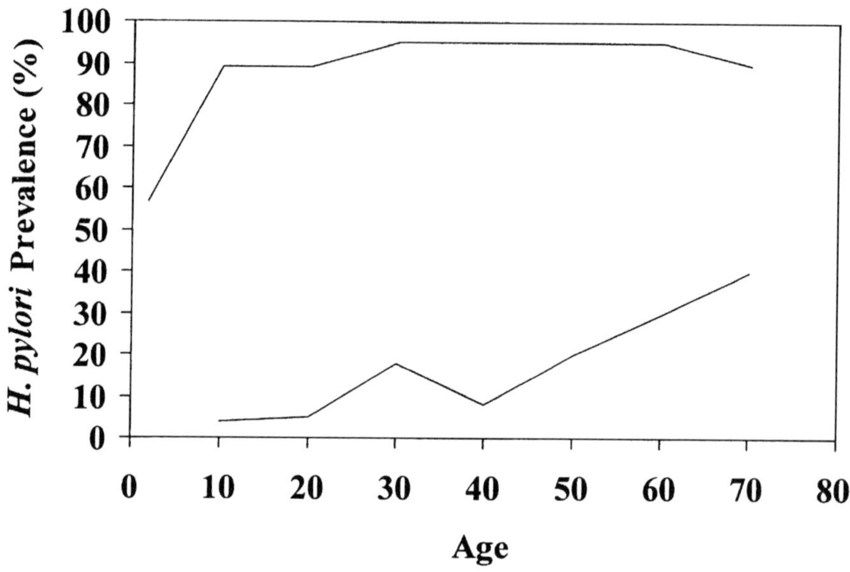

FIGURE 1. Prevalence of *Helicobacter pylori* infection in populations at high (Nariño-Colombia) and low (Australia) gastric cancer risks. In Nariño, the infection is acquired very early in life: 50% at age 2 and close to 90% at age 9. The high prevalence (over 90%) persists throughout life. In Australia the prevalence in children is very low. It increases with age and may reflect a cohort phenomen driven by the prevalence of infection in children.

number of older children in the family. Although the methods of transmission of the infection are not known, the above data strongly suggest that the infection is mainly transmitted from older to younger siblings.[20] Once acquired, the infection persists for life in developing populations of low socio-economic status. In affluent populations, the infection frequently clears "spontaneously".[21] The contrast between the prevalence of infection in high gastric cancer risk and low cancer risk populations is shown in Figure 1.[22] In children from the rural Andes of Colombia (Aldana), approximately 50% of children are infected at the age of 2 years and close to 90% are infected at 9 years of age. In such population, the infection persists for life, as seen by a prevalence of infection in adults of over 90%. In Australia, the prevalence of infection in childhood is very low and increases slightly in later years. It has been proposed that such a pattern reflects a cohort phenomenon: the prevalence in each age group of adults representing the prevalence in the community when they were children.

3. THE GASTRIC PRECANCEROUS PROCESS

It seems clear that the infection is generally acquired during childhood,[20] while cancer is diagnosed decades later. In most cases, gastric carcinoma in preceded by a pre-cancerous process lasting decades. *H. pylori* infection may lead to different outcomes, two of which behave very differently in terms of cancer risk (Figure 2). In most high risk populations the infection is associated with gland loss (atrophy) and intestinal metaplasia, a nosologic entity known as multifocal atrophic gastritis (MAG). In low risk populations the infection is predominantly antral and is not associated with atrophy or metaplasia: diffuse, antral predominant, non-atrophic gastritis (DAG). MAG is associated with gastric peptic ulcer while DAG is associated with duodenal peptic ulcer. A study in Sweden examined the cancer

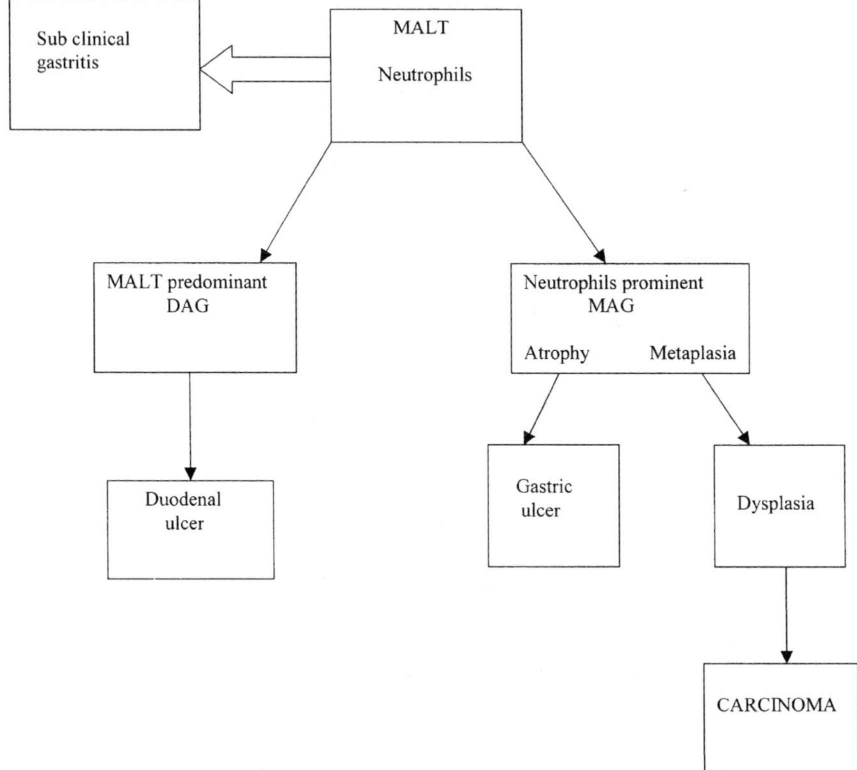

FIGURE 2. Outcomes of *Helicobacter pylori* infection. Outline of the possible paths of the host response to *Helicobacter pylori* infection and its relationship with white blood ell infiltration: mucosa associated lymphoid tissue (MALT) and polymorphonuclear neutrophils. Pathway A leads to subclinical infection. Pathway B leads to diffuse antral (nonatrophic) gastritis (DAG) and in some patients to duodenal ulcer. Pathway C leads to multifocal atrophic gastritis (MAG), gland loss (atrophy), in some patients to intestinal metaplasia, gastric ulcer and occasionally to gastric cancer epithelial cells. Attention to the inflammatory process as a possible carcinogen has concentrated in its potential as an inducer of oxidative damage, whose relevance is becoming more convincing in several anatomic sites. Neoplasms of the liver and the genital tract are associated with chronic infections.

risk of patients with gastric or duodenal ulcers diagnosed years previously and treated medically (not by gastrectomy). This study clearly confirmed previous clinical observations: gastric ulcers increase gastric cancer risk while duodenal ulcers do not.[23] Since both types of ulcer are etiologically linked to *H. pylori* infection, it becomes clear that the factors which modulate the infection determine the outcome.

Bacterial genotypes are important determinants of the outcome of the infection. *Cag* A positive strains carry a higher cancer risk than *Cag* A negative strains.[24] *Cag* A positive strains often carry other markers of virulence, especially the s_1 and m_1 variants of the *Vac* A gene.[25]

The host response to the infection, and especially the inflammatory process in the gastric mucosa, are the subject of considerable scientific scrutiny at the present time. As shown in Fig 2, most subjects infected with *H. pylori* have subclinical infections. It is not entirely clear which factors (bacterial and host) determine such outcome. Low virulence strains (*Cag* A negative) as well as adequate host defenses may result in very mild forms of chronic gastritis. In populations at high risk of gastric cancer, atrophy and metaplasia have been linked to *H. pylori* infection,[26] especially those with more virulent genotypes: Cag A positive, *Vac* A mosaicism s_1 m_1. Polymorphonuclear neutrophils are prominent in the inflammatory exudate. In low risk populations, mucosal-associated lymphoid tissue (MALT) is predominant, especially in the antrum.

4. POSSIBLE MECHANISMS OF CARCINOGENESIS

The mechanisms by which *H. pylori* induces gastric cancer are unknown. Before the rediscovery of the bacterium, epidemiologic studies had pointed to gastric irritants such as excessive dietary salt as pro-carcinogenic forces and adequate intake of fresh fruits and vegetables as protectors against carcinogenesis. No dietary pre-formed carcinogen as such has been identified. The intragastric formation of carcinogens was postulated because high levels of nitrite were reported in the gastric juice of subjects with multifocal atrophic gastritis, resulting from the reduction of dietary nitrates by anaerobic bacteria colonizing the atrophic gastric mucosa. Some common dietary items of high risk populations, such as Chinese cabbage in Asia and fava beans in Colombia yielded highly mutagenic nitroso-indoles when exposed to nitrite. (27) Whether such intraluminal carcinogens initiate or promote carcinogenesis in the human gastric mucosa has not been determined.

After the role of *H. pylori* in gastric carcinogenesis was proposed, attention has focused on the possible role of the inflammatory process in carcinogenesis. No convincing evidence of "carcinogens" in the bacterium itself has been reported. Cell damage by the bacteria, therefore, may not be by direct contact, the bacteria being separated from the target cells. The bacteria are located in the gastric lumen, overlying the original gastric foveolar epithelium, away from the metaplastic epithelium which is believed to be the Neoplastic precursor. The inflammatory neutrophils degenerate before they reach their bacterial target, but they may release their toxins (mutagens) in the vicinity of replicating.

H. pylori infection attracts polymorphonuclear neutrophils and monocytes to the human gastric mucosa, they express strongly the inducible form of nitric oxide synthase (iNOS).[28] This enzyme may lead to high concentrations of nitric oxide in epithelial cells. Although the chemistry of these nitration and nitrosation reactions is complex and not well understood, it is known that several compounds with considerable oxidative potential are formed: NO.; N_2O_3; ONOOH etc. Most of these nitric oxides and their byproducts react with DNA, cell membranes or mitochondria, which can lead to mutations and neoplastic transformations. Since the inflammatory process is chronic, it is presumed that small amounts of these oxidative radicals are formed over a very prolonged period of time. At the same time, cell replication is constantly taking place in the gastric mucosa.[29] Dividing cells may become a target for the mutagenic radicals.

Simultaneously with the above events, host defense mechanisms are active. Although poorly understood, it is widely believed that antioxidant forces of diverse origin are being activated. Several antioxidant enzymes are present in the gastric mucosa, mostly produced by inflammatory cells. Positive staining for catalase and superoxide dismutase, protectors from oxidative damage, has been shown in *H. pylori* infected mucosa.

It appears then that the carcinogenesis process represents a very prolonged conflict between oxidative and antioxidant forces. The final outcome may be determined by multiple interactions between such forces. In the case under consideration, inflammatory cells brought to the field by *H. pylori* constantly attack the gastric mucosal cells. Antioxidant forces (primarily protective enzymes such as catalase, superoxide dismutase and glutathione peroxidase) protect the cells. Suppressing the attackers or reinforcing the defenders are two routs toward prevention of subsequent cancer. This protracted "war" is outlined in the hypothetical scheme shown in Figure 3. Carcinogenesis via inflammation is depicted on the left. Similar results might hypothetically develop through the formation of intraluminal carcinogens as shown in the right side of the diagram as a result of chronic gastritis. *H. pylori* is the most frequent cause of chronic gastritis.

5. PREVENTION

Gastric cancer is the second most frequent malignant neoplasm in the world, second to lung cancer (excluding skin cancer).[30] The prognosis is generally very poor, largely due to late stage at diagnosis in most cases. Prevention then becomes

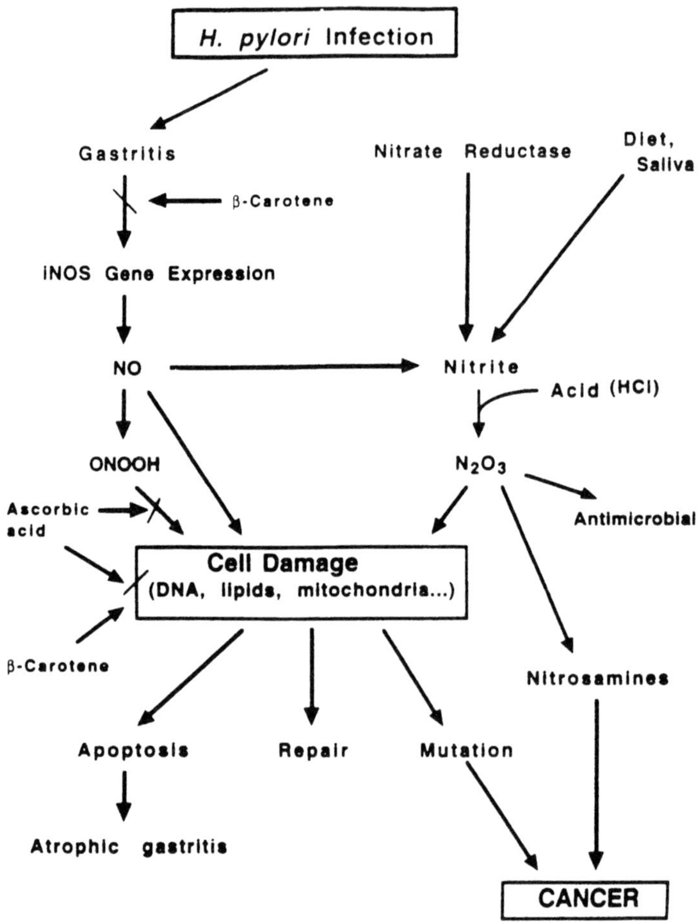

FIGURE 3. Hypothetical representation of events which might lead to neoplastic transformation in the gastric mucosa. On the left events connected with the inflammatory response to *Helicobacter pylori* are represented. Polymorphonuclear neutrophils and macrophages produce inducible nitric oxide synthase (iNOS), which leads to the formation of several nitric oxides (NO), peroxinitrite (ONOOH) and related species. They induce cell damage which can be repaired, lead to apoptosis or to mutations which might lead to eventual neoplastic transformation.

very important as a strategy for control of gastric cancer. The declining rates in most countries clearly suggest that prevention is taking place, an "unplanned triumph".[31] The challenge, therefore, is to identify the changes in modern societies which are responsible for the declining rates. Intervention to promote these changes should accelerate the decline in cancer rates. Some secular trends in modern societies are closely related to gastric cancer etiology, such as: a) the declining prevalence of *Helicobacter pylori* infection, b) the decrease in consumption of salt in foods and c) the increasing dietary consumption of fresh fruits and vegetables. These trends are mostly related to improved sanitation in the home environment and to technologic developments in refrigeration which allow better food preservation and transportation.

Testing adequately the effectiveness of interventions on the above mentioned etiologic factors would require controlled, randomized prospective prevention trials. A recent review discussed ongoing trials.[32] Five of them evaluate progression of the right side of the diagram events leading to intra luminal nitric oxides and nitrosamines are outlined.

Antioxidants such as β-carotene or ascorbic acid tend to interfere with such chain of events. On the precancerous process by means of follow up of precancerous lesions. They are being conducted in Europe (7 countries), and Latin America: Mexico, Venezuela and Colombia. Four such trials provide dietary vitamin supplements, mostly ascorbic acid and beta-carotene. With the exception of the Venezuela trial, all others attempt to eradicate *H. pylori* infection. Five trials rely on the diagnosis of cancer to evaluate progression of the disease. They are being conducted in Germany-Austria, Japan, China and the United Kingdom. These types of studies require large numbers of subjects followed up for a long time. Their results may not be available for several years.

The only trial completed and reported at the present time was conducted in the high risk population of Nariño, in the Colombian Andes.[33] Six hundred and thirty subjects with diagnosed multifocal atrophic gastritis (with or without intestinal metaplasia) completed a 6 year controlled randomized intervention trial. It followed a factorial design with anti-*Helicobacter* treatment and/or dietary supplementation with ascorbic acid and/or beta-carotene. Two sets of gastric biopsies, taken at baseline and 72 months, evaluated changes in the previously defined categories of the gastric precancerous process, namely atrophy, metaplasia and dysplasia. Forward (progression) and backward (regression) events were documented. Curing the infection (74% of treated subjects) increased markedly and significantly the rate of regression of precursor lesions (relative risk of regression 8.7, with 95% confidence intervals of 2.7–28.2) in subjects with atrophy. Figure 4 compares the effects of intervention in 8 categories. Compared with placebo, each of the three basic interventions significantly and independently increased the rate of regression: relative risks of 4.8 for anti-*Helicobacter* therapy, 5.1 for beta-carotene and 5.0 for ascorbic acid in patients with atrophic (not metaplastic) gastritis. Corresponding (significant) increased risk of regression was observed in patients with intestinal metaplasia (3.1; 3.4; 3.3). Combinations of treatments did not significantly increase the regression rates over those observed with any of the 3 basic interventions. The results of this study support the notion that curing *Helicobacter pylori* infection in high risk populations is a valid strategy for gastric cancer prevention. Antioxidant micronutrients are also effective. They may be taken as dietary supplements, as shown in the Colombian trial, or as fresh fruits and vegetables, as supported by previous epidemiologic studies.

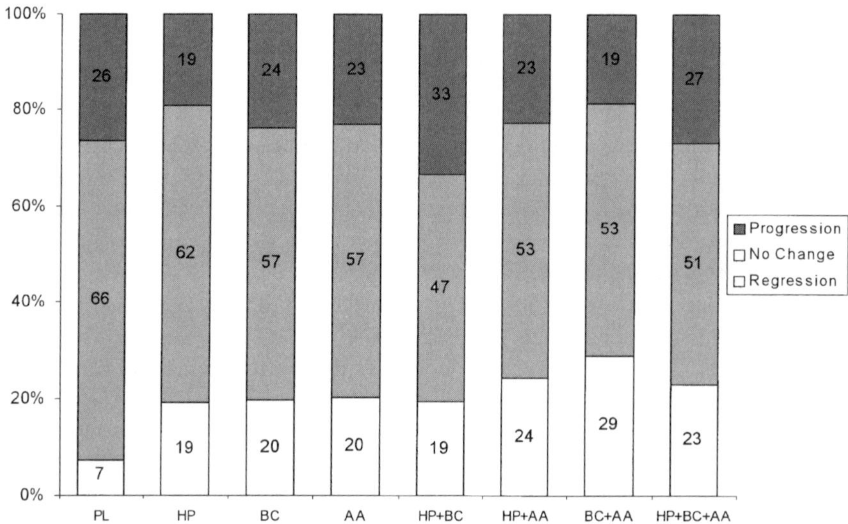

FIGURE 4. Rates of regression, no change and progression in a Colombian chemprevention trial of gastric dysplasia. Subjects on placebo (PL) had a significantly lower rate of regression than those on anti-*Helicobacter* treatment (HP), betacarotene supplementation (BC), ascorbic acid supplementation (AA) or combinations of such interventions.

6. MALT LYMPHOMA (MALTOMA)

Although totally different from carcinoma, lymphomas are neoplastic diseases of the stomach. Their association with *Helicobacter pylori* infection was yet another surprise for the medical community and followed upon the observation that most patients with gastric maltoma were infected with *Helicobacter pylori.*[34] When the infection was treated and cured, the investigators in a small study witnessed the unexpected gradual disappearance of the tumor mass in 5 out of 6 patients.[35] The observation was repeated in several countries and at present, a relatively large series of cases have documented the universality of the phenomenon.[36] Gastric maltomas are rare, and therefore, not amenable to the classic descriptive and analytical epidemiologic studies. The proof of causality came from what is generally considered one of the most robust techniques, namely the intervention.

Maltomas are known to be preceded by chronic gastritis and then by lymphoid hyperplasia. The lymphomas that are successfully treated for *Helicobacter pylori* infection revert to the precursor stages. Successive biopsies after treatment show histopathologic changes of lymphoid hyperplasia and then chronic gastritis. The successive steps seen in neoplastic development after treatment are seen in reverse order towards chronic gastritis.

The regression of lymphomas following anti-bacterial therapy revives old discussions about the nature of neoplasia. In the case of gastric maltomas, the issue is complex. Monoclonality has been used as a criterion to diagnose "true" neoplasia.[37] Monoclonality in gastric lymphocytes led to overdiagnosis of lymphoma. It was later realized that the monoclonality regularly observed in gastric lymphomas persists after "cure" of the tumors and may also be found in gastric lesions which do not meet histopathologic criteria for MALT lymphoma. In this situation, monoclonality cannot be equated with neoplasia.[38] Metastasis to other organs is an accepted criteria for malignancy. That is almost never seen in gastric maltoma. Before the era of *Helicobacter*, most of the lesions presently classified as MALT lymphomas were called "pseudolymphomas."

The etiopathogenesis of *H. pylori* related gastric maltomas is unknown. It has been postulated that specific strains of bacteria induce lymphomas. It is also probable (but unknown) that specific host genotypes confer special susceptibility to gastric lymphoma. If the hypothesis of DNA damage via oxidative stress is found to be correct, it could be speculated that the same oxidative radicals which induce mutations in epithelial cells would be able to induce similar damage in the gastric lymphoid tissue attracted by *H. pylori* as an inflammatory response.

7. EPILOGUE: A NEW PARADIGM

H. pylori induced carcinogenesis represents a new paradigm which may replace old paradigms based on "smoking guns" such as ionizing radiation and tobacco smoking. The old paradigm centered in the identification of "carcinogens." In the new molecular revolution the search is for "oncogenes," as if the similarities in the endings of both words implied similar mechanisms of actions.

The new paradigm calls for a prolonged conflict between forces which attack and forces which preserve the functional integrity of cells, tissues and organs. The inflammatory cells are at the center of the conflict. They are the carriers of the attackers, in the form of nitric oxides, and also carriers of the defense mechanisms, in the form of antioxidant enzymes. Our understanding of these complex phenomena is in its infancy.

Mother nature is showing us the way to cancer prevention. In the case of stomach cancer, suppressing (or controlling) the attackers, namely *Helicobacter pylori* infection, may reduce cancer risk. Reinforcing the defenders, namely providing abundant dietary antioxidants may accomplish similar results.

Theories of carcinogenesis based on chronic oxidative damage to cells fit very well the new paradigm. Long overdue emphasis should be given to the other side of the coin, namely the antioxidant forces. They may provide plausible hypotheses to answer some profound questions about human carcinogenesis, such as: Why does it take years or decades to develop clinical cancer? and Why most subjects escape the carcinogenic impact of oxidation?

REFERENCES

1. Bizzozero G., 1893, Ueber die schalauchferinger drusen des magendarmkanals und die baziehungen ihres epitihels zudem oberfacheniepithel der schleimhaur. *Arch. f. Mikr. Anat.* **42**:82–152.
2. Salomon H., 1896, Hueber das spirillum des sangetiermagens und sein verbalten zu deu belegzellen. *Zentralbl. Bakterial. Mikrobiol. Hyg.* **19**:433–442.
3. Warren J. R., 1983, Unidentified curved bacilli on gastric epithelium in active chronic gastritis (Letter to the Editor) *Lancet* **1**:1273.
4. Marshall B. J., 1983, Unidentified curved bacilli on gastric epithelium in active chronic gastritis (Letter to the Editor) *Lancet* **1**:1273–1275.
5. Marshall B. J., Armstrong J. A., McGechic D. B., *et al.*, 1985, Attempt to fulfill Koch's postulates for pylori campylobacter *Med. J. Austr.* **142**:436–439.
6. Marshall B. J., Goodwin C. S., Warner J. R., *et al.*, 1988, Prospective double-blind trial of duodenal ulcer relapse after eradication of *Helicobacter pylori Lancet ii*: 1437–1442.
7. International Agency for Research on Cancer, 1994, Monographs on the evaluation of carcinogenic risks to humans. Vol. 61 Schistosomes, liver flukes and *Helicobacter pylori*: *IARC*. Lyon.
8. Muñoz N., and Pisani P., 1994, *Helicobacter pylori* and gastric cancer *Europ. J. Gastroenterol. Hepatol.* **6**:1097–1103.
9. Huang J. Q., and Hunt R. H., 1998, An overview of *Helicobacter pylori* epidemiology Studies. In: *Helicobacter pylori*. Basic Mechanisms to Clinical Cure. Kluwer Academic Publishers Boston: 295–307.
10. Forman D., Sitas F., Newell D. G., *et al.*, 1990, Geographic association of *Helicobacter pylori* antibody prevalence and gastric cancer mortality in rural China. *Int. J. Cancer* **46**:608–611.
11. Forman D., Moeller D., and Coleman M., 1993, (on behalf of the Euro Gast Study Group) International Association between *Helicobacter pylori* and gastric cancer (Letter to the Editor) *Lancet* **342**:120–121
12. Huang J. Q., Sridhar S., Chen Y., *et al.*, 1998, Meta-analysis of the relationship between *Helicobacter pylori* seropositivity and gastric cancer. *Gastroenterology* **114**:1169–1179.
13. Hansson L. E., Engstrand L., Nyren O., *et al.*, 1993, *Helicobacter pylori* infection: independent risk indicator of gastric adenocarinoma. *Gastroeneterology* **105**:1098–1103.
14. Fukuda H., Saito D., Hayeshi S., *et al.*, 1995, *Helicobacter pylori* infection, serum pepsinogen level and gastric cancer. *Jpn. J. Cancer* **86**:64–71.
15. Nomura A., Stemmermann G. N., Chyou P. A., *et al.*, 1991, *Helicobacter pylori* infection gastric carcinoma among Japanese Americans in Hawaii. *New Engl. J. Med.* **325**:1132–1136.
16. Parsonnet J., Friedman G. D., Vandersteen D. F., *et al.*, 1991, *Helicobacter pylori* infection and the risk of gastric carcinoma. *New Engl. J. Med.* **320**:1127–1131.
17. Forman D., Newell D. G., Fullerton F., *et al.*, 1991, Association between infection with *Helicobacter pylori* and risk of gastric cancer: evidence from a prospective investigation. *Br. Med. J.* **302**: 1302–1305.
18. Forman D., Webb P., and Parsonnet J., 1994, *H. pylori* and gastric cancer (Letter to the Editor) *Lancet* **343**:243–244.
19. Blaser M. J., Chyou P. H., and Nomura A., 1995, Age at establishment of *Helicobacter pylori* infection and gastric carcinoma, gastric ulcer and duodenal ulcer risk. *Cancer Res.* **55**:562–565.
20. Goodman K., and Correa P., 2000, *Helicobacter pylori* transmission among Siblings. *Lancet* **355**:358–362.
21. Tindberg Y., Blennow M., and Grandstrom M., 1999, Clinical symptoms and social factors in cohort of children spontaneously clearing *Helicobacter pylori* infection. *Acta. Paediatr.* **88**:631–635.
22. Goodman K. J., Correa P., Tengana Aux H. J., *et al.*, 1996, *Helicobacter pylori* infection in the Colombian Andes: a population based study of transmission pathways. *Am. J. Epidemiol.* **144**:290–299.

23. Hansson L. E., Nyren O., Hsing A. W., *et al.*, 1996, The risk of stomach cancer in patients with gastric and duodenal ulcer disease. *New Engl. J. Med.* **335**:242–249.
24. Parsonnet J., Friedman G. D., Orentreich N., *et al.*, 1997, Risk of gastric cancer in people with Cag A positive or Cag A negative *Helicobacter pylori* infection. *Gut.* **40**:297–301.
25. Van Doorn L. J., Figurereido C., Megraud F., *et al.*, 1999, Geographic distribution of Vac A allelic types of *Helicobacter pylori. Gastroenterology* **116**:823–830.
26. Fontham E. T. H., Ruiz B., Perez A., *et al.*, 1995, Determinants of *Helicobacter pylori* infection and chronic gastritis. *Am. J. Gastroenterol.* **90**:1094–1101.
27. Yang D., Tannenbaum S. R., Buch C., *et al.*, 1984, 4-chloro-6-methoxyindole is the precursor of a potent mutagen that forms during nitrosation of fava beans (Vicia faba) *Carcinogenesis* **5**:1219–1224.
28. Mannick E. E., Bravo L. E., Zarama G., *et al.*, 1996, Inducable nitric oxide synthase, nitrotyrosine and apoptosis in *Helicobacter pylori* gastritis: effects of antibiotics and antioxidants. *Cancer Res.* **56**:323–343.
29. Correa P., and Miller M. J. S., 1998, Carcinogenesis, apoptosis and cell proliferation. *Brit. Med. Bull.* **54**:151–162.
30. Parkin D. M., Pisani P., and Ferlay, 1993, Estimates of the worldwide incidence of eighteen major cancers in 1985. *Int. J. Cancer* **54**:594–606.
31. Howson C. P., Hiyama T., and Wynder E. L., 1986, The decline in gastric cancer: epidemiology of an unplanned triumph. *Epi. Reviews* **8**:1–27.
32. Forman D., 1998, Lessons from ongoing intervention studies. In: Helicobacter pylori. Basic Mechanisms to Clinical Cure. RH Hunt and GNJ Tytgat, eds. Kluwer Academic Publishers, Boston 354–361.
33. Correa P., Fontham E., Ruiz, *et al.*, 1999, Chemoprevention of gastric dysplasia. Effect of anti-*Helicobacter pylori* treatment and antioxidant supplementation. (Abs) **45**(Suppl. III)A50.
34. Isaacson P. G., and Wright D. H., 1983, Malignant lymphoma of mucosa associated lymphoid tissue. A distinct type-B cell lymphoma. *Cancer* **52**:1410–1412.
35. Wotherspoon A. C., Doglioni C., Diss T. C., *et al.*, 1993, Regression of primary low grade gastric B-cell lymphoma of mucosa associated lymphoid tissue after eradication of *Helicobacter pylori. Lancet* **342**:575–577.
36. Stolte M., Morguer A., Meining A., *et al.*, 1966, Clincal presentation, diagnosis and treatment of *Helicobacter pylori* related gastric lymphoma. In: Hunt R and Tytgat GNJ eds. Helicobacter pylori: Basic mechanisms to Clinical Cure 1996. Kluwer Academic Press Derducht; 222–231.
37. Horsman D., Gascoyne R., Klasa R., *et al.*, 1992, t(11;18) q21; q21.1): a recurrent translocation in lymphomas of mucosa associated lymphoid tissue. *Gene Chromosome Cancer* **77**:74–78.
38. El-Zimaity, H. M. T., El-Zaatary F. A. K., Pina Dore M., *et al.*, 1999, The differential diagnosis of early gastric mucosa-associated lymphoma: polymerase chain reaction and paraffin section immunophenotyping. *Modern Path* **12**:885–893.

4

Risk Factors and Peptic Ulcer Pathology

BENJAMIN D. GOLD[1,2] and PHILIP M. SHERMAN[3]

1. INTRODUCTION

Acquisition of *Helicobacter pylori* infection occurs primarily in childhood, and ~50% of the world's population is infected.[1–4] The majority of individuals, both adults and children, who become infected never have symptoms or signs of definitive disease, and there is a broad spectrum of disease presentations.[5] Major areas lacking in current knowledge about this infection include; risk factors for the development of gastroduodenal disease, pathobiology of microbial-host interactions, the specific host and microbial factors which determine specific disease outcomes, and the natural history of *H. pylori* infection and the associated gastroduodenal diseases after initial acquisition in childhood.

A "screen and treat" policy has not been advocated in North America at the present time since less than 20% of infected people will develop peptic ulcers

BENJAMIN D. GOLD • Division of Pediatric Gastroenterology and Nutrition, Department of Pediatrics, Emory University School of Medicine, Children's Healthcare of Atlanta at Egleston Children's Hospital; Foodborne and Diarrheal Diseases Branch, Division of Bacterial and Mycotic Diseases, National Center for Infectious Diseases, Centers for Disease Control and Prevention, Atlanta, GA. PHILIP M. SHERMAN • Division of Pediatric Gastroenterology and Nutrition, The Hospital for Sick Children, Department of Pediatrics, University of Toronto, Toronto, Ontario, Canada.

Helicobacter pylori Infection and Immunity,
Edited by Yamamoto *et al.*, Kluwer Academic/Plenum Publishers, 2002.

TABLE 1

Percent of pediatric and adult *H. pylori*-infected patients with the different degrees of the various inflammatory cell components and the density of bacteria in antral biopsies

	Children (N = 42)			Adults (N = 40)			
Pathology	Mild	Moderate	Marked	Mild	Moderate	Marked	p
Density of *H. pylori*	19	29	52	36	29	35	0.05
Neutrophils	48	25	25	22	18	53	0.02
Plasma cells	24	36	40	5	31	64	0.005
Lymphocytes	13	31	56	9	33	58	NS
Eosinophils	42	38	12	16	20	62	0.001

NS = Not significant.

or gastric cancer during their lifetime. Moreover, the treatment itself has some risks, as well as promoting the development of antibiotic resistance in *H. pylori*.[6,7]

To date, a major impediment in the development of intervention strategies, particularly for use in children, has been a paucity of information regarding the evolution of inflammatory changes in the gastric and duodenal mucosa after childhood acquisition of *H. pylori*. This review will summarize current understanding of the pathogenesis and risks for peptic ulcer disease associated with childhood *H. pylori* infection.

Inflammation and ulcers in the duodenum and stomach have historically been classified either as primary or secondary (Table 1).[8] Until the mid-1980's, it was believed that most ulcers in the stomach or duodenum of children were a secondary phenomenon. Secondary ulcers generally occur due to systemic stresses like trauma, burns or septic shock, or as a result of drug ingestion (for example non-steroidal anti-inflammatory agents and corticosteroids).[9,10] In addition, secondary ulceration is associated with specific disease states such as Zollinger-Ellison syndrome and Crohn's disease.[8,11,12]

Duodenal and gastric ulcers in children who had no other systemic conditions were considered as primary in nature.[13,14] Family history of peptic ulcer disease is a common feature in the profile of these patients.[15] In virtually all of these children, inflammation of the gastric mucosa is present, and caused by *H. pylori*.[16,17] Further evidence for the familial nature of primary gastritis and peptic ulceration in children is the clustering of *H. pylori* infection amongst family members.[18–20] More recently, work by El-Omar *et al.*[21] has provided molecular evidence for the familial nature of gastric cancer associated with *H. pylori* infection. This group showed that there are interleukin-1 (IL-1) gene cluster polymorphisms suspected of enhancing production of IL-1β. These IL-1 polymorphisms are observed in family cohorts at increased risk of gastric atrophy and intestinal metaplasia induced by *H. pylori* and gastric cancer.[21]

Although small, single center case series observations indicate that there may be a rise in *H. pylori*-negative ulcers both in adults and children, this phenomena also could reflect mis-reporting or mis-diagnosis due to a rise in the use of proton pump inhibitors, which change the anatomic distribution of *H. pylori* in the human stomach.[22,23] Population-based epidemiological studies, involving multiple centers with the use of a standardized diagnostic protocol, are critically needed.

Mounting evidence demonstrates that there is a multifactorial process involved in the evolution of mucosal diseases following *H. pylori* infection. Both host factors and bacterial factors have been identified as potentially playing a role in gastroduodenal pathology associated with *H. pylori*.[5,24–26] The complex interaction between bacterial-specific and host-specific factors deserves critical appraisal because there are still many features of *H. pylori*-associated diseases in humans that remain undefined. An understanding of *H. pylori* as the etiologic agent in gastroduodenal inflammation and neoplasia is critical to define the pathobiology of gastritis and peptic ulcer disease.

2. PATHOBIOLOGY OF *H. pylori* INFECTION-INDUCED GASTRODUODENAL DISEASES

2.1. Bacterial Factors

Much controversy has ensued during the 18 years since the initial discovery of this organism and its link to human diseases. Two primary morphological shapes, bacillary and coccoid, have been described for the organism.[27] While the bacillary forms are the predominant, viable form of *H. pylori*, the coccoid morphology can be observed in culture as well as in some patients.[27] The biological relevance of the coccoid form is not clearly understood; it is either a nonviable dying bacterium or a form that protects the organism in dormancy. *H. pylori* produces many enzymes that facilitate colonization of the gastric mucosa including, for example, catalase, oxidase, phospholipase, thioredoxin reductase and urease.[28–31] In addition to being highly motile, to facilitate movement through the gastric mucus, it is the urease that allows this organism to metabolize urea to help to neutralize luminal acid in the immediate microenvironment during colonization.

Preliminary studies from our laboratory regarding *H. pylori* virulence gene alleles and corresponding gastroduodenal pathology in children demonstrate that specific correlations between *cagA*, *vacA* and *iceA* genes and severity of gastroduodenal mucosal inflammation in early infection cannot be made.[32] The *vacA* gene is present in all *H. pylori* strains and is made up of two variable regions. The "s" region (encoding the signal peptide) is located at the 5′ end of the gene and exists either as a s1 or s2 allele.[33] Within the s1 allele type, several subtypes have been found (s1a, s1b, and s1c).[34,35] The "m" (middle) region occurs as a m1 or m2 allele.[12] The combination of the s- and m-region allelic types determines the production of the cytotoxin.[33,36] Large amounts of vacuolating cytotoxin are produced from s1/m1 strains. *vacA* type s1a strains are isolated more frequently in adults with peptic ulcer disease and are associated with increased gastric epithelial damage.[34,37] In addition, van Doorn *et al.*[38,39] demonstrated that *vacA* alleles have a distinct distribution across different ethnic groups and geographic regions correlating with the distribution of gastroduodenal disease. In the adult population, certain *H. pylori* genotypes are associated with ethnicity and country of origin.[38] For example, vacA-s1c *H. pylori* strains are found exclusively in persons of Asian descent.[38] Studies of *H. pylori* strains isolated from the pediatric age group could prove to be very valuable to better understand transmission of the organism.

The *cag* pathogenicity island (cag-PI) contains the *cagA* gene (cytotoxin associated gene), which may be a marker for *H. pylori* infection associated with more severe disease outcome.[28,37,38,40] Proteins of genes on the cag-PI, other than Cag*A*, augment induction of pro-inflammatory chemokines in host gastric mucosal tissues.[28,41] There is also a close association between the presence of *cagA* and the *vacA* s1 genotype, with increased epithelial cell damage and mucosal inflammation.[42,43] The prevalence of CagA positivity among asymptomatic American children has been estimated to be 54% by Elitsur *et al.*[44] using serology to detect CagA antibodies, whereas the prevalence of CagA positivity among symptomatic children was estimated at 69%. Although there are a few small single center studies which have attempted to correlate *H. pylori* virulence genes with host disease in children,[3,45] no other epidemiological studies to date have been performed to determine the prevalence of cag pathogenicity island genes in *H. pylori*-infected children.[1,46,47]

An additional *H. pylori* virulence gene, iceA (*i*nduced by *c*ontact with *e*pithelium), has two mutually exclusive types *iceA*1 and *iceA2*.[48] The *iceA1* allele is more common in *H. pylori* strains isolated from adults with peptic ulcer disease compared to those with gastritis alone.[8,18,20,38,49] However, the prevalence of iceA alleles and their association with gastroduodenal disease in children is not known.

We evaluated the genotype of *H. pylori* strains isolated from children at four centers in North America (Miami, Fl.; Cleveland, Oh.; Atlanta, Ga.; Toronto, Canada) and compared *cagA*, *vacA*, and *iceA* genotypes to the clinical, demographic, endoscopic and histopathologic characteristics of these infected patients. *cag*A positive *H. pylori* strains were not more frequent in children with documented

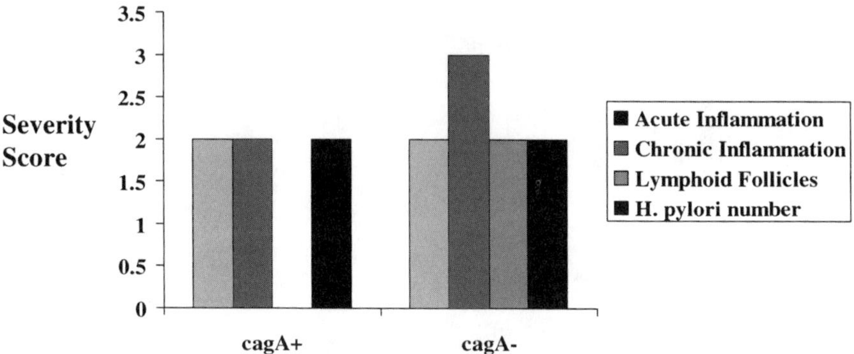

FIGURE 1. Lack of correlation between pediatric *H. pylori cag*A status and the severity of antral inflammation as assessed by the 4 parameters used by the Updated Sydney Classification of gastritis; acute inflammation, chronic inflammation, lymphoid follicles, and *H. pylori* number. Although not shown, a similar lack of correlation was seen between *vac*A or *ice*A genotype and inflammation severity scores.

ulcer disease compared to those infected by *cagA* negative strains. In addition, *cagA* status did not correlate with inflammation severity, as determined by the updated Sydney classification for gastritis (Figure 1). In addition, neither of the *vacA* s- and m-alleles were associated with ulcer disease or an increase in the severity of gastric mucosal inflammation. A lack of correlation to inflammation severity was also found with *iceA* alleles and *cagA* genotype in this pediatric cohort. However, as reported previously in adult studies, *H. pylori* strain genotype did cluster in association with geographic origin and ethnicity[32] (Figure 2).

In another study by Day *et al.*[1] *cagE*, formally called *picB*, was shown to be a genotype associated with more severe disease outcome; in particular, duodenal ulcer disease compared to gastritis alone. In this study, twelve (92%) of 13 children with duodenal ulcers were infected with *cag*E-positive isolates, compared with only 5 (31%) of 16 with gastritis alone ($p < 0.05$). Infection of gastric cells in tissue culture by *cagE*-positive *H. pylori* resulted in greater increments in IL-8 levels compared with *cagE*-negative strains.[1] At least in this tertiary care setting, *H. pylori* strains containing *cagE* are associated with the presence of duodenal ulceration in children and it appears that enhanced chemokine production following infection with *cagE*-positive *H. pylori* could affect disease outcome.

However, adult studies have shown that patients infected with *H. pylori* strains lacking these genetic markers can still develop peptic ulceration.[7,34,38,112] Moreover, we and others have shown that patients may be infected simultaneously with more than one strain that vary in their genotype, thereby making the study of *H. pylori* virulence markers with disease association extraordinarily difficult.[28,32] To date, no

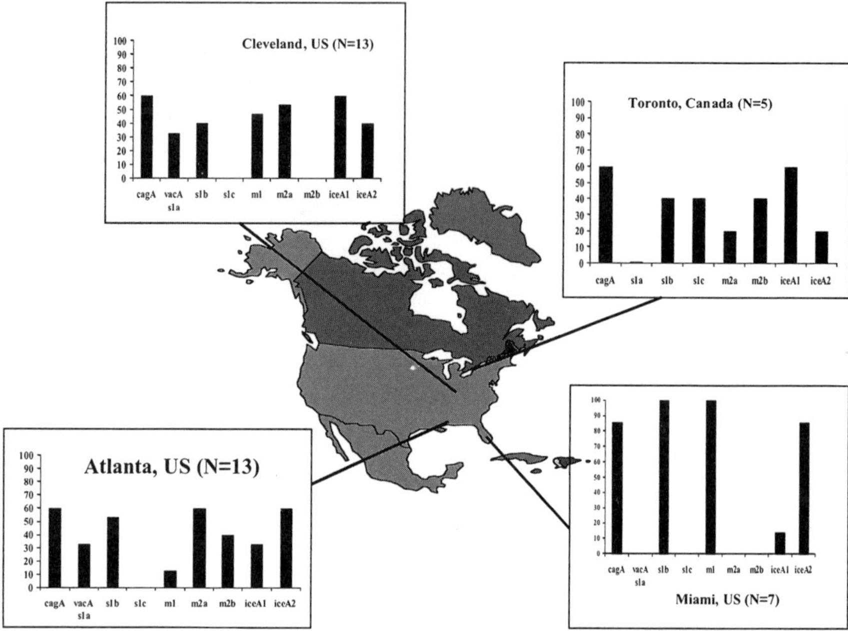

FIGURE 2. Map of North America, Canada and the United States depicting the location of the 4 participating centers (Miami, Florida, Atlanta, Georgia, Cleveland, Ohio and Toronto, Ontario, Canada), and the distribution of the *vac*A s and m-regions, *cag*A, and *ice*A1 and *ice*A2 genotypes of *H. pylori* strains obtained from the pediatric subjects. For each center, the prevalence of each type (s1a, s1b, s1c, s2, m1, m2a, and m2b; *cag*A positive, and *ice*A1, *ice*A2 genotypes) is given as a percentage of the total number of strains.

single gene or array of *H. pylori* genes has been identified that can serve as a precise marker for accurately predicting the development of gastroduodenal disease in an individual patient. Clinical sequelae also may be attributed to the role of other factors that govern disease expression. In particular, changes in gastric physiology and the host immune and inflammatory responses have been implicated in the pathogenesis of gastroduodenal disease.[50]

2.2. Host Factors

The quantity of gastric acid secretion has been long considered as the critical factor determining the development of mucosal ulceration in the stomach or duodenum. However, the effect of *H. pylori* colonization on gastric acid secretion remains a controversial subject. In particular, the impact of *H. pylori* infection on acid secretion in children is poorly defined. One study reported that there is a difference in acid secretion in children with gastric ulcers compared to those with duodenal ulcers.[51] The authors measured 24-hour intragastric pH as a determinant of acid secretion in 82 subjects; 10 children with gastric ulcers, 9 with duodenal ulcers, 58 non-ulcer patients, and 5 healthy adults. Gastric acid production was significantly reduced in patients with *Helicobacter pylori*-associated gastric ulcers. Conversely, gastric acidity was increased, or above adult levels, in children with duodenal ulcers.[51]

Other investigators have also demonstrated that 24 hour gastric acid output is different in ulcer patients and normal pediatric controls.[52] Intragastric pH monitoring was performed over a 48 hour period; the first 24 hours untreated, the second 24 hours with three doses of an H_2 receptor antagonist (cimetidine). Children with duodenal ulcers lacked the intragastric pH inversion that occurs in control subjects around midnight, and had persistent hypergastric acidity for the majority of the 24 hours. However, *H. pylori* infection status was not clearly defined in this study cohort.

The pathogenesis of gastroduodenal mucosal inflammation and ulceration due to *H. pylori* infection may also be contributed to by disturbances in mucus and bicarbonate secretion. The gastric mucus layer serves as a barrier to luminal pepsin and hydrochloric acid to prevent access to the apical surface of gastric epithelial cells. Bicarbonate secreted into the mucus layer serves as a barrier by neutralizing the acid, which diffuses into the mucus blanket. The mucus layer also provides protection for epithelial cell turnover both in normal and perturbed states, as well as from mechanical damage during the digestive state. Studies demonstrate that there is impaired rate of bicarbonate production in the proximal duodenum of patients with duodenal ulcerations in particular, those with *H. pylori* infection.[53] Further studies demonstrate that in human proximal duodenum, PGE_2 and cAMP activate distinct HCO_3-transport pathways likely involving a DIDS-sensitive Cl–/HCO_3-exchanger and a DIDS-insensitive HCO_3-conductance. These may be directly related to *H. pylori* colonization via either signal transduction or cell cytoskeletal rearrangements.[54] Studies of gastric acid and duodenal bicarbonate secretion in *H. pylori*-infected children compared to uninfected age-matched controls are lacking and needed in order to understand the evolution of gastroduodenal inflammation following the initial acquisition of infection in childhood.

Helicobacter infection in both humans and ferrets results in a decrease in gastroduodenal mucosal surface hydrophobicity. This change is believed to be due to disturbances in the gastric surface mucus layer content and character.[55,56] It is postulated that the mucus confers hydrophobicity to the stomach and decreased production leads to the exposure of gastric surface cells to pepsin, acid and other aggressive factors with eventual erosion of the epithelial cell layer. Studies in adults have demonstrated decreased polymerization of mucin glycoproteins in patients with duodenal ulcers.[57,58] More recent work has shown that *H. pylori* infection co-localizes with muc5AC mucin *in vivo*,[59] and alters mucin gene function *in vitro*.[60] Other investigators have reported that mucin alterations *in vivo* may be related to *H. pylori cagA* and *vacA* gene expression.[61] These investigators demonstrated that a greater effect on mucin occurred with *cagA*$^+$, *vacA*$^+$ *H. pylori* strains than with isolated lacking one or both genes. To date, however, comparable studies have not been performed in *H. pylori*-infected children.

Gastric hormones, specifically gastrin[62] and somatostatin, also likely play an important role in determining disease outcome after *H. pylori* infection. Children infected by *H. pylori* have decreased numbers of D-cells (somatostatin secreting cells), decreased circulating somatostatin levels, and increased circulating gastrin levels compared to uninfected controls.[63] This observation is more common in younger than older children and even more so than in adults; findings possibly a reflection of the evolving pathobiology associated with the infection. Following eradication of *H. pylori* in the infected child, D-cell numbers, D-cell to G-cell ratios, and circulating somatostatin and gastrin levels return to normal levels.[63]

In addition, pepsinogens I and II[64] have been implicated in mediating *H. pylori*-induced disease. Moreover, data suggesting the inherited nature of *H. pylori*-associated disease are provided by family cohort studies demonstrating increased serum pepsinogen levels.[65,66] These investigations showed that children with duodenal ulcers and their parents had increased levels of serum pepsinogen I.[65,66] Subsequent studies of *H. pylori*-infected children and family members demonstrate that chronic infection is associated with elevated levels of serum pepsinogen.[63]

More recent canine studies by Beales *et al.*[67] demonstrated that gastrin release could be achieved by *H. pylori*. *H. pylori* sonicates, water extract preparations, and lipopolysaccharide had no stimulatory actions on gastrin release, but the sonicates from two of four strains potentiated the effects of IL-8, leading to maximal gastrin release of 230% ± −130% and 232% ± −33% above basal, respectively ($P < 0.05$). The authors concluded that IL-8 stimulated gastrin release from isolated G cells, and the effect was potentiated by *H. pylori* products. Based on these findings, they postulated that the interaction of cytokines and *H. pylori* may contribute to the hypergastrinemia seen *in vivo*.[67] In summary, the overall impact of *H. pylori* on gastric acid physiology and the relationship thereof to disease expression deserves further study particularly in the initial infection occurring in childhood.

A vigorous local and systemic host immune response is observed after gastric colonization by *H. pylori* organisms, yet spontaneous clearance is rare.[68,69] Our lab, and others, have reported that *H. pylori* binds to glycosylated epithelial cell membrane-associated receptors.[56,70] One glycoconjugate receptor in particular, Lewis antigen phenotype of *H. pylori* has been reported to mirror that of the host.[70] In this case, it is possible that these antigens activate local T cells that secrete "anti-inflammatory" cytokines that could modulate the host response via a "bystander" effect, thereby conferring tolerance to a small population of T cells which then are activated and impair the immune reactivity to other local T cells.[71] However, this hypothesis has not been substantiated. Based on the cytokine analysis, it appears that most of the cytokines in the gastric mucosa during infection are pro-inflammatory rather than anti-inflammatory.[71] This may favor chronic infection, and explain the rare observations of spontaneous clearance of *H. pylori* infection. In addition, the predominant Th1 response observed during infection is unlikely to be effective against a pathogen within the lumen of the stomach, and more likely to have adverse effects on the host and thereby contribute to gastroduodenal disease.

Another possibility is that natural infection with *H. pylori* selectively inhibits antigen-specific responses. Recent studies describe the ability of *H. pylori* to induce apoptosis of host cells through Fas/FasL interactions.[72,73] Since cag PAI strains predominate in humans, it is possible that this ability to induce apoptosis in T cells confers a selective advantage that complements other mechanisms favoring the persistent growth and survival of these strains.[73]

H. pylori adherence to and interaction with the gastric epithelium provides a focal point to examine the induction of host responses. One potential interaction is through the bacterial BabA protein interacting with Lewis B-like carbohydrate structures on the host cell membrane.[74] However, to date, the only host cell receptor shown to be capable of signal transduction is the class II MHC molecule. As a consequence of binding these molecules expressed on the cell surface, gastric epithelial cells begin the process of programmed cell death.[75] Findings to date indicate that *H. pylori* strains with and without the cag PAI bind comparably and induce apoptosis of gastric epithelial cells.[76]

H. pylori first comes in contact with gastric epithelial cells *in vivo*. Therefore, the epithelial cell is likely to be centrally involved in the initiation of the host response. IL-8 is produced by gastric epithelium, both *in vitro* and *in vivo*, in response to cag PAI (+) *H. pylor.*[77] Other studies link infection with cag PAI strains to increased production of ENA-78 and RANTES by epithelial cells.[78–80] The cag PAI contains 31 genes including several that encode a type IV secretory apparatus.[28] Within this region, the *cag*E gene is a required element for the induction of IL-8.[81] The type IV secretory pathway permits the transfer of bacterial proteins into the infected host cell.[82,83] CagA has been identified as one bacterial protein that is transferred and tyrosine phosphorylated in the cytoplasm of the host cell. Other bacterial products may be similarly transported into the host cell where they can impact on signal transduction pathways and modify the host response to infection.

A monocyte and macrophage response is seen in infected gastric mucosa, particularly in children (Table 1 and 2). In adults, both polymorphonuclear cells and plasma cells are also present in the inflammatory infiltrate.[84–86] Our

TABLE 2
Lymphoid follicles in biopsy specimens of children and adults with *H. pylori* infection

Characteristic	Children	Adults
Total biopsies	52	45
No. (%) specimens without lymphoid follicles	20 (38)	19 (42)
No. (%) specimens with lymphoid follicles	32 (61)	26 (58)
Mean ± SD no. of lymphoid follicles per specimen (range)	2.00 ± 1.08 (1–5)	2.08 ± 1.48 (1–7)

$p > 0.05$

laboratory has performed comparative studies of *H. pylori*-infected children versus *H. pylori*-infected adults and demonstrated a chronic, macrophagic, monocytic inflammatory cell infiltrate in the early infection, and a lack of neutrophils compared to the polymorphonuclear inflammatory cell response that is observed in many infected adults (Table 1 and 2).[87]

A lymphofollicular gastritis has also been described particularly in childhood. However, the clonality of the T cells, macrophages and plasma cells contained in these lymphoid follicles remains poorly defined. It is still not clear if T-cells play a major role in the mucosal inflammation following *H. pylori* infection even though elevated levels of IL-1, IL-2, and tumor necrosis factor-alpha are detectable in the gastric epithelium of infected individuals.[88]

3. PATHOLOGIC SEQUELAE

3.1. Gastritis

Warren and Marshall first reported the association of *H. pylori* colonizing the gastric mucosa with antral gastritis in adults in 1983.[89] Shortly thereafter, Hill *et al.*[90] described four children with chronic mononuclear cell gastritis who were infected with *H. pylori*. The same year, Cadranel and colleagues[91] described organisms present in eight children with chronic, lymphocytic gastritis. Subsequently, Drumm *et al.* observed *Helicobacter*-like organisms in 70% of 67 pediatric patients with a chronic-active Gastritis.[16] Similar observations of gastric mucosal inflammatory cell infiltrates associated with spiral-shaped organisms colonizing the mucosa and in the mucus layer overlying gastric epithelium were also made Czinn and Carr[17] in 25 children. Additional studies confirm that *H. pylori* colonization of the gastric mucosa in children is virtually always associated with gastritis of a predominantly chronic inflammatory cell infiltrate.[18,92,93] Single center case series reports of eradication of *H. pylori* from the gastric mucosa demonstrate that there is an associated resolution of the antral gastritis.[93] However, multicenter randomized controlled eradication trials of *H. pylori*-infected children have not been performed and are critically needed.

Studies in adults established the presence of the organism in nearly all cases of chronic gastritis.[94] It was initially suggested that *H. pylori* colonized inflamed tissue rather than causing the inflammation, since gastritis is a common finding in adults.[94] However, the prevalence of gastritis is less frequent in children thereby enabling the investigation of *H. pylori* as a cause for gastritis rather than an opportunistic colonizer of inflamed tissue.[95] Studies also showed that *H. pylori* colonization is not a common finding on the gastric mucosa of children with secondary causes of gastritis, such as NSAID's, eosinophilic gastroenteritis and Crohn's disease.[96] Taken together, these observations provide compelling evidence for the pathogenic role of *H. pylori* infection in the development of chronic antral gastritis in children.

H. pylori associated gastritis is characterized by the presence of acute and chronic inflammation, with immature surface epithelial cells.[22,71] Depletion of mucus is often present in the epithelial cells, due to active cell renewal. The degree of mucosal inflammation varies in severity from a minimal inflammatory infiltrate in the lamina propria, with preserved architecture, to severe gastritis with dense mucosal inflammation. In severe cases, intraepithelial neutrophils can be detected both in the surface epithelium and in gastric pits as microabscesses.[68] However, we have found that *H. pylori*-infected children have lesser degrees of neutrophilic infiltrates compared to adults.[69,97]

Previously, it was believed that in *H. pylori* gastritis, fundic inflammation was less important than that of the antral mucosa.[98,99] However, the controversial relationship between *H. pylori* and the development, or concurrent presence, of gastroesophageal reflux disease may well be due to the anatomic location of the inflammatory cell infiltrate.[100] Moreover, patients who have been receiving a proton pump inhibitor for acid suppression frequently have colonization of fundic and cardia mucosa by *H. pylori*. Carditis, of both a chronic and active phenotype, is frequent in *H. pylori*-infected adults.[22,101] Studies are needed in children to more accurately determine the relationship between *H. pylori* infection, the sites of gastric inflammation, and long-term disease sequelae.

H. pylori-associated gastritis in children is commonly not apparent at endoscopy, thereby making biopsy essential for definitive diagnosis.[17,95] Nodularity of the antral mucosa has been described in association with *H. pylori* gastritis in children.[102] However, its significance still is not yet defined. Although, less common than in children, antral nodularity has also been observed in *H. pylori*-infected adults.[103–105]

3.2. Ulcers

Although there is a notable lack of good large population-based pediatric studies, rates of peptic ulcer disease during childhood seem to be low. Large pediatric endoscopy centers have reported an incidence of 5 to 7 children with gastric or duodenal ulcers per year.[106] More recent studies in United States Children's Hospitals showed that ulcers occurred in 1–2% of all hospitalizations.[107] There was a slight male predominance, and teenagers tended to have prevalence rates that were higher than younger ages. A trend was observed for an increased prevalence in black and Hispanic compared to white children, but these differences were not statistically significant. Although the ICD-9 diagnosis code for *H. pylori* did not become published until late 1995, there was a strong association between those children with duodenal ulcers and, to a lesser extent, gastric ulcers and *H. pylori* infection.

A strong correlation has also been demonstrated between duodenal ulceration, *H. pylori* gastritis and duodenal gastric metaplasia in children[108] Other studies have shown that *H. pylori* gastritis is found in 90% pediatric patients with duodenal ulcer disease.[92] In both adults and children, the presence of severe antral inflammation often will correlate with an increased frequency of duodenal ulceration.[22,109] In a more recent single center pediatric study, pre-pylori channel ulcers and duodenal ulcers were associated with severe antral gastritis and *cag*A+ *H. pylori* strains.[44,110] Similar to adults, duodenal ulceration in the absence of *H. pylori* infection is uncommon in childhood. However, there are single center small series that report an increase in *H. pylori*-negative ulcers both in the US and Canada (unpublished data). This observation may be due to a number of factors including, for example, missing the organism on biopsy due to a low density of colonization and a proximal shift in bacterial colonization due to the use of proton pump inhibitors or incidental use of antimicrobials.[22] Conversely, these *H. pylori*-negative ulcers may be due to other factors such as the surreptitious use of non-steroidal anti-inflammatory agents.

It has also been convincingly demonstrated that duodenal ulcer disease in children does not relapse if *H. pylori* is eradicated from the gastric mucosa.[6] In one study, 23 children with *H. pylori* gastritis associated with duodenal ulcers were treated using either cimetidine alone or a combination of cimetidine and amoxicillin.[93] Although, only a small portion of the children remained uninfected, when *H. pylori* was eradicated from the gastric mucosa using combination therapy, no recurrence of duodenal ulcer disease was detected 6 months after the end of treatment. In contrast, 50% of patients whose ulcers were originally healed but remained colonized by *H. pylori* (cimetidine only therapy) had a recurrence of their ulcer by 6 months. It has also been shown that healing of duodenal ulcers following eradication of *H. pylori* is often followed by re-epithelialization of the duodenal ulcer by gastric rather than intestinal mucosa.[111]

3.3. Gastric Cancer

The role of *H. pylori* in intestinal type gastric adenocarcinoma has been defined by a variety of sources: studies paralleling the epidemiological features of cancer with those of *H. pylori* infection,[112] cross-sectional studies of *H. pylori* infection in patients with cancer,[113] and prospective studies of *H. pylori* infection.[114,115] These data pose a difficult problem for the pediatrician managing a child infected with *H. pylori*. Evidence for the presence of gastric adenocarcinomas in children is limited to a handful of case reports. Thus, establishing causality and thereby treatment guidelines for infected children based on the role of *H. pylori* in gastric carcinoma cannot be done at the present time.[6,7]

Gastric cancer prevalence is higher in areas of poverty; afflicting people in developing nations and in lower socioeconomic classes in the industrialized world.[116] In many countries of Latin America and Asia, gastric cancer remains the most common malignancy among men and the second most common among women. Incidence rates as high as 80 per 100,000 population have been reported in Colombia and Japan. In contrast, gastric cancer affects less than 10 per 100,000 people per year in the United States and Western Europe.[117,118] However, within low-risk countries, there are ethnic groups with increased risk. In the United States, for example, the prevalence of gastric cancer among blacks, Asians, and Hispanics is almost double that among whites.[119] Interestingly, in all of these populations, prevalence rates of *H. pylori* are 2–10-fold higher than in the overall population.

H. pylori infection is a marker of increased gastric adenocarcinoma risk. Definite proof of cause, however, will be accomplished only when controlled trials demonstrate that elimination or prevention of infection prevents malignancy. Studies of *H. hepaticus* as a cause of liver cancer in mice and *H. mustelae* as an etiologic agent in gastric adenocarcinoma in ferrets add biological plausibility to the role of *H. pylori* in gastric cancer in humans[120–122] Moreover, studies in Mongolian gerbils infected by *H. pylori* demonstrate that *H. pylori* infection is carcinogenic in an unmanipulated animal host.[123–126] In addition, long term studies documenting reversal of pre-neoplastic conditions with anti-*H. pylori* therapy are needed to support the association of *H. pylori* and cancer. However, preliminary data in a large cohort of Chinese patients demonstrate that eradication of *H. pylori* does indeed arrest the progression of pre-neoplastic lesions.[127,128] Future studies should focus on the reversibility of intestinal metaplasia and, in particular, gastric epithelial cell dysplasia once *H. pylori* infection is eradicated.[129,130]

3.4. Gastric Lymphomas

In infancy and early childhood, the stomach mucosa contains only small number of immunocompetent lymphocytes and plasma cells. Chronic inflammation can develop, as the child gets older, lymphocytes accumulate in the submucosa and gradually increase their number. With the eradication of *H. pylori*, chronic inflammation decreases and the density of submucosal lymphocytes dramatically declines. Since most gastric lymphomas arise in areas of chronic inflammation, it seems plausible that prior *H. pylori* infection and gastric lymphomas are linked. Primary non-Hodgkin's lymphoma of the stomach is an uncommon cancer, accounting for only 10% of lymphomas and 3% of gastric neoplasms. Gastric non-Hodgkin's lymphoma remains, however, the most common extranodal form of this lymphoma, accounting for 20% of primary extranodal disease. In addition, immunological studies have shown these tumors to be of B-cell lineage.[131]

Low-grade B-cell lymphomas that arise in the stomach, lung, salivary gland, and thyroid recapitulate the structural features of mucosa-associated lymphoid tissue (MALT) as typified in Peyer's patches.[132] These lymphomas, together with the high-grade lesions that may evolve from them, are collectively known as MALT lymphomas.[132] MALT lymphomas were first described in the early 1980s when Isaacson and Wright[133] noted that the histology of certain low grade, B-cell gastrointestinal lymphomas were unlike that of comparable low-grade nodal lymphomas but was similar to that of mucosa-associated lymphoid tissue. Paradoxically, however, MALT is not present in either the normal stomach or other sites in which MALT lymphomas arise.

In the stomach, lymphoid tissue is acquired as a result of colonization of the gastric mucosa by *H. pylori*.[134] Wotherspoon and colleagues[135] demonstrated that this *H. pylori*-associated lymphoid tissue is of MALT type. They suggested that MALT acquired in response to *H. pylori* infection provides the background on which other, yet unidentified, factors act to result in the development of lymphoma in a small proportion of cases. Hussell and colleagues[136] demonstrated that cellular proliferation of low-grade B-cell gastric MALT lymphomas is dependent on *H. pylori*-specific T-cells. Multiple serological studies provide evidence indicate that infection with *H. pylori* increases the risk of gastric non-Hodgkin's lymphoma.[137,138]

Specific colonization of lymphoid follicle centers by neoplastic cells,[139] and the binding of specific antibodies indicate that MALT tumors are immunologically responsive.[140] Given the close association between gastric MALT lymphoma and *H. pylori*, this organism might evoke the immunological response, and eradication of *H. pylori* might thereby inhibit the tumor. In fact, studies suggest that anti-*H. pylori* therapy can eradicate MALT lymphoma in some cases.[141] More recently studies demonstrating regression of MALT lymphoma following eradication of *H. pylori*, provide additional evidence for initiation of eradication therapy in *H. pylori* infected patient with this disease outcome.[142–147] Studies in children are limited to case reports, but clearly demonstrate regression of the tumor following eradication therapy in the rare case of the *H. pylori*-infected child with MALT lymphoma.[148]

4. SUMMARY AND FUTURE DIRECTIONS

There have been major in-roads in our understanding of the pathogenesis of gastroduodenal disease since *H. pylori* first became recognized as a human pathogen. In particular, advances in molecular bacteriology including the complete sequencing of the *H. pylori* genome provide tools with which to better delineate the pathogenesis of disease.[149] More recent developments indicate that a better understanding of the microbial-host interaction is critical to furthering knowledge with respect to *H. pylori*-induced disease outcomes. Moreover, only recently has attention been applied to elucidating the role of the host response and the immunophysiological reactions both in the pathogenesis of *H. pylori* infection and as predictors of disease.

In vitro models that are biologically relevant, reproducible and represent chronic infection are critically needed. In addition, currently available animal models do not provide the ideal means to study the pathogenesis of disease outcomes, such as gastroduodenal ulceration and gastric cancer. Therefore, improvement in these *in vitro* and *in vivo* models along with validation of key observations in humans will be essential. Multicenter, multinational studies of *H. pylori* infection in the pediatric population, which include specific, randomized controlled eradication trials, are critically needed to extend current knowledge base and develop better predictors of disease outcome.

Acknowledgements. Dr. Gold is supported by a grant received from the National Institutes of Health, NIDDK, R01—DK53708

REFERENCES

1. Day A. S., Jones N. L., Lynett J. T., *et al.*, 2000, cagE is a virulence factor associated with *Helicobacter pylori*-induced duodenal ulceration in children. *J. Infect. Dis.* **181**(4):1370–1375.
2. Graham D. Y., Rakel R. E., Fendrick A. M., *et al.*, 1999, Recognizing peptic ulcer disease. Keys to clinical and laboratory diagnosis. *Postgrad. Med.* **105**(3):113–116, 121–123, 127–128 passim.
3. Miehlke S., Genta R. M., Graham D. Y., and Go M. F., 1999, Molecular relationships of *Helicobacter pylori* strains in a family with gastroduodenal disease. *Am. J. Gastroenterol.* **94**(2): 364–368.
4. Parsonnet J., Shmuely H., and Haggerty T., 1999, Fecal and oral shedding of *Helicobacter pylori* from healthy infected adults [see comments]. *Jama.* **282**(23):2240–2245.
5. Graham D. Y., and Yamaoka Y., 1998, *H. pylori* and cagA: relationships with gastric cancer, duodenal ulcer, and reflux esophagitis and its complications. *Helicobacter.* **3**(3):145–151.
6. Drumm B., Koletzko S., and Oderda G., 2000, *Helicobacter pylori* Infection in Children: a consensus statement. Medical Position Paper: report of the European Paediatric Task Force on *Helicobacter pylori* on a Consensus Conference, Budapest, Hungary, September 1998. *J. Pediatr. Gastroenterol. Nutr.* **30**(2):207–213.

7. Sherman P., Hassall E., Hunt R. H., Fallone C. A., Veldhuyzen van Zanten S., and Thomson A. B. R., 1999, Canadian Helicobacter Study Group Consensus Conference on the Approach to *Helicobacter pylori* infection in Children and Adolescents. *Can. J. Gastroenterol.* **13**(7): 553–559.
8. Gold B. D., 1999, Pediatric *Helicobacter pylori* infection: clinical manifestations, diagnosis, and therapy. *Curr. Top Microbiol. Immunol.* **241**:71–102.
9. Sonnenberg A., Schwartz J. S., Cutler A. F., Vakil N., and Bloom B. S., 1998, Cost savings in duodenal ulcer therapy through *Helicobacter pylori* eradication compared with conventional therapies: results of a randomized, double-blind, multicenter trial. Gastrointestinal Utilization Trial Study Group. *Arch. Intern. Med.* **158**(8):852–860.
10. Sonnenberg A., and Everhart J. E., 1996, The prevalence of self-reported peptic ulcer in the United States. *Am. J. Public. Health.* **86**(2):200–205.
11. Hirschowitz B. I., 1996, Nonsteroidal anti-inflammatory drugs and the gut. *South Med. J.* **89**(3):259–263.
12. Bourke B., Jones N., and Sherman P., 1996, *Helicobacter pylori* infection and peptic ulcer disease in children. *Pediatr. Infect. Dis. J.* **15**(1):1–13.
13. Sherman P. M., 1994, Peptic ulcer disease in children. Diagnosis, treatment, and the implication of *Helicobacter pylori. Gastroenterol. Clin. North Am.* **23**(4):707–725.
14. Mitchell H. M., and Hazell S. L., 1996, *Helicobacter pylori*, gastric ulcer, and duodenal ulcer [letter; comment]. *N. Engl. J. Med.* **335**(24):1841; discussion 1842–1843.
15. Malaty H. M., Graham D. Y., Isaksson I., Engstrand L., and Pedersen N. L., 2000, Are genetic influences on peptic ulcer dependent or independent of genetic influences for *Helicobacter pylori* infection? *Arch. Intern. Med.* **160**(1):105–109.
16. Drumm B., O'Brien A., Cutz E., and Sherman P., 1987, Campylobacter pyloridis-associated primary gastritis in children. *Pediatrics.* **80**(2):192–195.
17. Czinn S. J., Dahms B. B., Jacobs G. H., Kaplan B., and Rothstein F. C., 1986, Campylobacter-like organisms in association with symptomatic gastritis in children. *J. Pediatr.* **109**(1):80–83.
18. Drumm B., Perez-Perez G. I., Blaser M. J., and Sherman P. M., 1990, Intrafamilial clustering of *Helicobacter pylori* infection. *N. Engl. J. Med.* **322**(6):359–363.
19. Malaty H. M., Graham D. Y., Klein P. D., Evans D. G., Adam E., and Evans D. J., 1991, Transmission of *Helicobacter pylori* infection. Studies in families of healthy individuals. *Scand. J. Gastroenterol.* **26**(9):927–932.
20. Rowland M., Kumar D., Daly L., O'Connor P., Vaughan D., and Drumm B., 1999, Low rates of *Helicobacter pylori* reinfection in children. *Gastroenterology.* **117**(2):336–341.
21. El-Omar E. M., Carrington M., Chow W. H., *et al.*, 2000, Interleukin-1 polymorphisms associated with increased risk of gastric cancer. *Nature.* **404**(6776):398–402.
22. Genta R. M., 1999, Atrophy, acid suppression and *Helicobacter pylori* infection: a tale of two studies. *Eur. J. Gastroenterol. Hepatol.* 11 Suppl **2**:S29–33; discussion S43–45.
23. Genta R. M., and Graham D. Y., 1996, *Helicobacter pylori* in a Gastric Pit. *N. Engl. J. Med.* **335**(4):250.
24. Blaser M. J., 1997, The versatility of *Helicobacter pylori* in the adaptation to the human stomach. *J. Physiol. Pharmacol.* **48**(3):307–314.
25. Blaser M. J., 1997, Ecology of *Helicobacter pylori* in the human stomach. *J. Clin. Invest.* **100**(4):759–762.
26. Blaser M. J., 1997, Not all *Helicobacter pylori* strains are created equal: should all be eliminated? [see comments]. *Lancet.* **349**(9057):1020–1022.
27. Chan W. Y., Hui P. K., Leung K. M., Chow J., Kwok F., and Ng C. S., 1994, Coccoid forms of *Helicobacter pylori* in the human stomach. *Am. J. Clin. Pathol.* **102**(4):503–507.
28. Covacci A., Telford J. L., Del Giudice G., Parsonnet J., and Rappuoli R., 1999, *Helicobacter pylori* virulence and genetic geography. *Science.* **284**(5418):1328–1333.

29. Dorrell N., Martino M. C., Stabler R. A., *et al.*, 1999, Characterization of *Helicobacter pylori* PldA, a phospholipase with a role in colonization of the gastric mucosa. *Gastroenterology.* **117**(5): 1098–1104.
30. Windle H. J., Fox A., Ni Eidhin D., and Kelleher D., 2000, The thioredoxin system of *Helicobacter pylori. J. Biol. Chem.* **275**(7):5081–5089.
31. Weeks D. L., Eskandari S., Scott D. R., and Sachs G., 2000, A H+-gated urea channel: the link between *Helicobacter pylori* urease and gastric colonization. *Science.* **287**(5452):482–485.
32. Gold B. D., Owens M. L., van Doorn L. J., *et al.*, 1999, Correlation of *Helicobacter pylori* genotype with clinical and demographic characteristics of infected children. *Gastroenterology.* **116**(4, part 2):174.
33. Atherton J. C., Cao P., Peek R. M., Jr., Tummuru M. K., Blaser M. J., and Cover T. L., 1995, Mosaicism in vacuolating cytotoxin alleles of *Helicobacter pylori*. Association of specific vacA types with cytotoxin production and peptic ulceration. *J. Biol. Chem.* **270**(30):17771–17777.
34. Atherton J. C., Peek R. M., Jr., Tham K. T., Cover T. L., and Blaser M. J., 1997, Clinical and pathological importance of heterogeneity in vacA, the vacuolating cytotoxin gene of *Helicobacter pylori. Gastroenterology.* **112**(1):92–99.
35. Miehlke S., Meining A., Morgner A., *et al.*, 1998, Frequency of vacA genotypes and cytotoxin activity in *Helicobacter pylori* associated with low-grade gastric mucosa-associated lymphoid tissue lymphoma. *J. Clin. Microbiol.* **36**(8):2369–2370.
36. Cover T. L., 1996, The vacuolating cytotoxin of *Helicobacter pylori. Mol. Microbiol.* **20**(2):241–246.
37. Xiang Z., Censini S., Bayeli P. F., *et al.*, 1995, Analysis of expression of CagA and VacA virulence factors in 43 strains of *Helicobacter pylori* reveals that clinical isolates can be divided into two major types and that CagA is not necessary for expression of the vacuolating cytotoxin. *Infect. Immun.* **63**(1):94–98.
38. van Doorn L. J., Figueiredo C., Sanna R., *et al.*, 1998, Clinical relevance of the cagA, vacA, and iceA status of *Helicobacter pylori. Gastroenterology.* **115**(1):58–66.
39. van Doorn L. J., Figueiredo C., Rossau R., *et al.*, 1998, Typing of *Helicobacter pylori* vacA gene and detection of cagA gene by PCR and reverse hybridization. *J. Clin. Microbiol.* 36(5): 1271–1276.
40. Karaolis D. K., Somara S., Maneval D. R., Jr., Johnson J. A., and Kaper J. B., 1999, A bacteriophage encoding a pathogenicity island, a type-IV pilus and a phage receptor in cholera bacteria [see comments]. *Nature.* **399**(6734):375–379.
41. Mobley H. L., 1997, *Helicobacter pylori* factors associated with disease development [see comments]. *Gastroenterology.* **113**(6 Suppl):S21–28.
42. Li L., Kelly L. K., Ayub K., Graham D. Y., and Go M. F., 1999, Genotypes of *Helicobacter pylori* obtained from gastric ulcer patients taking or not taking NSAIDs. *Am. J. Gastroenterol.* **94**(6):1502–1507.
43. Peek R. M., Jr., Vaezi M. F., Falk G. W., *et al.*, 1999, Role of *Helicobacter pylori* cagA(+) strains and specific host immune responses on the development of premalignant and malignant lesions in the gastric cardia. *Int. J. Cancer.* **82**(4):520–524.
44. Elitsur Y., Neace C., Werthammer M. C., and Triest W. E., 1999, Prevalence of CagA, VacA antibodies in symptomatic and asymptomatic children with *Helicobacter pylori* infection. *Helicobacter.* **4**(2):100–105.
45. Kolho K. L., Karttunen R., Heikkila P., Lindahl H., and Rautelin H., 1999, Gastric inflammation is enhanced in children with CagA-positive *Helicobacter pylori* infection. *Pediatr. Infect. Dis. J.* **18**(4):337–341.
46. Day A. S., and Sherman P. M., 2000, *Helicobacter pylori* infection, host genes, and disease outcome [news] [In Process Citation]. *Pediatr. Res.* **47**(6):703.
47. Day A. S., and Sherman P. M., 1999, Understanding disease outcome following acquisition of *Helicobacter pylori* infection during childhood. *Can. J. Gastroenterol.* **13**(3):229–234.

48. Figueiredo C., Quint W. G., Sanna R., *et al.*, 2000, Genetic organization and heterogeneity of the iceA locus of *Helicobacter pylori*. *Gene*. **246**(1–2):59–68.
49. Censini S., Lange C., Xiang Z., *et al.*, 1996, cag, a pathogenicity island of *Helicobacter pylori*, encodes type I-specific and disease-associated virulence factors. *Proc. Natl. Acad. Sci. USA*. **93**(25):14648–14653.
50. Graham D. Y., 1997, *Helicobacter pylori* infection in the pathogenesis of duodenal ulcer and gastric cancer: a model. *Gastroenterology*. **113**(6):1983–1991.
51. Nagita A., Amemoto K., Yoden A., *et al.*, 1996, Diurnal variation in intragastric pH in children with and without peptic ulcers. *Pediatr. Res.* **40**(4):528–532.
52. Yamashiro Y., Shioya T., Ohtsuka Y., *et al.*, 1995, Patterns of 24 h intragastric acidity in duodenal ulcers in children: the importance of monitoring and inhibiting nocturnal acidity. *Acta. Paediatr. Jpn.* **37**(5):557–561.
53. Isenberg J. I., Selling J. A., Hogan D. L., and Koss M. A., 1987, Impaired proximal duodenal mucosal bicarbonate secretion in patients with duodenal ulcer. *N. Engl. J. Med.* **316**(7): 374–379.
54. Nyberg L., Pratha V., Hogan D. L., Rapier R. C., Koss M. A., and Isenberg J. I., 1998, Human proximal duodenal alkaline secretion is mediated by Cl-/HCO3-exchange and HCO3-conductance. *Dig. Dis. Sci.* **43**(6):1205–1210.
55. Lichtenberger L. M., and Romero J. J., 1994, Effect of ammonium ion on the hydrophobic and barrier properties of the gastric mucus gel layer: implications on the role of ammonium in *H. pylori*-induced gastritis. *J. Gastroenterol. Hepatol.* **9**(Suppl 1):S13–19.
56. Gold B. D., Islur P., Policova Z., Czinn S., Neumann A. W., and Sherman P. M., 1996, Surface properties of *Helicobacter mustelae* and ferret gastrointestinal mucosa. *Clin. Invest. Med.* **19**(2): 92–100.
57. Asante M., Ahmed H., Patel P., *et al.*, 1997, Gastric mucosal hydrophobicity in duodenal ulceration: role of *Helicobacter pylori* infection density and mucus lipids. *Gastroenterology*. **113**(2): 449–454.
58. Goggin P. M., Marrero J. M., Spychal R. T., Jackson P. A., Corbishley C. M., and Northfield T. C., 1992, Surface hydrophobicity of gastric mucosa in *Helicobacter pylori* infection: effect of clearance and eradication. *Gastroenterology*. **103**(5):1486–1490.
59. Van den Brink G. R., Tytgat K. M., Van der Hulst R. W., *et al.*, 2000, H pylori colocalises with MUC5AC in the human stomach. *Gut*. **46**(5):601–607.
60. Byrd J. C., Yunker C. K., Xu Q. S., Sternberg L. R., and Bresalier R. S., 2000, Inhibition of gastric mucin synthesis by *Helicobacter pylori*. *Gastroenterology*. **118**(6):1072–1079.
61. Beil W., Enss M. L., Muller S., Obst B., Sewing K. F., and Wagner S., 2000, Role of vacA and cagA in *Helicobacter pylori* inhibition of mucin synthesis in gastric mucous cells [In Process Citation]. *J. Clin. Microbiol.* **38**(6):2215–2218.
62. Taylor I. L., 1984, Gastrointestinal hormones in the pathogenesis of peptic ulcer disease. *Clin. Gastroenterol.* **13**(2):355–382.
63. Oderda G., Vaira D., Dell'Olio D., *et al.*, 1990, Serum pepsinogen I and gastrin concentrations in children positive for *Helicobacter pylori*. *J. Clin. Pathol.* **43**(9):762–765.
64. Westerveld B. D., Pals G., Lamers C. B., *et al.*, 1987, Clinical significance of pepsinogen A isozymogens, serum pepsinogen A and C levels, and serum gastrin levels. *Cancer*. **59**(5):952–958.
65. Rotter J. I., Sones J. Q., Samloff I. M., *et al.*, 1979, Duodenal-ulcer disease associated with elevated serum pepsinogen I: an inherited autosomal dominant disorder. *N. Engl. J. Med.* **300**(2):63–66.
66. Rotter J. I., Petersen G., Samloff I. M., *et al.*, 1979, Genetic heterogeneity of hyperpepsinogenemic I and normopepsinogenemic I duodenal ulcer disease. *Ann. Intern. Med.* **91**(3):372–377.
67. Beales I., Blaser M. J., Srinivasan S., *et al.*, 1997, Effect of *Helicobacter pylori* products and recombinant cytokines on gastrin release from cultured canine G cells. *Gastroenterology*. **113**(2):465–471.

68. Wyatt J. I., 1995, Histopathology of gastroduodenal inflammation: the impact of *Helicobacter pylori*. *Histopathology*. **26**(1):1–15.
69. Ashorn M., 1995, What are the specific features of *Helicobacter pylori* gastritis in children? *Ann. Med.* 27(5):617–620.
70. Wirth H. P., Yang M., Peek R. M., Jr., Hook-Nikanne J., Fried M., and Blaser M. J., 1999, Phenotypic diversity in Lewis expression of *Helicobacter pylori* isolates from the same host. *J. Lab. Clin. Med.* **133**(5):488–500.
71. Ernst P. B., and Gold B. D., 1999, *Helicobacter pylori* in childhood: new insights into the immunopathogenesis of gastric disease and implications for managing infection in children [In Process Citation]. *J. Pediatr. Gastroenterol. Nutr.* **28**(5):462–473.
72. Wang J., Fan X., Lindholm C., *et al.*, 2000, *Helicobacter pylori* modulates lymphoepithelial cell interactions leading to epithelial cell damage through Fas/Fas ligand interactions. *Infect. Immun.* **68**(7):4303–4311.
73. Jones N. L., Day A. S., Jennings H. A., and Sherman P. M., 1999, *Helicobacter pylori* induces gastric epithelial cell apoptosis in association with increased Fas receptor expression. *Infect. Immun.* **67**(8):4237–4242.
74. Ilver D., Arnqvist A., Ogren J., *et al.*, 1998, *Helicobacter pylori* adhesin binding fucosylated histo-blood group antigens revealed by retagging. *Science*. **279**(5349):373–377.
75. Fan X., Crowe S. E., Behar S., *et al.*, 1998, The effect of class II major histocompatibility complex expression on adherence of *Helicobacter pylori* and induction of apoptosis in gastric epithelial cells: a mechanism for T helper cell type 1-mediated damage. *J. Exp. Med.* **187**(10):1659–1669.
76. Wagner S., Beil W., Westermann J., *et al.*, 1997, Regulation of epithelial cell growth by *Helicobacter pylori*: Evidence for a major role of apoptosis. *Gastroenterology.* **113**:1836–1847.
77. Bodger K., and Crabtree J. E., 1998, *Helicobacter pylori* and gastric inflammation. *Br. Med. Bull.* **54**:139–150.
78. Shimoyama T., and Crabtree J. E., 1997, Mucosal chemokines in *Helicobacter pylori* infection. *J. Physiol. Pharmacol.* **48**(3):315–323.
79. Crowe S. E., Alvarez L., Dytoc M., *et al.*, 1995, Expression of interleukin 8 and CD54 by human gastric epithelium after *Helicobacter pylori* infection in vitro. *Gastroenterology.* **108**(1):65–74.
80. Crabtree J. E., Covacci A., Farmery S. M., *et al.*, 1995, *Helicobacter pylori* induced interleukin-8 expression in gastric epithelial cells is associated with CagA positive phenotype. *J. Clin. Pathol.* **48**(1):41–45.
81. Tummuru M. K., Sharma S. A., and Blaser M. J., 1995, *Helicobacter pylori* picB, a homologue of the Bordetella pertussis toxin secretion protein, is required for induction of IL-8 in gastric epithelial cells. *Mol. Microbiol.* **18**(5):867–876.
82. Stein M., Rappuoli R., and Covacci A., 2000, Tyrosine phosphorylation of the *Helicobacter pylori* CagA antigen after cag-driven host cell translocation. *Proc. Natl. Acad. Sci. U.S.A.* **97**:1263–1268.
83. Odenbreit S., Puls J., Sedlmaier B., Gerland E., Fischer W., and Haas R., 2000, Translocation of *Helicobacter pylori* CagA into gastric epithelial cells by type IV secretion. *Science.* **287**(5457):1497–1500.
84. Genta R. M., and Graham D. Y., 1994, Comparison of biopsy sites for the histopathologic diagnosis of *Helicobacter pylori*: a topographic study of *H. pylori* density and distribution [see comments]. *Gastrointest. Endosc.* **40**(3):342–345.
85. Genta R. M., and Hamner H. W., 1994, The significance of lymphoid follicles in the interpretation of gastric biopsy specimens. *Arch. Pathol. Lab. Med.* **118**(7):740–743.
86. Genta R. M., and Graham D. Y., 1994, *Helicobacter pylori*: the new bug on the (paraffin) block. *Virchows. Arch.* **425**(4):339–347.
87. Whitney A. E., Guarner J., Hutwagner L., and Gold B. D., 1998, A331 HDBHpGoCaAG. Histopathological differences between *Helicobacter pylori* gastritis of children and adults. *Gastroenterology.* **114**(4):331.

88. Ernst P. B., and Gold B. D., 1999, *Helicobacter pylori* in childhood: new insights into the immunopathogenesis of gastric disease and implications for managing infection in children. *J. Pediatr. Gastroenterol. Nutr.* **28**(5):462–473.
89. Warren J. R., and Marshall B. J., 1983, Unidentified curved bacilli on gastric epithelium in active chronic gastritis. *Lancet.* **1**:1273–1275.
90. Hill R., Pearman J., Worthy P., Caruso V., Goodwin S., and Blincow E., 1986, Campylobacter pyloridis and gastritis in children [letter]. *Lancet.* **1**(8477):387.
91. Cadranel S., Goossens H., De Boeck M., Malengreau A., Rodesch P., and Butzler J. P., 1986, Campylobacter pyloridis in children [letter]. *Lancet.* **1**(8483):735–736.
92. Kilbridge P. M., Dahms B. B., and Czinn S. J., 1988, Campylobacter pylori–associated gastritis and peptic ulcer disease in children [see comments]. *Am. J. Dis. Child.* **142**(11):1149–1152.
93. Yeung C. K., Fu K. H., Yuen K. Y., *et al.*, 1990, *Helicobacter pylori* and associated duodenal ulcer. *Arch. Dis. Child.* **65**(11):1212–1216.
94. Peterson W. L., 1991, *Helicobacter pylori* and peptic ulcer disease [see comments]. *N. Engl. J. Med.* **324**(15):1043–1048.
95. Drumm B., Sherman P., Cutz E., and Karmali M., 1987, Association of Campylobacter pylori on the gastric mucosa with antral gastritis in children. *N. Engl. J. Med.* **316**(25):1557–1561.
96. Drumm B., 1990, *Helicobacter pylori* [see comments]. *Arch. Dis. Child.* **65**(11):1278–1282.
97. Quieroz D. M. M., Rocha G. A., Mendes E. N., *et al.*, 1991, Differences in the distribution and severity of *Helicobacter pylori* gastritis in children and adults with duodenal ulcer disease. *J. Pediatr. Gastroenterol. Nutr.* **12**:178–181.
98. Loffeld R. J., Potters H. V., Arends J. W., Stobberingh E., Flendrig J. A., and van Spreeuwel J. P., 1988, Campylobacter associated gastritis in patients with non-ulcer dyspepsia. *J. Clin. Pathol.* **41**(1):85–88.
99. Louw J. A., Falck V., van Rensburg C., Zak J., Adams G., and Marks I. N., 1993, Distribution of *Helicobacter pylori* colonisation and associated gastric inflammatory changes: difference between patients with duodenal and gastric ulcers. *J. Clin. Pathol.* **46**(8):754–756.
100. Peters F. T., Kuipers E. J., Ganesh S., *et al.*, 1999, The influence of *Helicobacter pylori* on oesophageal acid exposure in GERD during acid suppressive therapy. *Aliment. Pharmacol. Ther.* **13**(7):921–926.
101. Genta R. M., Huberman R. M., and Graham D. Y., 1994, The gastric cardia in *Helicobacter pylori* infection. *Hum. Pathol.* **25**(9):915–919.
102. Hassall E., and Dimmick J. E., 1991, Unique features of *Helicobacter pylori* disease in children. *Dig. Dis. Sci.* **36**(4):417–423.
103. Goodwin C. S., Armstrong J. A., and Marshall B. J., 1986, Campylobacter pyloridis, gastritis, and peptic ulceration. *J. Clin. Pathol.* **39**(4):353–365.
104. Marshall B. J., 1986, *Campylobacter pyloridis* and gastritis. *J. Infect. Dis.* **153**(4):650–657.
105. Sbeih F., Abdullah A., Sullivan S., and Merenkov Z., 1996, Antral nodularity, gastric lymphoid hyperplasia, and *Helicobacter pylori* in adults. *J. Clin. Gastroenterol.* **22**(3):227–230.
106. Drumm B., Rhoads J. M., Stringer D. A., Sherman P. M., Ellis L. E., and Durie P. R., 1988, Peptic ulcer disease in children: etiology, clinical findings, and clinical course. *Pediatrics.* **82**(3 Pt 2):410–414.
107. Gold B. D., Kennedy M., Stockwell J., and Friedman C. R., 1999, Epidemiology of Peptic Ulcer Disease and *Helicobacter pylori* (Hp) in Hospitalized Children using the Pediatric Hospital Information System. *J. Pediatr. Gastroenterol. Nutr.* **29**(4):491.
108. Shabib S. M., Cutz E., Drumm B., and Sherman P. M., 1994, Association of gastric metaplasia and duodenitis with *Helicobacter pylori* infection in children. *Am. J. Clin. Pathol.* **102**(2):188–191.
109. Genta R. M., and Franceschi F., 1999, Treating biopsies to cure patients: the management of histological findings in mucosa-associated lymphoid tissue (MALT) [editorial; comment]. *J. Clin. Gastroenterol.* **29**(2):116–117.

110. Elitsur Y., 1999, *H. pylori*-CagA serum antibody and RAP in children [letter; comment]. *Am. J. Gastroenterol.* **94**(2):539.
111. Kim N., Lim S. H., Lee K. H., and Choi S. E., 1998, Long-term effect of *Helicobacter pylori* eradication on gastric metaplasia in patients with duodenal ulcer. *J. Clin. Gastroenterol.* **27**(3): 246–252.
112. Correa P., 1995, *Helicobacter pylori* and gastric carcinogenesis. *Am. J. Surg. Pathol.* **19**(Suppl 1):S37–43.
113. Parsonnet J., Friedman G. D., Vandersteen D. P., *et al.*, 1991, *Helicobacter pylori* infection and the risk of gastric carcinoma [see comments]. *N. Engl. J. Med.* **325**(16):1127–1131.
114. Parsonnet J., Vandersteen D., Goates J., Sibley R. K., Pritikin J., and Chang Y., 1991, *Helicobacter pylori* infection in intestinal- and diffuse-type gastric adenocarcinomas [published erratum appears in J Natl Cancer Inst 1991 Jun 19;83(12):881]. *J. Natl. Cancer. Inst.* **83**(9):640–643.
115. Forman D., Newell D. G., Fullerton F., *et al.*, Association between infection with *Helicobacter pylori* and risk of gastric cancer: evidence from a prospective investigation [see comments]. *Bmj.* **302**(6788):1302–1305.
116. Forman D., 1991, The etiology of gastric cancer. *IARC Sci. Publ.* **105**:22–32.
117. Chiba N., Thomson A. B., and Sinclair P., 2000, From bench to bedside to bug: An update of clinically relevant advances in the care of persons with *Helicobacter pylori*- associated diseases. *Can. J. Gastroenterol.* **14**(3):188–198.
118. Hansson L. E., 2000, Risk of stomach cancer in patients with peptic ulcer disease. *World J. Surg.* **24**(3):315–320.
119. El-Omar E. M., Oien K., Murray L. S., *et al.*, 2000, Increased prevalence of precancerous changes in relatives of gastric cancer patients: critical role of *H. pylori* [see comments]. *Gastroenterology.* **118**(1):22–30.
120. Ward J. M., Anver M. R., Haines D. C., and Benveniste R. E., 1994, Chronic active hepatitis in mice caused by *Helicobacter hepaticus. Am. J. Pathol.* **145**(4):959–968.
121. Ward J. M., Fox J. G., Anver M. R., *et al.*, 1994, Chronic active hepatitis and associated liver tumors in mice caused by a persistent bacterial infection with a novel Helicobacter species. *J. Natl. Cancer Inst.* **86**(16):1222–1227.
122. Fox J. G., Dewhirst F. E., Tully J. G., *et al.*, 1994, *Helicobacter hepaticus* sp. nov., a microaerophilic bacterium isolated from livers and intestinal mucosal scrapings from mice. *J. Clin. Microbiol.* **32**(5):1238–1245.
123. Ikeno T., Ota H., Sugiyama A., *et al.*, 1999, *Helicobacter pylori*-induced chronic active gastritis, intestinal metaplasia, and gastric ulcer in Mongolian gerbils. *Am. J. Pathol.* **154**(3):951–960.
124. Watanabe T., Tada M., Nagai H., Sasaki S., and Nakao M., 1998, *Helicobacter pylori* infection induces gastric cancer in mongolian gerbils [see comments]. *Gastroenterology.* **115**(3):642–648.
125. Honda S., Fujioka T., Tokieda M., Satoh R., Nishizono A., and Nasu M., 1998, Development of *Helicobacter pylori*-induced gastric carcinoma in Mongolian gerbils. *Cancer. Res.* **58**(19):4255–4259.
126. Fujioka T., Honda S., and Tokieda M., 2000, *Helicobacter pylori* infection and gastric carcinoma in animal models. *J. Gastroenterol. Hepatol.* 15 Suppl:D55–59.
127. Saito K., Arai K., Mori M., Kobayashi R., and Ohki I., 2000, Effect of *Helicobacter pylori* eradication on malignant transformation of gastric adenoma [In Process Citation]. *Gastrointest. Endosc.* **52**(1):27–32.
128. Sung J. J., Lin S. R., Ching J. Y., *et al.*, 2000, Atrophy and intestinal metaplasia one year after cure of *H. pylori* infection: a prospective, randomized study [see comments]. *Gastroenterology.* **119**(1):7–14.
129. Correa P., Haenszel W., Cuello C., *et al.*, 1990, Gastric precancerous process in a high risk population: cohort follow-up. *Cancer. Res.* **50**(15):4737–4740.

130. Chen V. W., Abu-Elyazeed R. R., Zavala D. E., *et al.*, 1990, Risk factors of gastric precancerous lesions in a high-risk Colombian population. II. Nitrate and nitrite. *Nutr. Cancer.* **13**(1–2):67–72.
131. Villar H. V., Wong R., Paz B., *et al.*, 1991, Immunophenotyping in the management of gastric lymphoma. *Am. J. Surg.* **161**(1):171–175; discussion 175–176.
132. Isaacson P. G., and Spencer J., 1987, Malignant lymphoma of mucosa-associated lymphoid tissue. *Histopathology.* **11**(5):445–462.
133. Isaacson P., and Wright D. H., 1983, Malignant lymphoma of mucosa-associated lymphoid tissue. A distinctive type of B-cell lymphoma. *Cancer.* **52**(8):1410–1416.
134. Stolte M., and Eidt S., 1989, Lymphoid follicles in antral mucosa: immune response to Campylobacter pylori? *J. Clin. Pathol.* **42**(12):1269–1271.
135. Wotherspoon A. C., Ortiz-Hidalgo C., Falzon M. R., and Isaacson P. G., 1991, *Helicobacter pylori*-associated gastritis and primary B-cell gastric lymphoma [see comments]. *Lancet.* **338**(8776):1175–1176.
136. Hussell T., Isaacson P. G., and Spencer J., 1993, Proliferation and differentiation of tumour cells from B-cell lymphoma of mucosa-associated lymphoid tissue in vitro. *J. Pathol.* **169**(2):221–227.
137. Forman D., Webb P., and Parsonnet J., 1994, H pylori and gastric cancer [letter]. *Lancet.* **343**(8891):243–244.
138. Parsonnet J., Hansen S., Rodriguez L., *et al.*, 1994, *Helicobacter pylori* infection and gastric lymphoma [see comments]. *N. Engl. J. Med.* **330**(18):1267–1271.
139. Isaacson P. G., 1999, Mucosa-associated lymphoid tissue lymphoma. *Semin. Hematol.* **36**(2):139–147.
140. Isaacson P. G., 1999, Gastrointestinal lymphomas of T- and B-cell types. *Mod. Pathol.* **12**(2): 151–158.
141. Wotherspoon A. C., 1998, *Helicobacter pylori* infection and gastric lymphoma. *Br. Med. Bull.* **54**(1):79–85.
142. Du M. Q., and Isaacson P. G., 1998, Recent advances in our understanding of the biology and pathogenesis of gastric mucosa-associated lymphoid tissue (malt) lymphoma. *Forum (Genova).* **8**(2):162–173.
143. Nobre-Leitao C., Lage P., Cravo M., *et al.*, 1998, Treatment of gastric MALT lymphoma by *Helicobacter pylori* eradication: a study controlled by endoscopic ultrasonography. *Am. J. Gastroenterol.* **93**(5):732–736.
144. Steinbach G., Ford R., Glober G., *et al.*, 1999, Antibiotic treatment of gastric lymphoma of mucosa-associated lymphoid tissue. An uncontrolled trial. *Ann. Intern. Med.* **131**(2):88–95.
145. Thiede C., Wundisch T., Neubauer B., *et al.*, 2000, Eradication of *Helicobacter pylori* and stability of remissions in low-grade gastric B-cell lymphomas of the mucosa-associated lymphoid tissue: results of an ongoing multicenter trial. *Recent. Results. Cancer. Res.* **156**:125–133.
146. Yamashita H., Watanabe H., Ajioka Y., Nishikura K., Maruta K., and Fujino M. A., 2000, When can complete regression of low-grade gastric lymphoma of mucosa-associated lymphoid tissue be predicted after *Helicobacter pylori* eradication? [In Process Citation]. *Histopathology.* **37**(2):131–140.
147. Go M. F., and Smoot D. T., 2000, *Helicobacter pylori*, gastric MALT lymphoma, and adenocarcinoma of the stomach [In Process Citation]. *Semin. Gastrointest. Dis.* **11**(3):134–141.
148. Blecker U., McKeithan T. W., Hart J., and Kirschner B. S., 1995, Resolution of *Helicobacter pylori*-associated gastric lymphoproliferative disease in a child. *Gastroenterology.* **109**(3):973–977.
149. Alm R. A., Ling L. S., Moir D. T., *et al.*, 1999, Genomic-sequence comparison of two unrelated isolates of the human gastric pathogen *Helicobacter pylori* [published erratum appears in Nature 1999 Feb 25;397(6721):719]. *Nature.* **397**(6715):176–180.

5

Helicobacter pylori Eradication Therapy

JIA-QING HUANG and RICHARD H. HUNT

1. INTRODUCTION

Helicobacter pylori (*H. pylori*) infection is a well recognized upper gastrointestinal pathogen. Eradication of the infection heals type B chronic active gastritis, peptic ulcer disease and virtually abolishes ulcer recurrence.[1–5] Cure of the infection also results in a complete histological regression of gastric MALT lymphoma in 80% of the patients and prevents recurrence in almost all cases[6–8] and may prevent metachronous occurrence of gastric adenocarcinoma following endoscopic resection of early gastric cancer.[9]

It has been more than 14 years since the first randomized, placebo controlled clinical trial of bismuth and erythromycin for the eradication of *H. pylori* infection was published.[10] Treatment to eradicate the infection has evolved from single agents to combination therapies consisting of either a bismuth salt and two antibiotics, or an antisecretory agent and one or more antibiotics.[11,12] Treatments that achieve an eradication rate of greater than 80%, on an intent-to-treat basis, have been recommended by most recent consensus conferences and authorities.[13–16] These include bismuth-based triple therapies, triple therapies involving a proton pump

JIA-QING HUANG and RICHARD H. HUNT • Division of Gastroenterology, Department of Medicine, McMaster University Medical Center, 1200 Main Street West, Room 4W8, Hamilton, Ontario, Canada L8N 3Z5.

Helicobacter pylori Infection and Immunity,
Edited by Yamamoto *et al.*, Kluwer Academic/Plenum Publishers, 2002.

inhibitor (PPI) and two antibiotics, quadruple therapies, or more recently combinations with ranitidine bismuth citrate (RBC) and two antibiotics. Over the past 10 years and numerous trials, several factors determining treatment success have been identified. These include the components of a treatment regimen, treatment duration, patient compliance, strains of *H. pylori* and possibly the patient's gastric secretory status.[17,18] This chapter will discuss these issues together with several newly emerging treatment regimens for the management of *H. pylori* infection.

2. TREATMENT-RELATED FACTORS

The components of a treatment regimen are the most important factor for determining the outcome of *H. pylori* eradication therapy. This includes the drugs selected, and which doses and what dose frequency is given and the treatment duration. Early studies with single antibiotics or dual therapies have proved ineffective for treating *H. pylori* infection.[19] PPI based triple therapies are significantly more effective for eradicating *H. pylori* infection than dual therapies consisting of two antibiotics or a PPI plus a single antibiotic.[20–22] The superiority of PPI triple therapies over dual therapies has been confirmed by numerous comparative clinical trials.[23,24] For example, in a French study, the eradication rate achieved with lansoprazole 30 mg, amoxicillin 1 g and clarithromycin 500 mg all given bid for 14 days was 57.7% higher than with a dual therapy consisting of lansoprazole and amoxicillin.[23] Similar results also were reported in a multicenter study involving 352 patients from the US.[24] Moreover, the eradication rate achieved with one week PPI based triple therapy was significantly better than dual therapy given for 2 weeks,[25,26] indicating that PPI-based triple therapies are the choice for the eradication treatment of *H. pylori* infection.

The importance and rationale for combining antibiotics with a PPI for *H. pylori* eradication has been extensively discussed elsewhere.[11,27,28] In brief, PPIs may have synergistic effects on the eradication of *H. pylori* infection with several currently used antibiotics by offering an optimal intragastric pH environment under which the effect of acid-labile antimicrobials will be maximized.[11,27,28] PPIs also have a direct inhibitory effect on *H. pylori* growth *in vitro* through a urease independent pathway.[29] Moreover, the successful clinical results of PPI-based treatment regimens support the view of synergism.[21,30,31] The synergistic effect between PPI and antibiotics on *H. pylori* eradication has been confirmed by a recent large multicenter study involving 539 patients from 7 countries, also known as the MACH 2 study.[21] In this study, dual therapies consisting of clarithromycin (C) 250 mg or 500 mg bid and amoxicillin (A) 1 g bid or metronidazole (M) 400 mg bid were compared with triple therapies involving the same dose of antibiotics plus omeprazole (O) 20 mg bid. All medications were given for 7 days. By intent-to-treat analysis, the eradication rates were 94%, and 87% for patients treated with OAC and OMC, respectively, whereas the cure rates were only 26% for patients receiving AC and 69% for patients treated with the MC regimen.[21] These results emphasize the importance of a properly controlled intragastric environment to facilitate the effect of the antimicrobial agents.[27,28]

3. DOSE, DOSE FREQUENCY AND TREATMENT DURATION

The dose, dose frequency and treatment duration play an important role in determining the success of *H. pylori* eradication treatment. In a comprehensive review of the literature, consisting of 55 treatment arms and 3221 patients, we have shown that the dose of clarithromycin has a significant impact on the efficacy of the 7-day PAC regimen.[31] By intent-to-treat analysis, the eradication rate achieved with the clarithromycin 500 mg bid-containing regimens was 86.6% (95% CI 81–89.3), whereas the cure rate was only 78.2% (95% CI 71.2–85.2) for clarithromycin 250 mg bid-containing regimens, irrespective of the dose frequency of the PPI ($p < 0.0001$). Similar results were also seen when the dose frequency of the PPI was taken into account (Table 1). The dose frequency of the PPI also affects the efficacy of both the PAC and PMC combination regimens.[31] As shown in Table 1, *H. pylori* eradication rates were significantly higher in studies when the PPI was dosed twice daily than in studies using a once daily dose of PPI. The difference was seen consistently irrespective of the dose of clarithromycin.

TABLE 1
Pooled analysis of combination therapies for *H. pylori* eradication with a PPI, clarithromycin and metronidazole or amoxicillin given for 7 days

Regimen	N. arms	Per-protocol N/N. evaluated	% cure (95%CI)	Intent-to-treat N/N. treated	% cure (95%CI)
PMC	55	2388/2676	89.2 (86.8–91.7)	2522/2893	87.2 (84.8–89.5)
C250 mg	40	1621/1831	88.5 (85.5–91.5)	1784/2057	86.7 (83.9–89.6)
PPI qd	13	483/581	83.1 (76.7–89.6)	478/585	81.7 (75.5–87.9)
PPI bid	27	1138/1250	91 (88.4–93.6)[a]	1306/1472	88.7 (86.1–91.3)[a]
C500 mg*	15	767/845	90.9 (87–94.5)[b]	738/836	88.3 (84–92.5)[c]
PAC	55	2649/3010	88 (85.3–90.7)	2726/3221	84.6 (81.6–87.7)
C250 mg	16	593/712	83.3 (77.4–89.1)	599/766	78.2 (71.2–85.2)
PPI qd	5	136/181	75.1 (60.5–89.7)	136/195	69.7 (51.9–87.6)
PPI bid	11	457/531	86.1 (81.9–90.4)[a]	463/571	81.1 (75.3–86.9)[a]
C500 mg	39	2056/2298	89.5 (86.9–92)[d]	2127/2455	86.6 (81–89.3)[d]
PPI qd	1	23/28	82.1 NA	23/28	82.1 NA
PPI bid	38	2033/2270	89.6 (87–92.1)	2104/2427	86.7 (84–89.4)

P, PPI; M, metronidazole; C, clarithromycin; A, amoxicillin; qd, once daily; bid, twice daily; N. arm, number of treatment arms; N/N. evaluated, number/number evaluated; N/N. treated, number/number treated; NA, not available. *PPI bid was used in all studies.
[a]$p \leq 0.001$ vs PPI qd; [b]$p = 0.082$ vs C250 mg; [c]$p = 0.259$; [d]$p < 0.0001$ vs C250 mg.

PPI-based triple therapies are given for 7 days most commonly around the world with the exception of the USA where eradication treatments are given for 14 days.[13–16] In an analysis of 380 studies and 15,971 patients, we have shown that three 7-day treatment regimens were able to achieve an eradication rate of 90% by intent-to-treat analysis.[32] These included PAC and PMC, when clarithromycin 500 mg bid is used and PPI plus yield poor eradication rates, especially for metronidazole-containing regimens given in areas where the prevalence of metronidazole-resistant strains is high.[33] However, few US studies have evaluated the difference in *H. pylori* eradication between 7- and 14-days or 10- and 14-days.[34,35] Fennerty *et al.*, showed no difference in eradication rates (84% vs 85%) at 10- and 14-days when patients were treated with the standard doses of lansoprazole, amoxicillin and clarithromycin.[34] In another study reported by Laine *et al.*, the standard doses of omeprazole, amoxicillin and clarithromycin were given for 7, 10 and 14 days.[35] No statistically significant differences were seen in the eradication rates among the three treatment durations (86%, 90% and 92% for 7, 10, and 14 days, respectively).[35] Although PPI-based triple therapies are recommended for 14 days in the US, it has been suggested that this may be at the expense of poor patient compliance and higher initial cost compared to 7-day treatment.[35]

4. PATIENT-RELATED FACTORS

Poor patient compliance has been considered a major factor contributing to treatment failure, especially in patients treated with bismuth-based triple therapies.[36] In a recent meta-analysis of the discontinuation rates associated with *H. pylori* eradication treatment, Buring *et al.*, have shown that, among 63 articles involving 5996 patients, bismuth-containing regimens were associated with a 46% higher drop-out rate compared to non-bismuth treatments.[37] The discontinuation rate increased with the increasing number of doses taken per day. In contrast, treatments containing a PPI had the lowest dropout rates compared to non-PPI treatment regimens with an odds ratio of 0.89 (95% CI 0.73–1.09).[37] This is consistent with our earlier analysis in which we have shown that the adverse events-related dropout rates with 7-day PAC and PMC were only 0.2% and 2.2%, respectively.[32]

5. BACTERIAL RESISTANCE

Bacterial resistance to metronidazole or clarithromycin plays an important role in determining the success of *H. pylori* eradication treatments. There is a good correlation between bacterial resistance to clarithromycin and treatment failure,[38] however, the clinical relevance of *H. pylori* resistance to nitroimidazoles detected *in vitro* has been controversial, especially in studies using PMC combination.[17]

TABLE 2

Groups (N.a.)	Patients	Overall	M-R	M-S
7-d PAC (6)	319	90.0%[a]	89.2%[e]	86.4%[i]
7-d PMC (21)	1540	83.8[b]	78.7%[f]	93.0%[j]
7-d PAM (6)	406	75.9%[c]	50.5%[g]	91.7%[l]
10–14 PAM (11)	819	85.7%[d]	66.8%[h]	90.4%[m]

N.a. = number of treatment arms; d = day. p = 0.0064 a vs b; p < 0.0001 a vs c, f vs j, g vs l, h vs m; p = 0.062 a vs d; p = 0.0263 e vs f; p < 0.0001 e vs g, e vs h, f vs g, f vs h; p = 0.0268 i vs j; p = ns between j, l, m and between i & l, i & m and e & i. M-R = metronidazole resistant and M-S metronidazole sensitive.

Several factors might be contributing to the inconsistent results seen across studies. These include different methods used for determining metronidazole resistance, different cut-off values for the minimum inhibitory concentrations (MIC) and probably different locations within the stomach from which biopsies were taken.[17]

We have performed a meta-analysis of 44 studies consisting of 44 treatment arms and 3084 patients treated with three different PPI-based triple therapies. The efficacy of PMC and PAM combinations was significantly reduced in the presence of metronidazole resistance, whereas, the efficacy of the PAC regimen was, of course, not affected by the status of bacterial resistance to metronidazole,[39] (Table 2). When treatments were given to patients harboring metronidazole-sensitive strains of *H. pylori*, the eradication rates, by intent-to-treat analysis, were 93% for the 7-day PMC, 92% for 7-day PAM and 90% for 10–14-day PAM regimens, respectively. However, in the presence of metronidazole resistance, the efficacy was reduced by 14%, 41%, and 24%, respectively. Based on these results, we developed a model to predict the likelihood of treatment failure for the PMC and PAM regimens in the presence of metronidazole resistance using the PAC regimen as a reference[40] (Table 3). As shown in Table 3, when metronidazole resistance is present, the relative risk for treatment failure increases by 2.2, 4 and 7.9-fold when

TABLE 3

Regimen	Overall cure (%)	Re-treatment needed (%)	Increased risk (%)[a]*	Relative risk (95% CI)*
7-d PAC	89.2	10.8	–	–
7-d PMC	78.7	21.3	13.09	2.19 (1.00–4.81)
10–14d PAM	66.8	33.2	32.84	3.99 (1.88–8.44)
7-d PAM	50.5	49.5	76.24	7.93 (3.8–16.54)

d = day; a = increased risk for treatment failure; *in comparison with patients treated with PAC; CI = confidence interval with Mantel-Haenszel method.

patients are treated with the 7-day PMC, 10–14-day PAM and 7-day PAM, respectively. The results strongly suggest that metronidazole-containing regimens should be avoided when metronidazole resistance is suspected or proven.

6. *H. pylori* STRAINS

Results from several recent studies suggest that *H. pylori* infection is easier to eradicate in patients harboring *cagA* positive strains than in those infected with *cagA* negative strains of *H. pylori*.[41,42] This may explain, at least in part, the difference in *H. pylori* eradication rates seen between patients with peptic ulcer and those with non-ulcer dyspepsia (NUD), when patients are treated with the same regimens.[18] Virulent strains of *H. pylori* are reported to be more prevalent in patients with duodenal ulcer than in those with NUD.[43]

There may be a genetic difference in the strains of *H. pylori* between patients with duodenal ulcer and those with asymptomatic gastritis.[44] However, whether these differences contribute to the differences in *H. pylori* eradication rates remains to be further studied.

7. NEWER TREATMENT REGIMENS

Ranitidine bismuth citrate (RBC) was developed specifically for *H. pylori* eradication by incorporating bismuth into the ranitidine molecule. Studies have shown that RBC has synergism with clarithromycin for inhibiting *H. pylori* growth *in vitro*.[45] When given with clarithromycin for 2 weeks, eradication rates range from 55–96% by intent-to-treat analysis.[46] The results from a recent large comparative study (n = 530) have shown that dual therapy with RBC 400 mg bid and clarithromycin 500 mg bid (RBCC) given for 14 days was significantly more effective for treating *H. pylori* infection than 2-week dual therapy with omeprazole 20 mg bid and clarithromycin 500 mg bid (OC).[47] By intent-to-treat analysis, the eradication rate was 77% for the RBCC and 60% for the OC combinations ($p < 0.001$) with adverse event-related drop out rates being 3% for the RBCC and 1% for the OC regimens, respectively.[47] Another large study (n = 383) compared the efficacy of two different doses of clarithromycin (500 mg bid vs tid), but did not find any statistically significant difference in *H. pylori* eradication rates between the two doses of clarithromycin (63% vs 65%, p = ns),[48] suggesting that a dose of clarithromycin higher than 500 mg bid is not necessary in the RBCC combination.

Because of the suboptimal eradication rate and relatively longer treatment duration with the RBC dual regimen, RBC-based triple therapies have been developed and increasingly studied over the last two years. Pipkin and Williamson reviewed published studies of RBC-based triple therapies up to May 1998 and found no significant difference in the pooled eradication rates between the three most commonly used RBC-based triple therapies and the corresponding PPI-based triple regimens.[49] However, this review article can be criticized for its methodology because the authors did not take into account the impact of different doses of the PPI and/or clarithromycin on *H. pylori* eradication.[50]

More recently, Sung and colleagues reported a large randomized study comparing the effects of four different RBC-based combinations on *H. pylori* eradication.[51] Four hundred patients with dyspepsia were randomized to receive a one week treatment with RBC 400 mg combined with either two of the following antibiotics: amoxicillin (A) 1 g, clarithromycin (C) 500 mg and tetracycline (T) 1 g. The fourth group received dual therapy consisting of RBC 400 mg and clarithromycin 500 mg for 2 weeks. All medications were given twice daily and a follow-up urea breath test was done 4 weeks after stopping the medications. The eradication rates, by intent-to-treat analysis, were 86% for the RBCAC, 90% for the RBCMC, 79% for the RBCMT, and 82% for the RBCC, respectively. There was a trend towards a statistically significant difference in *H. pylori* eradication rate in favor of the RBCAC and RBCMC regimens. The important finding of this study is that metronidazole resistance had no impact on the efficacy of either RBCMC or RBCMT. In patients harboring metronidazole resistant strains of *H. pylori*, the cure rate was 94% for the RBCMC and 74% for the RBCMT regimens, indicating that the clarithromycin containing regimen was superior to the tetracycline containing regimen. However, the eradication rates were not significantly different from those achieved in patients infected with metronidazole sensitive strains when patients were treated with the RBCMC and RBCMT regimens (79% and 84%, respectively).[51] Another study from the same group also showed that one-week RBCMT was very effective for treating patients harboring metronidazole-resistant strains of *H. pylori* with a cure rate of 100% (25/25 patients).[52] The excellent effect of RBC and metronidazole containing regimens on metronidazole-resistant strains may reflect the synergistic effect between RBC and metronidazole on *H. pylori in vitro* as shown by Lopez-Brea *et al.*[53] This warrants further clinical investigation.

8. FURAZOLIDONE-CONTAINING REGIMENS

Although PPI-based triple therapies are effective for treating *H. pylori* infection in the majority of patients, bacterial resistance to metronidazole and/or clarithromycin has begun to impair the effects of these regimens.[54] Several newer agents such as furazolidone and rifabutin have been used as a substitute for metronidazole for *H. pylori* eradication in bismuth- or PPI-based triple therapies in regions where the prevalence of metronidzole resistant strains is high.[55–58]

Xiao and colleagues compared the efficacy of three different *H. pylori* eradication treatments consisting of bismuth (B) 240 mg bid, furazolidone (F) 100 mg bid, clarithromycin (C) 250 mg bid, amoxicillin (A) 1 g bid, or josamycin (J) 1 g bid.[56] A total of 180 *H. pylori*-infected patients were randomly assigned to one of the following treatments for one week: BFC, BCA and BFJ. By intent-to-treat analysis, *H. pylori* eradication was achieved in 88%, 58% and 77% of the patients treated with the BFC, BCA and BFJ combination regimens, respectively. Both furazolidone-containing regimens were significantly more effective than the BCA therapy for eradicating *H. pylori* infection.[56] Treatment-related adverse events were generally mild in nature and seldom resulted in withdrawals. Although patients in the furazolidone-containing groups reported more treatment-related adverse events, there were no significant differences in the rates of adverse events between the three groups (11.7%, 13.3% and 5.0%, respectively).[56] Another study from the same group compared the efficacy of four different triple therapies in two comparative trials.[55] In trial 1, seventy patients were randomly assigned to the following one-week treatment combinations: clarithromycin 250 mg bid and furazolidone 100 mg bid either with bismuth 240 mg bid or lansoprazole (L) 30 mg bid. By intent-to-treat analysis, *H. pylori* eradication was successful in 91% (32/35) of the patients in both groups. The second trial was designed to evaluate the impact of metronidazole-resistant strains of *H. pylori* on the efficacy of furazolidone- and metronidazole-containing regimens. In this trial, lansoprazole 30 mg bid in the LFC combination was substituted by omeprazole (O) 20 mg od. Seventy patients were randomly assigned to OFC or omeprazole, metronidazole and clarithromycin (OMC) for one week. *H. pylori* eradication was achieved in 86% (30/35) and 74% (26/35) of the patients treated with OFC and OMC, respectively ($p > 0.05$). The prevalence of metronidazole-resistant strains of *H. pylori* was comparable in both groups (47% in the OFC and 38% in the OMC). Although a breakdown analysis by the status of bacterial resistance to metronidazole was not provided for patients treated with the OFC regimen, the overall high eradication rate (86%) suggests that OFC was effective for treating patients harboring metronidazole-resistant strains. In contrast, the efficacy of OMC was markedly reduced when metronidazole resistance was present. The eradication rate was 67% for patients harboring metronidazole-resistant strains of *H. pylori* compared to 86% for those infected with metronidazole-sensitive strains.[55]

Furazolidone-containing regimens also have several other advantages over metronidazole-containing regimens such as low cost and virtually no reports of bacterial resistance.[55,56] However, compared to the currently recommended PPI-based triple therapies, treatment-related adverse events are common, which can lead to high dropout rates as shown in a recent small study from the US.[59]

9. BISMUTH BASED SINGLE CAPSULE TRIPLE THERAPY

Bismuth based triple therapies are the oldest, probably least expensive, but highly effective treatment regimens for the eradication of *H. pylori* infection.[19,37]

The wide acceptance of these treatment regimens has been limited because of the complexity of the drug administration and poor patient compliance due to treatment-related adverse events. Recently, a single capsule, containing colloidal bismuth subcitrate 40 or 60 mg (B), metronidazole 125 mg (M) and tetracycline 125 mg (T), has been developed and proven to be highly effective for eradicating *H. pylori* infection.[60,61] In a pilot study reported by de Boer *et al.*, 53 *H. pylori* infected patients were treated with two capsules given four times a day for 10 days.[60] Eradication of *H. pylori* infection was confirmed by histology and culture 5 weeks after the end of treatment. In an all-patient-treated analysis, *H. pylori* eradication was achieved in 94.4% of patients. Forty-seven patients (47/52, 90.4%) reported 100% compliance with the treatment with only two treatment related dropouts.

The second study was an interim report of an on-going multicenter parallel randomized clinical trial conducted in North America comparing 10-day OBMT and OAC.[61] The OBMT consisted of omeprazole 20 mg bid and 3 capsules of BMT qid. The OAC included omeprazole 20 mg, amoxicillin 500 mg and clarithromycin 500 mg, given twice daily. By intent-to-treat analysis, *H. pylori* eradication was achieved in 85.5% and 73.4% of patients treated with OBMT (65/76) and OAC (58/79), respectively. Furthermore, the efficacy of OBMT was not affected by metronidazole-resistant strains of *H. pylori*. In contrast, the efficacy of OAC has been significantly affected by clarithromycin resistant strains. Further clinical trials with a large sample size are needed to confirm the excellent results reported in these two studies.

10. MANAGEMENT OF TREATMENT FAILURES

With the currently recommended first-line treatment regimens, *H. pylori* eradication can be achieved in over 85% of patients at the first attempt. However, between 19% and 21% of patients would be expected to fail the most commonly used PPI- and RBC-based triple therapies and thus, will require re-treatment for persisting infection.[17] Several steps are important in the management of patients with a prior treatment failure. These include the determination of bacterial resistance to metronidazole, and/or clarithromycin (or much less likely, amoxicillin) depending on what antibiotics were used previously, and the assessment of patient compliance with previous treatments. This information is helpful for selecting a proper re-treatment regimen. Treatment should be given with full doses of the medications for two weeks treatment duration with the same combination, or with different combinations to avoid the antibiotic previously used when bacterial resistance is suspected or proven.

PPI-based triple therapies are usually used when any dual or bismuth-based triple therapies fail. However, dual combination regimens are no longer recommended for treating *H. pylori* infection. PPI-based triple therapies are the most commonly recommended first-line treatments used worldwide.[62–65] Patients who fail PPI-based triple regimens pose a challenge to management since secondary bacterial resistance to metronidazole or clarithromycin often follows when metronidazole- or clarithromycin-containing regimens have failed.[17]

Recommendations for re-treatment of *H. pylori* infection are available from several major consensus conferences worldwide.[13–16] The European *Helicobacter pylori* Study Group has recommended that, in the case of treatment failure, a re-treatment regimen should be selected after consideration of previous treatment combinations or microbial sensitivities, or both. PPI-based quadruple therapy can be used in the event of failure of triple therapy.[15] The Asian-Pacific Consensus conference suggested that, following treatment failure with a PCA or RBC-based clarithromycin and amoxicillin combination, the same regimen could be repeated.[16] Following one eradication failure with a regimen containing metronidazole, treatment may be repeated, substituting amoxicillin for metronidazole. Seven days PPI-based quadruple therapy was also recommended as a backup treatment by this group.[16] In the United States, the recommended treatment duration is longer than that recommended in Europe, the Asian-Pacific region or in Canada. Two weeks treatment duration was recommended by the US consensus meeting.[13] More recent data suggest that PPI-based quadruple therapy is effective for treating patients who have failed both RBC-based triple therapies and second attempt treatment with PCA.[62]

Since previous treatment failure leads to the development of secondary bacterial resistance to both metronidazole and clarithromycin[63] and the efficacy of re-treatment is significantly decreased with the increasing number of previous treatment attempts,[64] it is understandable that the higher success rate with the first-line treatment, the lower will be the rate of treatment failures. Thus, choosing the best available first-line treatment regimen should be considered to be the best approach to "rescue" treatment. In this respect, it is logical to use the PPI based amoxicillin and clarithromycin combination to avoid using the two most effective antibiotics, metronidazole and clarithromycin together, for the eradication of *H. pylori* infection at the initial treatment.[65]

11. CONCLUSION

After more than a decade of trial and error, several factors determining the success of *H. pylori* eradication treatment have been identified. These include the components of a treatment regimen, the treatment duration, patient compliance, and the presence of resistant strains of *H. pylori*. Treatment regimens consisting of a PPI at the recommended dose, clarithromycin 500 mg, amoxicillin 1 g or metronidazole 400 mg, all given bid for 7 days, are the most commonly used combination regimens for *H. pylori* eradication. In the US, the recommended treatment duration is 14 days. More recent data suggest that RBC-based triple therapies and furazolidone-containing regimens may provide an alternative approach to PPI-based triple therapies especially in areas where the prevalence of metronidazole-resistant strains is high. Most literature suggests that PPI-based quadruple therapies are the most effective rescue treatment for patients who have failed PPI-based triple therapies although this has still not been formally evaluated. Since treatment failure is closely correlated with the development of secondary bacterial resistance to metronidazole or clarithromycin, use of the best available first-line treatment regimen is the most effective approach to the management of treatment failure.

REFERENCES

1. Hunt R. H., and Lam S. K., 1998, *Helicobacter pylori*: from art to a science. *J. Gastroenterol. Hepatol.* **13**(1):21–28.
2. Genta R. M., Lew G. M., and Graham D. Y., 1993, Changes in the gastric mucosa following eradication of *Helicobacter pylori*. *Modern Pathol.* **6**(3):281–289.
3. Labenz J., and Borsch G., 1994, Highly significant change of the clinical course of relapsing and complicated peptic ulcer disease after cure of *Helicobacter pylori* infection. *Am. J. Gastroenterol.* **89**(10):1785–1788.
4. Huang J. Q., Sridhar S., Wilkinson J., Chen Y., and Hunt R. H., 1996, Antibiotics accelerate healing of duodenal ulcer (DU) when combined with proton pump inhibitors (PPI) or H_2-receptor antagonists (H_2RAs). *Gastroenterol.* **110**(4):A137.
5. Huang J. Q., and Hunt R. H., 1996, Does initial choice of *Helicobacter pylori* treatment regimen influence the recurrence rate of duodenal ulcer? A meta-analysis. *Gut.* **39**(suppl 3):A142(808).
6. Huang J. Q., Sheldon A., and Hunt R. H., 1997, Is there a causal relationship between *H. pylori* infection and gastric maltoma? A meta-analysis of the evidence from epidemiological studies and clinical trials. *Gut.* **41**(suppl 1):A49(04/179).
7. Stolte M., Morgner A., Meining A., Thiede C. H., Wündisch T. H., Bayerdörffer E., and Neubauer A., 1998, Early and long-term results of Helicobacter pylori cure of MALT lymphoma What are the pitfalls. In: Hunt R. H., Tytgat G. N. J. eds. *Helicobacter pylori*: Basic Mechanisms to Clinical Cure. Kluwer Academic Publishers, London, pp 373–382.
8. Neubauer A., Thiede C., Morgner A., Alpen B., Ritter M., Neubauer B., Wundisch T., Ehninger G., Stolte M., and Bayerdörffer E., 1997, Cure of *Helicobacter pylori* infection and duration of remission of low-grade gastric mucosa-associated lymphoid tissue lymphoma. *J. Natl. Cancer Inst.* Sep 17;**89**(18):1350–1355.
9. Uemura N., Mukai T., Okamoto S., Yamaguchi S., Mashiba H., Taniyama K., Sasaki N., Haruma K., Sumii K., and Kajiyama G., 1997, Effect of *Helicobacter pylori* eradication on subsequent development of cancer after endoscopic resection of early gastric cancer. *Cancer Epidemiol. Biomarkers Prev.* **6**(8):639–642.
10. McNulty C. A. M., Gearty J. C., Crump B., Davis M., Donovan I. A., Melikian V., Lister D. M., and Wise R., 1986, *Campylobacter pyloridis* and associated gastritis: investigator blind, placebo controlled trial of bismuth salicylate and erythromycin ethylsuccinate. *BMJ* **293**(6548):645–649.
11. Huang J. Q., and Hunt R. H., 1997, Review: eradication of *Helicobacter pylori*: problems and recommendations. *J. Gastroenterol. Hepatol.* **12**:590–598.
12. Hunt R. H., 1996, Eradication of *Helicobacter pylori* infection. *Am. J. Med.* **100**(suppl 5A):42S–51S.

13. Peura D. A., and the American Digestive Health Foundation, 1997, The report of the Digestive Health Initiative[SM] international update conference on *Helicobacter pylori. Gastroenterol.* **113**:S4–S8.
14. Hunt R. H., and Thomson A. B. R., 1998, Canadian *Helicobacter pylori* consensus conference. *Can. J. Gastroenterol.* **12**(1):31–41.
15. Current European concepts in the management of *Helicobacter pylori* infection. The Maastricht Consensus Report. European *Helicobacter Pylori* Study Group. *Gut.* Jul. **41**(1):8–13.
16. Lam S. K., and Talley N. J., 1998, *Helicobacter pylori* consensus: Report of the 1997 Asia Pacific consensus conference on the management of *Helicobacter pylori* infection. *J. Gastroenterol. Hepatol.* **13**:1–12.
17. Huangand J. Q., and Hunt R. H., 1999, Treatment after failure: the problem of "non-responders". *Gut.* **45**(suppl 1):40–44.
18. Huang J. Q., and Hunt R. H., 1998, Are one week anti-*H. pylori* treatments more effective in patients with peptic ulcer disease (PUD) than in those with non-ulcer dyspepsia (NUD)? A meta-analysis. *Am. J. Gastroenterol.* **93**(9):1639(abstract 119).
19. Chiba N., Rao B. V., Rademaker J. W., and Hunt R. H., 1992, Meta-analysis of the efficacy of antibiotic therapy in eradicating *Helicobacter pylori. Am. J. Gastroenterol.* **87**(12):1716–1727.
20. Chiba N., and Hunt R. H., 1999, Drug therapy of *Helicobacter pylori* infection: A meta-analysis. In: Scarpignato C., Bianchi Porro G. (eds), Clinical Pharmacology and Therapy of *Helicobacter pylori* Infection. *Prog. Basic Clin. Pharmacol.* Basel, Karger, vol 11, pp 227–268.
21. Lind T., Megraud F., Unge P., Bayerdorffer E., O'morain C., Spiller R., Veldhuyzen Van Zanten S., Bardhan K. D., Hellblom M., Wrangstadh M., Zeijlon L., and Cederberg C., 1999, The MACH2 study: role of omeprazole in eradication of *Helicobacter pylori* with 1-week triple therapies. *Gastroenterol.* **116**(2):248–253.
22. Schmid C. H., Whiting G., Cory D., Ross S. D., and Chalmers T. C., 1999, Omeprazole plus antibiotics in the eradication of Helicobacter pylori infection: a meta-regression analysis of randomized, controlled trials. *Am. J. Ther.* **6**(1):25–36.
23. Lamouliatte H., Cayla R., Zerbib F., Forestier S., de Mascarel A., Joubert-Collin M., and Megraud F., 1998, Dual therapy using a double dose of lansoprazole with amoxicillin versus triple therapy using a double dose of lansoprazole, amoxicillin, and clarithromycin to eradicate *Helicobacter pylori* infection: results of a prospective randomized open study. *Am. J. Gastroenterol.* **93**(9): 1531–1534.
24. Schwartz H., Krause R., Sahba B., Haber M., Weissfeld A., Rose P., Siepman N., and Freston J., 1998, Triple versus dual therapy for eradicating Helicobacter pylori and preventing ulcer recurrence: a randomized, double-blind, multicenter study of lansoprazole, clarithromycin, and/or amoxicillin in different dosing regimens. *Am. J. Gastroenterol.* **93**(4):584–590.
25. Wong B. C., Xiao S. D., Hu F. L., Qian S. C., Huang N. X., Li Y. Y., Hu P. J., Manan C., Lesmana, Carpio R. E., Perez J. Y., Fock K. M., Kachintorn U. K., Phornphutkul M., Kullavanijaya, Ho J., and Lam S. K., 2000, Comparison of lansoprazole-based triple and dual therapy for treatment of *Helicobacter pylori*-related duodenal ulcer: an Asian multicentre double-blind randomized placebo controlled study. *Aliment. Pharmacol. Ther.* **14**(2):217–224.
26. Calvet X., Lopez-Lorente M., Cubells M., Bare M., Galvez E., and Molina E., 1999, Two-week individual vs. one-week triple therapy for cure of *Helicobacter pylori* infection in primary care: a multicentre, randomized trial. *Aliment. Pharmacol. Ther.* **13**(6):781–786.
27. Hunt R. H., 1993, pH and Hp—gastric acid secretion and *Helicobacter pylori*: implications for ulcer healing and eradication of the organism. *Am. J. Gastroenterol.* **88**(4):481–483.
28. Hunt R. H., 1993, Hp and pH: implications for the eradication of *Helicobacter pylori. Scand. J. Gastroenterol.* Suppl. **196**:12–16.
29. Nagata K., Takagi E., Tsuda M., Nakazawa T., Satoh H., Nakao M., Okamura H., Tamura T., 1995, Inhibitory action of lansoprazole and its analogs against *Helicobacter pylori*: inhibition of growth is not related to inhibition of urease. *Antimicrob. Agents Chemother.* **39**(2):567–570.

30. Houben M. H., Van Der Beek D., Hensen E. F., Craen A. J., Rauws E. A., and Tytgat G. N., 1999, A systematic review of Helicobacter pylori eradication therapy—the impact of antimicrobial resistance on eradication rates. *Aliment. Pharmacol. Ther.* **13**(8):1047–1055.
31. Huang J., and Hunt R. H., 1999, The importance of clarithromycin dose in the management of *Helicobacter pylori* infection: a meta-analysis of triple therapies with a proton pump inhibitor, clarithromycin and amoxycillin or metronidazole. *Aliment. Pharmacol. Ther.* **13**(6): 719–729.
32. Huang J. Q., Chiba N., Wilkinson J. M., and Hunt R. H., 1997, Which combination therapy can eradicate 90% *Helicobacter pylori* infection? A meta-analysis of amoxicillin, metronidazole, tetracycline and clarithromycin containing regimens. *Gastroenterol.* **112**(4):A19.
33. de Boer W. A., 1999, Quadruple therapy: second- or first-line eradication regimen? In: Scarpignato C., and Bianchi Porro G. (eds), Clinical Pharmacology and Therapy of *Helicobacter pylori* Infection. *Prog. Basic Clin. Pharmacol.* Basel, Karger, vol 11, pp 212–226.
34. Fennerty M. B., Kovacs T. O., Krause R., Haber M., Weissfeld A., Siepman N., Rose P., 1998, A comparison of 10 and 14 days of lansoprazole triple therapy for eradication of *Helicobacter pylori*. *Arch. Intern. Med.* 10–24;**158**(15):1651–1656.
35. Laine L., Estrada R., Trujillo M., Fukanaga K., and Neil G., 1996, Randomized comparison of differing periods of twice-a-day triple therapy for the eradication of *Helicobacter pylori*. *Aliment. Pharmacol. Ther.* **10**(6):1029–1033.
36. Graham D., Lew G. M., Malaty H. M., *et al.*, 1992, Factors influencing the eradication of *Helicobacter pylori* with triple therapy. *Gastroenterol.* **102**:493–496.
37. Buring S. M., Winner L. H., Hatton R. C., and Doering P. L., 1999, Discontinuation rates of *Helicobacter pylori* treatment regimens: A meta-analysis. *Pharmacotherapy* **19**(3):324–332.
38. Houben M. H. M. G., van de Beek D., Hensen E. F., de Craen A. J. M., Rauws E. A. J., and Tytgat G. N. J., 1999, A systematic review of *Helicobacter pylori* eradication therapy—the impact of antimicrobial resistance on eradication rates. *Aliment. Pharmacol. Ther.* **13**:1047–1055.
39. Huang J. Q., and Hunt R. H., 1999, Impact of metronidazole-resistant (M-R) *H. pylori* strains on proton pump inhibitor (PPI)-based triple therapies: A meta-analysis. *Am. J. Gastroenterol.* **94**(9):2752 (abstract 702).
40. Huang J. Q., and Hunt R. H., 1999, Predicting treatment failure with PPI-based triple therapies in metronidazole-resistant *H. pylori* infections: A model based on trial meta-analysis data. *Am. J. Gastroenterol.* **94**(9):2753 (abstract 703).
41. Marais A., Monteiro L., Lamouliatte H., Samoyeau R., and Mégraud F., 1998, Cag negative status of *Helicobacter pylori* is a risk factor for failure of PPI-based triple therapies in non-ulcer dyspepsia. *Gastroenterol.* **114**(4):A214.
42. van Doorn L.-J., Schneeberger P. M., Nouhan N., Plaisier A. P., Quint W. G. V., deBoer W. A., 2000, Importance of *Helicobacter pylori cagA* and *vacA* status for the efficacy of antibiotic treatment. *Gut.* **46**:321–326.
43. Go M. F., and Graham D. Y., 1996, Presence of the cagA gene in the majority of *Helicobater pylori* strains is independent of whether the individual has duodenal ulcer or asymptomatic gastritis. *Helicobacter* **1**(2):107–111.
44. Yoshimura H. H., Evans D. G., and Graham D. Y., 1993, DNA-DNA hybridization demonstrates apparent genetic differences between *Helicobacter pylori* from patients with duodenal ulcer and asymptomatic gastritis. *Dig. Dis. Sci.* **38**:1128–1131.
45. Williamson R., and Pipkin G. A., 1998, Does bismuth prevent antimicrobial resistance of *Helicobacter pylori*? In: Hunt R. H., Tytgat G. N. J. eds. *Helicobacter pylori*: Basic Mechanisms to Clinical Cure. Kluwer Academic Publishers, London, pp 416–425.
46. Chiba N., and Hunt R. H., 1999, Ulcer disease and *Helicobacter pylori* infection: etiology and treatment. In: McDonald J. W. D., Burroughs A., and Feagan B. (eds), Evidence Based Gastroenterology and Hepatology. Chapter 2, 66–90. *B.M.J. Books*.

47. Pare P., Farley A., Romaozinho J. M., Bardhan K. D., French P. C., Roberts P. M., 1999, Comparison of ranitidine bismuth citrate plus clarithromycin with omeprazole plus clarithromycin for the eradication of *Helicobacter pylori. Aliment. Pharmacol. Ther.* **13**(8):1071–1078.
48. Schwartz H. I., Perschy T. B., McSorley D. J., and Sorrells S. C., 1999, Twice-daily versus thrice-daily clarithromycin in combination with ranitidine bismuth citrate in the eradication of *Helicobacter pylori. Helicobacter* **4**(2):121–127.
49. Pipkin G. A., Williamson R., and Wood J. R., 1998, Review article: one-week clarithromycin triple therapy regimens for eradication of *Helicobacter pylori. Aliment. Pharmacol. Ther.* **12**(9):823–837.
50. Huang J. Q., and Hunt R. H., 1999, Letter: Clarithromycin-based triple therapies. *Aliment. Pharmacol. Ther.* **13**(3):437–438.
51. Huang J. Q., and Hunt R. H., 1999, Letter: Clarithromycin-based triple therapies. *Aliment. Pharmacol. Ther.* **13**(3):437–438.
52. Sung J. J., Chan F. K., Wu J. C., Leung W. K., Suen R., Ling T. K., Lee Y. T., Cheng A. F., and Chung S. C., 1999, One-week ranitidine bismuth citrate in combinations with metronidazole, amoxycillin and clarithromycin in the treatment of *Helicobacter pylori* infection: the RBC-MACH study. *Aliment. Pharmacol. Ther.* **13**(8):1079–1084.
53. Kung N. N., Sung J. J., Yuen N. W., Li T. H., Ng P. W., Lai W. M., Lui Y. H., Lam K. N., Choi H., and Leung E. M., 1999, One-week ranitidine bismuth citrate vs. colloidal bismuth subcitrate-based anti-*Helicobacter* triple therapy: a prospective randomized controlled trial. *Am. J. Gastroenterol.* **94**(3):721–724.
54. Lopez-Brea M., Domingo D., Sanchez I., Prieto N., and Alarcon T., 1998, Study of the combination of ranitidine bismuth citrate and metronidazole against metronidazole-resistant *Helicobacter pylori* clinical isolates. *J. Antimicrob. Chemother.* **42**(3):309–314.
55. Megraud F., 1999, Resistance of *Helicobacter pylori* to antibiotics: the main limitation of current-proton-pump inhibitor triple therapy. *Eur. J. Gastroenterol. Hepatol.* **11** Suppl 2:S35–S37; discussion S43–S45.
56. Liu W. Z., Xiao S. D., Shi Y., Wu S. M., Zhang D. Z., Xu W. W., and Tytgat G. N., 1999, Furazolidone-containing short-term triple therapies are effective in the treatment of *Helicobacter pylori* infection. *Aliment. Pharmacol. Ther.* **13**(3):317–322.
57. Xiao S. D., Liu W. Z., Hu P. J., Xia D. H., and Tytgat G. N., 1999, High cure rate of *Helicobacter pylori* infection using tripotassium dicitrato bismuthate, furazolidone and clarithromycin triple therapy for 1 week. *Aliment. Pharmacol. Ther.* Mar. **13**(3):311–315.
58. Dani R., Queiroz D. M., Dias M. G., Franco J. M., Magalhaes L. C., Mendes G. S., Moreira L. S., De Castro L. P., Toppa N. H., Rocha G. A., Cabral M. M., and Salles P. G., 1999, Omeprazole, clarithromycin and furazolidone for the eradication of *Helicobacter pylori* in patients with duodenal ulcer. *Aliment. Pharmacol. Ther.* Dec. **13**(12):1647–1652.
59. Perri F., Festa V., Andriulli A., 1998, Treatment of antibiotic-resistant *Helicobacter pylori. N. Engl. J. Med.* Jul. 2;**339**(1):53.
60. Graham D. Y., Osato M. S., Hoffman J., Opekun A. R., Anderson S., and El-Zimaity H. M., 2000, Furazolidone combination therapies for *Helicobacter pylori* infection in the United States. *Aliment Pharmacol. Ther.* Feb;**14**(2):211–215.
61. De Boer W. A., van Etten R. J. X. M., Schneeberger P. M., and Tytgat G. N. J., 2000, A single drug for *Helicobacter pylori* infection: first results with a new bismuth triple monocapsule. *Am. J. Gastroenterol.* **95**(3):641–645. Laine L., Riff D., Stanton D., Lamet M., Farley A., Korcek W., Schuman R., Piotrowski J., Dallaire C., Fallone C., Archambault A., Cockeram C., Fay D., Olsheski W., Barkun A., Bradette M., Gaddam S., Lahaie R., Ponich T., van Zanten S., Pulverman S., Chiba N., Thomson A., Bianchi T., Graham D., Murali N., Bernstein C., Zidel B., McHattie J., Provenza M., Rapier R., Taub W., Taunk J., Watier A., Hunt R. *et al.*, 2000, Bismuth based single capsule triple therapy in North America: interim results of a North American study of OBMT vs OAC. *Helicobacter pylori*: Basic mechanisms to clinical cure 2000, Bermuda, March 26–29.

62. Chan F. K., Sung J. J., Suen R., Wu J. C., Ling T. K., and Chung S. C., 2000, Salvage therapies after failure of *Helicobacter pylori* eradication with ranitidine bismuth citrate-based therapies. *Aliment. Pharmacol. Ther.* Jan. **14**(1):91–95.
63. Miyaji H., Azuma T., Ito S., Suto H., Ito Y., Yamazaki Y., Sato F., Hirai M., Kuriyama M., Kato T., and Kohli Y., 1997, Susceptibility of Helicobacter pylori isolates to metronidazole, clarithromycin and amoxycillin in vitro and in clinical treatment in Japan. *Aliment. Pharmacol. Ther.* Dec. **11**(6):1131–1136.
64. Moshkowitz M., Konikoff F. M., Peled Y., Brill S., Hallak A., Tiomny E., Santo M., Bujanover Y., and Gilat T., 1996, One week triple therapy with omeprazole, clarithromycin and tinidazole for *Helicobacter pylori*: differing efficacy in previously treated and untreated patients. *Aliment. Pharmacol. Ther.* Dec. **10**(6):1015–1019.
65. de Boer W. A., and Tytgat G. N. J., Treatment of *Helicobacter pylori* infection. *B.M.J.* **320**:31–34. From Huang J., and Hunt R. H., 1999, The importance of clarithromycin dose in the management of *Helicobacter pylori* infection: a meta-analysis of triple therapies with a proton pump inhibitor, clarithromycin and amoxycillin or metronidazole. *Aliment. Pharmacol. Ther.* Jun. **13**(6): 719–729.

6

Mechanism of Antibiotic Resistance in *Helicobacter pylori*

GE WANG and DIANE E. TAYLOR

1. INTRODUCTION

Helicobacter pylori is an important human gastric pathogen, infecting over half of the world population and causing gastritis, ulcers and gastric cancer. Current standard therapy regimens for treating these diseases are multiple antibiotics in combination with proton pump inhibitors (PPIs). Antibiotics that are frequently included in triple therapy regimens are clarithromycin, metronidazole and amoxicillin. In addition to the lack of compliance of the patient with the treatment, emergence of antibiotic resistance has become an increasing problem leading to the therapy failure. In this chapter we will summarize currently available data concerning the mechanisms of antibiotic resistance in *H. pylori*.

2. SUSCEPTIBILITY AND RESISTANCE

From a bacteriological viewpoint, a bacterial strain is defined as resistant to an antibiotic if it can tolerate significantly higher drug concentration than

GE WANG and DIANE E. TAYLOR • Department of Medical Microbiology and Immunology, University of Alberta, Edmonton, Alberta, Canada T6G 2H7.

Helicobacter pylori Infection and Immunity,
Edited by Yamamoto *et al.*, Kluwer Academic/Plenum Publishers, 2002.

TABLE 1
Variability in MIC (μg/ml) breakpoints used to define resistance to metronidazole and clarithromycin in *H. pylori*[42]

Geographic origin of strains	Metronidazole	Clarithromycin
Peru	≥4	≥0.125
Canada/Europe	>4	≥2
United States	≥64	≥2
Canada (joint study)	≥16	≥4
Montreal and Halifax, Canada	>8	>2
Italy	>8	>8

the concentration inhibiting the growth of other strains of the same species. Pharmacological resistance describes a situation when a bacterial strain can tolerate drug concentration higher than those achieved *in vivo* at the site of infection. In laboratory susceptibility testing, the activity of an antibiotic on bacteria is usually measured by its minimal inhibitory concentration (MIC), and sometimes by its minimal bactericidal concentration (MBC). Variable results could be obtained because of different growth states of strains, different methods used and variations in laboratory techniques. Another significant difficulty encountered in comparing incidence of antibiotic resistance in *H. pylori* is lack of clear breakpoints. Table 1 lists some examples of MIC breakpoints used to define resistance to clarithromycin and metronidazole by different laboratories throughout the world.[42] Clearly, the decision on what MIC level defines resistance has a significant impact on the assessment of prevalence of resistance. This is particularly true for metronidazole resistance because it does not exhibit a bimodal distribution but rather shows a continuous spectrum of MICs. According to the Guide to Antimicrobial Therapy,[31] the peak serum level achievable for metronidazole is 2.5 to 13 μg/ml (mean 6.2 μg/ml) for a 250 mg oral dose, whereas it is 2 to 3 μg/ml for clarithromycin at an oral dose of 500 mg. Therefore, cut-off values of 8 μg/ml for metronidazole and 2 or 4 μg/ml for clarithromycin to define resistance appear to be appropriate in relation to treatment response.[42]

By conventional antibiotic susceptibility testing *in vitro*, *H. pylori* is normally highly susceptible to the majority of antibiotics (Table 2).[40] However, monotherapy with a number of these drugs proved uniformly unsuccessful. This could be because *H. pylori* lives in an environment where the diffusion of antibiotics is limited and where the pH is lower than required for the drug to be effective. Slow growth of *H. pylori* may also provide a survival advantage because most antibiotics are effective only on actively multiplying organisms. Furthermore, even if a particular antibiotic were able to kill the majority of the infecting *H. pylori*,

TABLE 2
Antibiotic susceptibilities of *H. pylori*

Normally susceptible to:		*Intrinsically resistant to:*
Erythromycin	Tetracycline	Trimethoprim
Clarithromycin	Kanamycin	Vancomycin
Metronidazole	Chloramphenicol	Polymyxin B
Penicillins	Ciprofloxacin	Nalidixic acid
Cephalosporins	Bismuth salts	Sulfonamides
Streptomycin	Rifampicin	

the remaining viable cells would soon re-populate the stomach when antibiotic pressure was removed. Therefore, the susceptibility determined *in vitro* does not always reflect the situation *in vivo*.

H. pylori is intrinsically resistant to several antibiotics (Table 2). Resistance to trimethoprim, vancomycin and polymyxin B is also characteristic of related *Campylobacter spp.* These antibiotics have been useful for selection and maintenance of *H. pylori* in culture to avoid contamination by other bacteria and fungi.

3. CLINICALLY RELEVANT RESISTANCE

Resistance to several groups of antibiotics has been reported in *H. pylori* isolates from gastric biopsy specimens. These include resistance to clarithromycin (a macrolide), metronidazole (a nitroimidazole), ciprofloxacin (a fluoroquinolone), amoxicillin (a beta-lactam), rifampicin (a rifamycin) and tetracycline. The mechanisms of resistance to clarithromycin and metronidazole have been extensively studied which will be the focus of this review. The available information on mechanisms of resistance to other antibiotics will also be summarized.

4. CLARITHROMYCIN RESISTANCE

Clarithromycin (Cla) is often a component of modern *H. pylori* triple therapy because it has excellent *in vitro* activity, and it is less affected than other macrolides by a decrease in pH. Use of clarithromycin in combination with a PPI and either metronidazole amoxicillin gave an eradicating effectiveness of 85%–95%.[17] The prevalence of *H. pylori* resistant to clarithromycin varies with geographic location, with a range from <1% to >10% reported.[41]

Macrolides act by binding to bacterial ribosomes, and more precisely, to the peptidyl transferase loop of domain V of the 23S rRNA. The binding leads to dissociation of peptidyl tRNA from the ribosome during the elongation reaction,

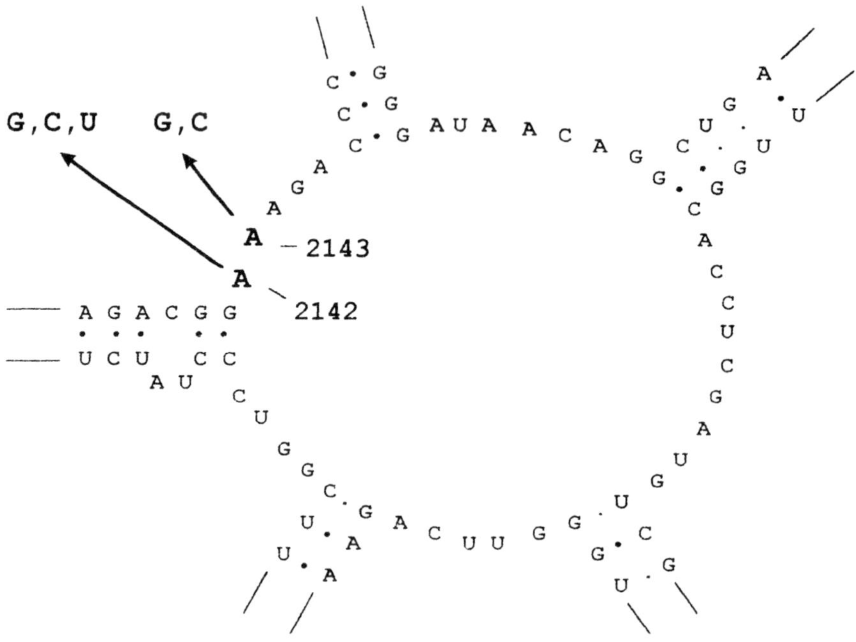

FIGURE 1. Structure of the central part of domain V (peptidyltransferase loop) of *H. pylori* 23S rRNA. The region covering positions 2142 and 2143 is clarithromycin-binding site. Arrows show the point mutations that confer clarithromycin resistance *in vitro*. In clinical isolates only A-to-G transition mutations are predominantly observed (see text).

thus blocking bacterial protein synthesis. Several mechanisms have been described in bacteria that confer macrolide resistance, such as inhibition of drug uptake by impermeability of the cell membrane, active drug efflux, inactivation of the drug by enzymes, and change (mutation or modification) of the drug-binding site in ribosomes.[51]

Versalovic *et al.*[45] reported for the first time that point mutations in the 23S rRNA gene were associated with clarithromycin resistance in *H. pylori.* Several studies examined Cla^R *H. pylori* isolates from various geographic locations,[8,29,38,40] and confirmed that point mutations in the 23S rRNA gene is the only mechanism of clarithromycin resistance in *H. pylori.* Specifically, adenine (A) to guanine (G) mutations at either of the two nucleotides (corresponding to positions 2058 and 2059 in *Escherichia coli* coordinate) in the peptidyl transferase region of the 23S rRNA were in most cases associated with clarithromycin resistance (Figure 1). The positions of these two nucleotides were shown to be 2142 and 2143 in *H. pylori* coordinate, according to the determination of the transcriptional start site of *H. pylori* 23S rRNA gene.[41] Recently, many simple and rapid methods have been developed to detect the point mutations in 23S rRNA gene for monitoring clarithromycin resistance, which are beyond the scope of this review.

It has been shown that clarithromycin has a strong binding affinity to the ribosomes of *H. pylori*.[13] Binding experiment using ^{14}C labeled erythromycin (a member of the macrolides) showed loss of drug binding to the ribosomes of Cla^R *H. pylori* strains compared to that of the susceptible parent strains.[29] This suggests that the point mutations in 23S rRNA change the ribosomal structure, thus inhibiting the binding of macrolide antibiotics.

Mutations at position 2142 usually confer a higher level of resistance than mutations at position.[38,46] Moreover, mutations at position 2142 were associated with a high level cross resistance to macrolide, lincosamide, and streptogramin B antibiotics (MLS phenotype), whereas mutations at position 2143 conferred an intermediate level resistance to macrolide and lincosamide, but no resistance to streptogramin.[46] In a variety of bacteria, a common mechanism for macrolide resistance is methylation of a specific adenine (equivalent to A2142 in *H. pylori*) by methylases encoded by *erm* genes.[51] Methylation of this adenine residue also confers an MLS phenotype. A study using a conserved PCR assay examined 10 Cla^R *H. pylori* isolates that showed MLS phenotype and did not reveal any evidence of *erm*-like genes in *H. pylori*.[7] In addition, mutations at some sites other than 2058 and 2059 in *E. coli* 23S rRNA also confer macrolide resistance (for example, at positions 2032, 2057, 2611). Mutations in the equivalent sites of *H. pylori* 23S rRNA gene have not been found in Cla^R isolates.[29]

Genomic mapping and gene cloning revealed that *H. pylori* has two copies of 23S rRNA gene,[41] and this has been confirmed by the whole genome sequences.[2] Most of the Cla^R *H. pylori* isolates as well as *in vitro* created mutants were found to carry mutations at both copies of the gene (homozygous).[46] This may reflect a high efficiency of DNA recombination in *H. pylori*. The mutation in one copy of the gene (heterozygous) may be easily recombined into the other 23S rRNA gene under the selection pressure to produce a diploid mutation that would confer a higher level of resistance.

While A-to-G transitions were observed in the majority of Cla^R isolates, a few cases were reported to be A-to-C transversion mutations,[29,38] and A-to-T mutation has never been found. *In vitro* site-directed mutagenesis data,[6,46] indicated that A-to-C mutations confer a similar level of resistance compared to A-to-G mutations, and A2142-to-T mutation also confers an intermediate level of resistance. Further examination of these site-directed mutants demonstrated that the A-to-G mutants grow significantly faster than the A-to-C or A-to-T mutants. Using a special multiplex sequence assay, the competitive growth advantage of the A-to-G mutants over the A-to-C mutants was quantitatively determined.[48] The order of competitive growth advantage, A2142G > A2143G >>> A2142C > A2143C (A2142T), provided a rational explanation for the mutation pattern observed in clinical isolates.

5. METRONIDAZOLE RESISTANCE

Metronidazole (Mtz) was among the first drugs used for eradicating *H. pylori* infection. Although the MIC is not particularly low (0.1 to 4 μg/ml), Mtz can become concentrated in the gastric compartment and has a rather stable activity at low pH. When used in combination with other antibiotics and PPIs, it is a highly effective therapy for eradication of *H. pylori* infection.[17]

Mtz is a pro-drug because it is not toxic to bacteria until it is reduced to a hydroxylamine derivative (Figure. 2). Hydroxylamine is a DNA-damaging agent and appears to cause cell death by breaking down bacterial DNA. In anaerobic bacteria and protozoa, Mtz is reduced (activated) by the ferredoxin-linked pyruvate and other ketoacid oxidoreductase enzyme complex. Mtz is commonly used in monotherapy for the treatment of many bacterial and protozoan infections, although this monotherapy is not usually successful in eradicating *H. pylori*. In contrast to anaerobic bacteria, where resistance to Mtz is rare, in microaerophiles such as *H. pylori*, the incidence of Mtz resistance is high, ranging from 10% to >90% depending on geographic region and patient group.[17]

Susceptibility testing demonstrated that patients can be infected with both Mtz^S and Mtz^R *H. pylori*. Co-infection of multiple strains in one patient may contribute to this phenomenon. Moreover, even within the same strain different patterns of susceptibility to metronidazole have been found.[11] These results might be explained by the existence of different subpopulations within the *H. pylori* isolates[20,43] (van der Wouden *et al.*, Jenks *et al.* determined the proportion of the Mtz^R isolates that emerged in mice originally infected with a single susceptible strain. After metronidazole monotherapy, the ratio of Mtz^R to Mtz^S isolates was 1 in 100, while it was 1 in 25 in the mice that were treated with metronidazole monotherapy followed by a triple therapy.

Several possible mechanisms have been proposed for metronidazole resistance in *H. pylori*. For example, a cloned *recA* gene from a Mtz^R *H. pylori* strain increased the already very high level of resistance in *E. coli*,[5] implying that the elevated DNA repair capacity may confer metronidazole resistance. A promising

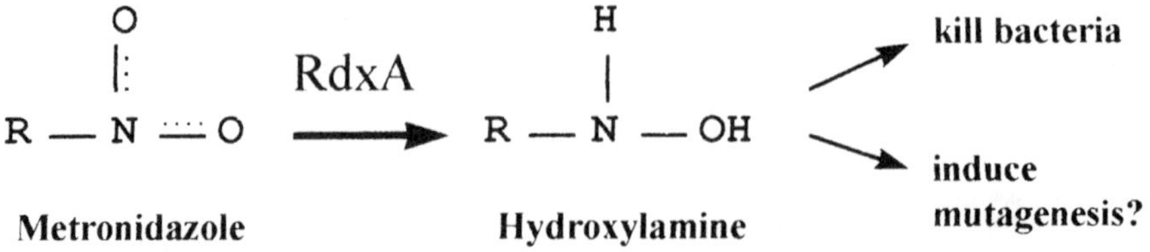

O
|:
R — N ⋯ O —RdxA→ R — N(H) — OH → kill bacteria / induce mutagenesis?
Metronidazole Hydroxylamine

FIGURE 2. Mechanism of action of metronidazole against *H. pylori*. Metronidazole itself is not toxic to bacteria. Wild type *H. pylori* have a functional nitroreductase (RdxA) that reduces metronidazole to hydroxylamine, which is responsible for killing the bacteria. Mutational inactivation of RdxA results in no reduction of metronidazole to hydoxylamine, conferring *H. pylori* resistant to metronidazole.

hypothesis was that the resistance results from the inability to reduce metronidazole to the active form. Cederbrant *et al.*[4] proposed that some Mtz^R *H. pylori* strains are unable to achieve a sufficiently low redox potential necessary for metronidazole reduction. Smith and Edwards[36] showed that Mtz^R *H. pylori* strains had a decreased oxidoreductase activity and that they were unable to remove intracellular oxygen from the site of metronidazole, thus preventing reduction of metronidazole.

Goodwin *et al.*[14] provided convincing evidence showing that metronidazole resistance in *H. pylori* is due to null mutations in a gene called *rdxA* that encodes an oxygen-insensitive NADPH nitroreductase. They proposed that *H. pylori* cells containing mutated (inactivated) *rdxA* gene are unable to transform metronidazole to the toxic form, exhibiting a resistance phenotype (Fig. 2). This hypothesis was verified with the following evidence. Disruption of the *rdxA* gene by insertion of a chloramphenicol resistance cassette resulted in a Mtz^R phenotype. Conversely, introduction of a functional (wild type) *H. pylori rdxA* gene carried on a shuttle vector plasmid into *E. coli* (normally Mtz^R) or into Mtz^R *H. pylori* rendered them Mtz^S, suggesting that expression of wild type *rdxA* (metronidazole-susceptibility) is the dominant phenotype. Compared to the parent susceptible strains, metronidazole-resistant mutants had 1 to 3 base substitutions at different positions that resulted in several types of amino acid substitution or truncation of the encoded protein. Another study[6] showed that the Mtz resistance in *H. pylori* NCTC11637 is due to the insertion of the mini-*IS605* and deletion of adjacent sequences in the *rdxA* gene.

The role of the *rdxA* gene in metronidazole resistance was further evaluated in other studies. Jenks *et al.*[20] determined the sequences of *rdxA* genes from a series of Mtz^S and Mtz^R isolates derived from single, Mtz^S strains using an *H. pylori* mouse model. The *rdxA* genes from most (25 out of 27), but not all, of the Mtz^R isolates contained 1 to 3 mutations (missense or framshift), compared to that of parental susceptible strains. Similarly, by determining the sequences of *rdxA* genes of paired Mtz^R and Mtz^S isolates from French and North African patients, Tankovic *et al.*[39] identified a variety of mutations within the *rdxA* gene that are associated with Mtz resistance. These mutations included missense mutations, deletion of a fragment, insertion of a variant *IS605*, and most frequently the frameshift mutations in the simple nucleotide repeat poly(A) sequences. However, in 1 of the 13 Mtz^R–Mtz^S pairs the *rdxA* gene did not appear to be involved in resistance. These results suggested that Mtz resistance in *H. pylori* is frequently associated with mutational inactivation of the *rdxA* gene, but other mechanisms are likely to exist. In another study, sequence analysis of the *rdxA* genes from 30 Mtz^R isolates also indicated that mutations within the *rdxA* gene are frequently responsible for resistance.[37] Due to the lack of the isogenic susceptible strains for comparison, however, a clear conclusion could not be drawn to ascribe particular missense mutations to the resistance phenotype. The types of mutations in *rdxA* that confer Mtz resistance observed in these studies are summarized in Table 3.

TABLE 3
Types of mutation in *rdxA* in metronidazole-resistant *H. pylori*

No. of strains	Nucleotide mutation	Protein change	References
1	A → G	Arg200 → Gly	Goodwin *et al.*, 1998
1	A → G	Tyr47 → Cys, Ala143 → Thr	
1	A → G	Gln50 → Arg, Lys63 → Glu	
1	G → A	Ala80 → Thr	
1	A → G, C → T, & other	Gly145 → Val	
1	A → G, C → T, & other	change of 8 amino acids	
	T → C, C → T	Tyr46 → His, Pro51 → Leu	Jenks *et al.*, 1991
brdrw	C → T	Pro51 → Leu	
15 1	C → T	Ala67 → Val	
2	+A	truncation at codon 22	
1	+A, G → A, G → C	truncation at codon 73	
1	+A	truncation at codon 73	
1	−A	truncation at codon 76	
6	+2T	truncation at codon 76	
2	−T	truncation at codon 90	
1	−T, −AT	truncation at codon 90	
1	−TC	truncation at codon 111	
1	−A	truncation at codon 114	
1	−T	truncation at codon 153	
1	−AT	truncation at codon 159	
1	+T	truncation at codon 166	
1	−G	truncation at codon 167	
1	−G	truncation at codon 193	
1			
2			
1	+A	truncation at codon 22	Tankovic *et al.*, 2000
1	+T	truncation at codon 22	
1	+GGCT	truncation at codon 35	
4	+A	truncation at codon 73	
1	+CG	C-terminus changed	
1	−206 bp	truncation at codon 81	
1	TG → CA	Cys16 → His	
1	C → T	Ser43 → Leu	
1	GC → TA	Ser79 → Ile	
1	+T	truncation at codon 59	
1	G → T	truncation at codon 74	
1	insertion of *IS605*	truncation at codon 99	
1	−6 bp	loss of 2 amino acids	
1	A → G	Thr58 → Ala	
1	C → T	Ala67 → Val	
1	C → A	Ala187 → Asp	
1	+A	truncation at codon 175	Solca *et al.*, 2000
2	C → T	truncation at codon 148	
1	G → T	truncation at codon 223	
1	G → T	truncation at codon 523	

More extensive studies on Mtz resistance have been performed using large numbers of clinical isolates from all over the world,[23,25] which confirmed the primary role of *rdxA* inactivation in the Mtz resistance. In the Mtz^R isolates, there was marked heterogeneity in the MIC of Mtz, ranging from 8 to 256 μg/ml, implicating that additional genes are involved. The two independent studies by Kwon *et al.*[28] and Jeong *et al.*[29] demonstrated that *frxA* is such an additional gene, which codes for an NAD(P)H-flavin oxidoreductase and is a paralog of *rdxA* (~25% amino acid sequence identity). Their results showed that inactivation of *rdxA* alone usually resulted in a moderate level Mtz resistance (MIC = 16–32 μg/ml), whereas double mutations in *rdxA* and *frxA* conferred a high-level resistance (MIC > 64 μg/ml). However, there still is a controversy between the two studies as to whether the *frxA* inactivation alone (namely, in a $rdxA^+$ background) confers a significant level of resistance. In a further study,[30] Jeong and Berg showed that the expression of the *frxA* gene in the mouse-colonizing strain SS1 is at a high level, while the *frxA* gene in most other Mtz^S *H. pylori* strains seems not to be well expressed. The high level expression of *frxA* along with *rdxA* renders the strain SS1 highly susceptible to Mtz, and inactivation of either gene alone did not result in Mtz-resistance in this strain. The results of Kwon *et al.*[28] showed that a ferredoxin-like protein (FdxB) is also involved in a low-level Mtz resistance.

6. AMOXICILLIN RESISTANCE

Amoxicillin (Amx) is a beta-lactam antibiotic. MIC values of amoxicillin against *H. pylori* are usually uniformly low (<0.01–0.1 μg/ml).[42] As resistance to metronidazole becomes more prevalent, metronidazole is increasingly being replaced by amoxycillin in triple therapy. Even though beta-lactams have been extensively used in the community for treating other infectious diseases, emergence of resistance to amoxicillin in *H. pylori* has been reported rarely. Dore *et al.*, identified some Amx^R isolates.[12] Interestingly, these isolates lost their resistance after storage at −80°C, but the resistance phenotype could be restored by plating these strains on to amoxicillin gradient plates. The molecular mechanisms for this behavior are unknown, but the same phenomenon has been described in other bacteria. Thus, the term "tolerance" was used to describe the situation in which the bacteria are inhibited but not killed by the antibiotic.[12] Recently, there were also reports on identification of a few stable Amx^R *H. pylori* isolates.[15,44]

Production of beta-lactamase is a frequent mechanism of resistance to beta-lactams in many bacterial species. However, beta-lactamase activity was not detected in the Amx^R *H. pylori* isolates, suggesting this is not the mechanism in *H. pylori*.[9,12,44] Another mechanism of bacterial resistance to beta-lactams is modification of the bacterial cell wall target, i.e., penicillin binding proteins (PBPs). PBPs are a set of enzymes responsible for the terminal stages of biosynthesis of peptidoglycan. Modification of PBPs leading to decreased affinity for antibiotics accounts for a relatively low level resistance and a stepwise increase over time in the MIC values. Dore *et al.*,[10] found that one of four PBPs that are normally present in Amx^S strains was missing in the Amx^R strains, suggesting that modification of a PBP may be responsible for the amoxicillin resistance. Kusters *et al.*,[24] found that a single amino acid change (S414R) in a PBP (PBP-1A, gene HP0597) causes amoxicillin resistance. Recently, Deloney and Schiller[9] selected a stable Amx^R strain. PBP profiles generated by labeling isolated *H. pylori* membrane fractions showed significantly decreased bio-Amx labeling of PBP1 in the Amx^R strain compared to that of the Amx^S strain. In addition, uptake analysis of ^{14}C-labeled penicillin G showed a significant decrease in uptake of the labeled antibiotic by the Amx^R strain compared to the Amx^S strain. These results demonstrated that alteration in PBP1 and in the uptake of β-lactam antibiotics account for amoxicillin resistance in this Amx^R strain.[9]

7. CIPROFLOXACIN RESISTANCE

Ciprofloxacin (Cip) is an antibiotic belonging to the fluroquinolones. Resistance to fluroquinolones was acquired very rapidly in *Campylobacter jejuni*, a close relative of *H. pylori*. Therefore, this antibiotic likely would not be appropriate to be used for eradication of *H. pylori*.[41] Indeed, Cip^R *H. pylori* isolates were obtained from patients enrolled in the clinical trial examining the efficacy of ciprofloxacin in treating *H. pylori* infection.[28] This is the only report on ciprofloxacin resistance in *H. pylori*.

Ciprofloxacin resistance is due to a mutation in the *gyrA* gene, which encodes the A subunit of DNA gyrase. This enzyme, consisting of two A and two B subunits, is required for DNA replication and RNA transcription since it introduces negative superhelical turns into DNA. The GyrA protein contains a quinolone resistance-determining region (QRDR) at the amino-terminus (amino acid residue 67–106). Mutations in this region of GyrA in many bacteria gave a high level of resistance to quinolone. Similarly, in the Cip^R *H. pylori* isolates, several types of base substitutions leading to the amino acid changes in the QRDR region of GyrA were identified.[28] These mutations were associated with an increase in the MIC of ciprofloxacin from $<0.25\,\mu g/ml$ to $8\,\mu g/ml$, and with cross resistance to all other fluroquinolone compounds.

8. RIFAMPICIN RESISTANCE

As resistance to clarithromycin and metronidazole in *H. pylori* appears to increase, there has been a continuous search for new drugs with activity against

H. pylori. For example, new rifamycin derivatives KRM1648 and KRM1657 have been recently developed. Determination of the antimicrobial activities against *H. pylori* showed that they have lower MIC's than those of amoxicillin, clarithromycin, metronidazole and rifampicin, suggesting that they might be useful for the eradication of *H. pylori* infections.[1]

Rifampicin (Rif) is a traditional representative of rifamycin group antibiotics. Rifampicin resistance in *E. coli* and other bacteria is known to be a result of mutation in the *rpoB* gene encoding the beta subunit of RNA polymerase, which is the rifampicin-binding target. The report of Heep *et al.*,[16] showed that the same mechanism is used in *H. pylori* to confer rifampicin resistance. Several types of point mutations, similar to those identified in *E. coli* and *Mycobacterium tuberculosis*, were observed in the *rpoB* genes of Rif^R *H. pylori* strains. It should be noted that the Rif^R strains they studied were laboratory-created mutants, because no Rif^R clinical isolates had been identified, presumably because rifampicin is not used in therapy regimens.

9. TETRACYCLINE RESISTANCE

Tetracyclines (Tet) are a family of broad-spectrum antibiotics that have been widely used for the treatment of bacterial infections, and tetracycline resistance has emerged in almost all bacterial genera.[32]

Currently tetracycline is not used extensively in *H. pylori* therapy. *H. pylori* resistance to tetracycline appears to be uncommon. Tetracycline has been used as a part of *H. pylori* triple therapy in Australia in the early 1990s, and a Tet^R *H. pylori* isolate was detected from a patient in whom the triple therapy had failed.[27] A Tet^R isolate was also reported by Han *et al.*[15] Recently, twenty-nine Tet^R strains were isolated from Korean and Japanese patients.[26] Interestingly, all of the 29 strains exhibited cross-resistance to metronidazole. The underlying mechanism for this cross-resistance is currently unknown.

Tetracycline inhibits bacterial protein synthesis by interacting with the ribosome. Bacterial resistance to tetracycline commonly arises through one of the four identified mechanisms: efflux of tetracycline, modification of tetracycline, ribosomal protection, or mutation of the 16S rRNA gene(s). Which of these resistance mechanisms is operative in *H. pylori* remains to be determined.

10. GENETIC PATHWAYS

Antibiotic resistance arises and is transmitted between bacterial species through different genetic pathways. Here we describe these pathways and discuss their roles in the development of antibiotic resistance in *H. pylori*.

11. GENE TRANSFER

Antibiotic resistance can arise through acquiring resistance genes from other bacterial species. Often, resistance genes encode enzymes that inactivate a particular antibiotic. Resistance genes can be either carried on a plasmid or incorporated into the chromosome by recombination. *In vitro* introduction of several resistance genes into *H. pylori* has been successfully performed in many genetic studies. For example, a gene from *Campylobacter coli* encoding chloramphenicol acetyltransferase (CAT) was inserted *in vitro* into an *H. pylori* plasmid.[50] When the recombinant plasmid was transferred back into *H. pylori* by electroporation or transformation it conferred chloramphenicol resistance. The CAT cassette can also be inserted within a cloned *H. pylori* gene *in vitro* and then introduced into *H. pylori* by transformation. In this case, the CAT gene is incorporated into chromosome by homologous recombination, resulting in disruption of the gene where it is inserted. This technology has been extensively used in *H. pylori* genetic studies to construct knock-out mutants.[14,30] For the same purpose, a kanamycin resistance gene cassette from *C. coli* encoding a kanamycin phosphotransferase has also been frequently used. As another example, beta-lactamase genes that confer ampicillin resistance have been transferred into *H. pylori* to study virulence factors by shuttle mutagenesis.[30]

Although resistance genes can be transferred into *H. pylori in vitro*, these mechanisms of antibiotic resistance have never been found in *H. pylori* clinical isolates (*in vivo*).

12. DNA TRANSFORMATION

Most of *H. pylori* strains are naturally competent for DNA transformation.[19,50] The majority of antibiotic resistance determinants from resistant *H. pylori* strains can be transferred to susceptible strains by natural transformation *in vitro*. Table 4 shows transformation frequencies for certain clinically-relevant antibiotic resistance markers, which were obtained using different *H. pylori* strains.

Normally, the transformation process includes uptake of DNA into the cell and subsequent incorporation of DNA into the chromosome by homologous recombination. Recently, several genes involved in natural competence and DNA uptake have been identified,[3,18,34,35] but the precise uptake mechanism and the subsequent DNA recombination process are not understood.

Currently, *in vivo* frequency of DNA transformation between different *H. pylori* strains or between cells of the same strain is not known. DNA recombination between different strains could occur in the stomach of a patient colonized by more than one *H. pylori* strain. Alternatively, if there is an environmental reservoir for *H. pylori*, genetic exchange between bacterial strains could occur outside

TABLE 4
Natural transformation of *H. pylori* with homologous chromosomal DNA

		Transformation		
DNA donor strain	Recipient Strain	Antibiotic Resistance marker	Frequency per viable cell	Reference
8091	UA841	Rif^R	4.0×10^{-4}	Wang *et al.*, 1993
JAH60	UA841	Mtz^R	3.0×10^{-5}	
UC970	UC165	Cip^R	3.6×10^{-4}	Moore *et al.*, 1995
UC079	UC165	Cip^R	7.3×10^{-4}	
Hp-F	UA802	Cla^R	1.9×10^{-6}	Taylor *et al.*, 1997
Hp-B	UA802	Cla^R	2.4×10^{-6}	
?	?	Amx^R	1×10^{-5}	van Zwet *et al.*, 1998

Abbreviations for antibiotics: Rif, rifampicin; Mtz, metronidazole; Cip, ciprofloxacin; Cla, clarithromycin; Amx, amoxicillin.

the human body. DNA transformation from the antibiotic-resistant cells to the susceptible cells of the same strain, if occurring at a high frequency *in vivo*, could increase the resistant population to a great extent, hence playing an important role in the rapid development of antibiotic resistance. However, this role of recombination depends on the availability of resistance determinants that normally arise from mutations in *H. pylori*.

13. MUTATION

Remarkably, the known mechanisms of antibiotic resistance in *H. pylori* are all due to mutations of chromosomal genes. No evidence is available to indicate that an antibiotic resistance determinant is acquired *in vivo* by plasmid- or transposon-mediated gene transfer from other bacterial species. It also appears that DNA recombination between different strains does not contribute much to antibiotic resistance. For example, the *rdxA* genes from different *H. pylori* strains can be easily distinguished from each other because they have an overall 5% nucleotide divergence. Comparing the Mtz^R strains to the parent susceptible strains, only one or a few bases in the *rdxA* gene have been changed (Table 3). This indicated that the resistance resulted from *de novo* mutation of the *rdxA* gene rather than acquiring a DNA fragment containing the mutation from an unrelated Mtz^R strain.[14,20]

Important roles of DNA mutation in antibiotic resistance prompted us to ask if *H. pylori* has evolved specialized mechanisms that either continuously or sporadically increase mutagenesis.[47] Recently, we have systematically examined the *in vitro* frequencies and spectra of the spontaneous mutations conferring resistance to clarithromycin, metronidazole, amoxycillin, ciprofloxacin, and rifampicin in *H. pylori*. The mutation rate of Rif^R or Cip^R determined in a fluctuation assay is 1–2 $\times 10^{-8}$ per cell per generation. In contrast, the spontaneous mutation rates of Cla^R, Mtz^R, or Amx^R are much lower ($<10^{-9}$).[51] The low frequency of Cla^R could be explained by its narrow spectrum of mutations (only mutations at two bases of the 23S rRNA gene). The low frequency of Amx^R suggests that cooperative mutations (modifications) in more than one target may be required for Amx^R in *H. pylori*, as indicated in the study of Deloney and Schiller.[9] The low frequency of Mtz^R *in vitro* is in sharp contrast to its high prevalence *in vivo*, and the possible reasons for this is currently under investigation. Nevertheless, by serial passages on media with increasing sublethal doses of Mtz, the Mtz^R mutants could be readily selected *in vitro*, suggesting that the mutagenic and selective effects of a sublethal dose of Mtz contribute to the rapid development of Mtz^R.[49]

Given the formation of hydroxylamine, a potent mutagen, by the RdxA nitroreductase of *H. pylori* (Fig. 2), it has been suggested that many of the mutations to Mtz^R were induced by the Mtz therapy (even that used for treatment of other infections), and the mutagenic and carcinogenic effects of the widespread use of Mtz may be a significant concern in public health.[14] Recently, the mutagenic effect of Mtz activation was experimentally demonstrated.[33] A sublethal dose of Mtz stimulates forward mutation to rifampin.resistance in *rdxA*$^+$ (Mtz^S) and also in *rdxA*$^-$ (Mtz^R) *H. pylori* strains, and the expression of *rdxA* in *E. coli* resulted in equivalent Mtz-induced mutation. As shown by alkaline gel electrophoretic tests, Mtz at concentrations near or higher than the MIC caused DNA breakage in *H. pylori* as well as in *E. coli* carrying the cloned *H. pylori rdxA*$^+$ gene.[33] If the mutation frequency increases in general, it could contribute to the development of resistance not only to metronidazole itself (through mutation in the *rdxA* gene) but also to other antibiotics such as clarithromycin (through mutation in 23S rRNA gene) (Figure 3). Therefore, these findings have implications for the emergency of resistance to various antibiotics and more generally to the evolution of virulence and the adaptation of *H. pylori* to individual hosts.

Many mutations *in vivo* are generated from DNA damage inflicted by a large number of endogenous and exogenous mutagens. Another genetic pathway leading to increased mutation rate is impaired function of DNA repair. Homologues of a number of *E. coli* genes that function in DNA damage reduction or repair, such as *mutT*, *mutY*, *ung*, and *nth* have been found in the *H. pylori* genomes,[2] but no supportive experimental evidence is available to confirm functional equivalence. Other repair genes present in *E. coli* such as *mutM*, *nfo*, *vsr*, *oxyR*, *ada*, and *ogt*, are not found in *H. pylori*, suggesting that *H. pylori* may have a lower DNA repair capacity than *E. coli*. Information from the genome sequences also

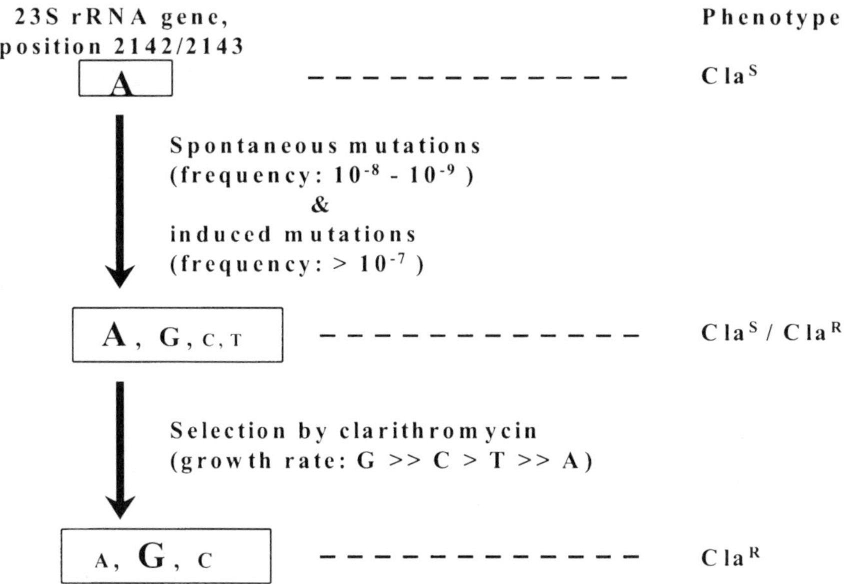

FIGURE 3. Dissecting occurrence of antibiotic resistance using clarithromycin resistance in *H. pylori* as an example. In wild type *H. pylori* 23S rRNA genes, the nucleotide residues at position 2142 and 2143 are adenine. As bacteria grow, there is a probability for mutation to occur. Although the spontaneous mutation rate could be as low as 10^{-9} per cell per generation, elevated exposure to DNA damaging agents and/or reduced DNA repair activity can significantly elevate mutagenesis above the background level. Nevertheless, in the absence of the antibiotic pressure (before drug therapy), the fraction of the mutated cells in the population is very small. In the presence of the antibiotic, the growth of wild type cells is inhibited, and the mutated cells that are resistant to the antibiotic are selectively accumulated to become the majority of the population.

implies that *H. pylori* lacks *E. coli mutHLS*-like DNA mismatch repair system.[47] Loss of *mutHLS* function in *E. coli* is known to increase mutation frequency about 100-fold and specifically elevate transition mutations (A:T $\rightarrow$ G:C and G:C $\rightarrow$ A:T). In *H. pylori*, homologous genes from different strains exhibit a high level of diversity within their nucleotide sequences, and transition mutations account for the majority of this diversity.[47] Investigating the mutagenic pathways in *H. pylori* will ultimately help us to understand more clearly how resistance to antibiotics occurs.

Acknowledgments. This work is supported by grants from the Canadian Bacterial Diseases Network and The National Cancer Institute of Canada with funds from the Terry Fox Run to D.E.T., who is a Medical Scientist with the Alberta Heritage Foundation for Medical Research (AHFMR).

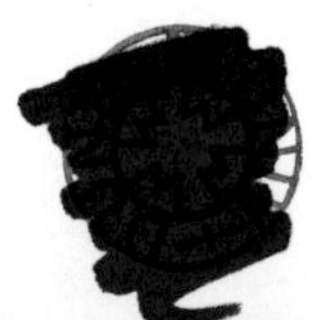

REFERENCES

1. Akada J. K., Shirai M., Fujii K., Okita K., and Nakazawa T., 1999, In vitro anti-*Helicobacter pylori* activities of new rifamycin derivatives, KRM1648 and KRM-1657. *Antimicrob. Agents Chemother.* **43**:1072–1076.
2. Alm R. A., Ling L. S., Moir D. T., King B. L., Brown E. D., Doig P. C., Smith D. R., Noonan B., Guild B. C., deJonge B. L., Carmel G., Tummino P. J., Caruso A., Uria-Nickelsen M., Mills D. M., Ives C., Gibson R., Merberg D., Mills S. D., Jiang Q., Taylor D. E., Vovis G. F., and Trust T. J., 1999, Genomic-sequence comparison of two unrelated isolates of the human gastric pathogen *Helicobacter pylori*. *Nature* **397**:176–180.
3. Ando T., Israel D. A., Kusugami K., and Blaser M. J., 1999, HP0333, a member of the *dprA* family, is involved in natural transformation in *Helicobacter pylori*. *J. Bacteriol.* **181**:5572–5580.
4. Cederbrant G., Kahlmeter G., and Ljungh A., 1992, A proposed mechanism for metronidazole resistance in *Helicobacter pylori*. *J. Antimicrob. Chemother.* **29**:115–120.
5. Chang K. C., Ho S. W., Yang J. C., and Wang J. T., 1997, Isolation of a genetic locus associated with metronidazole resistance in *Helicobacter pylori*. *Biochem. Biophys. Res. Commun.* **236**: 785–788.
6. Debets-Ossenkopp Y. J., Brinkman A. B., Kuipers E. J., Vandenbroucke-Grauls C. M., Kusters J. G., 1998, Explaining the bias in the 23S rRNA gene mutations associated with clarithromycin resistance in clinical isolates of *Helicobacter pylori*. *Antimicrob. Agents Chemother.* **42**:2749–2751.
7. Debets-Ossenkopp Y. J., Pot R. G., van Westerloo D. J., Goodwin A., Vandenbroucke-Grauls C. M., Berg D. E., Hoffman P. S., and Kusters J. G., 1999, Insertion of mini-IS605 and deletion of adjacent sequences in the nitroreductase (*rdxA*) gene cause metronidazole resistance in *Helicobacter pylori* NCTC11637. *Antimicrob. Agents Chemother.* **43**:2657–2662.
8. Debets-Ossenkopp Y. J., Sparrius M., Kusters J. G., Kolkman J. J., Vandenbroucke-Grauls C. M., 1996, Mechanism of clarithromycin resistance in clinical isolates of *Helicobacter pylori*. *FEMS Microbiol. Lett.* **142**:37–42.
9. DeLoney C. R., and Schiller N. L., 2000, Characterization of an In vitro-selected amoxicillin-resistant strain of *Helicobacter pylori*. *Antimicrob. Agents Chemother.* **44**:3368–3373.
10. Dore M. P., Graham D. Y., and Sepulveda A. R., 1999a, Different penicillin-binding protein profiles in amoxicillin-resistant *Helicobacter pylori*. *Helicobacter* **4**:154–61.
11. Dore M. P., Osato M. S., Kwon D. H., Graham D. Y., and El-Zaatari F. A., 1998, Demonstration of unexpected antibiotic resistance of genotypically identical *Helicobacter pylori* isolates. *Clin. Infect. Dis.* **27**:84–89.
12. Dore M. P., Osato M. S., Realdi G., Mura I., Graham D. Y., and Sepulveda A. R., 1999b, Amoxycillin tolerance in *Helicobacter pylori*. *J. Antimicrob. Chemother.* **43**:47–54.
13. Goldman R. C., Zakula D., Flamm R., Beyer J., and Capobianco J., 1994, Tight binding of clarithromycin, its 14-(R)-hydroxy metabolite, and erythromycin to *Helicobacter pylori* ribosomes. *Antimicrob. Agents Chemother.* **38**:1496–1500.
14. Goodwin A., Kersulyte D., Sisson G., Veldhuyzen van Zanten S. J., Berg D. E., and Hoffman P. S., 1998, Metronidazole resistance in *Helicobacter pylori* is due to null mutations in a gene (*rdxA*) that encodes an oxygen-insensitive NADPH nitroreductase. *Mol. Microbiol.* **28**:383–393.
15. Han S. R., Bhakdi S., Maeurer M. J., Schneider T., and Gehring S., 1999, Stable and unstable amoxicillin resistance in *Helicobacter pylori*: Should antibiotic resistance testing be performed prior to eradication therapy? *J. Clin. Microbiol.* **37**:2740–2741.
16. Heep M., Beck D., Bayerdorffer E., and Lehn N., 1999, Rifampin and rifbutin resistance mechanism in *Helicobacter pylori*. *Antimicrob. Agents Chemother.* **43**:1497–1499.
17. Hoffman P. S., 1999, Antibiotic resistance mechanisms of *Helicobacter pylori*. *Can. J. Gastroenterol.* **13**:243–249.

18. Hofreuter D., Odenbreit S., Henke G., and Haas R., 1998, Natural competence for DNA transformation in *Helicobacter pylori*: identification and genetic characterization of the *comB* locus. *Mol. Microbiol.* **28**:1027–1038.
19. Israel D. A., Lou A. S., and Blaser M. J., 2000, Characteristics of *Helicobacter pylori* natural transformation. *FEMS Microbiol. Lett.* **186**:275–280.
20. Jenks P. J., Ferrero R. L., and Labigne A., 1999a, The role of the *rdxA* gene in the evolution of metronidazole resistance in *Helicobacter pylori*. *J. Antimicrob. Chemother.* **43**:753–758.
21. Jenks P. J., Labigne A., and Ferrero R. L., 1999b, Exposure to metronidazole *in vivo* readily induces resistance in *Helicobacter pylori* and reduces the efficacy of eradication therapy in mice. *Antimicrob. Agents Chemother.* **43**:777–781.
22. Jeong J. Y., and Berg D. E., 2000, Mouse-colonizing *Helicobacter pylori* SS1 is unusually susceptible to metronidazole due to two complementary reductase activities. *Antimicrob. Agents Chemother.* **44**:3127–3132.
23. Jeong J. Y., Mukhopadhyay A. K., Dailidiene D., Wang Y., Velapatino B., Gilman R. H., Parkinson A. J., Nair G. B., Wong B. C., Lam S. K., Mistry R., Segal I., Yuan Y., Gao H., Alarcon T., Brea M. L., Ito Y., Kersulyte D., Lee H. K., Gong Y., Goodwin A., Hoffman P. S., and Berg D. E., 2000, Sequential inactivation of *rdxA* (HP0954) and *frxA* (HP0642) nitroreductase genes causes moderate and high-level metronidazole resistance in *Helicobacter pylori*. *J. Bacteriol.* **182**:5082–5090.
24. Kusters J. G., Schuijffel D. F., Gerrits M. M., van Zwet A. A., and Vandenbroucke-Grauls C. M. J. E., 1999, A single amino acid change in PBP-1A causes amoxicillin resistance in *Helicobacter pylori*. Gut **45**(Suppl. III):A5.
25. Kwon D. H., El-Zaatari F. A., Kato M., Osato M. S., Reddy R., Yamaoka Y., and Graham D. Y., 2000a, Analysis of *rdxA* and involvement of additional genes encoding NAD(P)H flavin oxidoreductase (FrxA) and ferredoxin-like protein (FdxB) in metronidazole resistance of *Helicobacter pylori*. *Antimicrob. Agents Chemother.* **44**:2133–2142.
26. Kwon D. H., Kim J. J., Lee M., Yamaoka Y., Kato M., Osato M. S., El-Zaatari F. A., and Graham D. Y., 2000b, Isolation and characterization of tetracycline-resistant clinical isolates of *Helicobacter pylori*. *Antimicrob. Agents Chemother.* **44**:3203–3205.
27. Midolo P. D., Korman M. G., Turnidge J. D., and Lambert J. R., 1996, *Helicobacter pylori* resistance to tetracycline. *Lancet* **347**:1194–1195.
28. Moore R. A., Beckthold B., Wong S., Kureishi A., and Bryan L. E., 1995, Nucleotide sequence of the gyrA gene and characterization of ciprofloxacin-resistant mutants of *Helicobacter pylori*. *Antimicrob. Agents Chemother.* **39**:107–111.
29. Occhialini A., Urdaci M., Doucet-Populaire F., Bebear C. M., Lamouliatte H., and Megraud F., 1997, Macrolide resistance in *Helicobacter pylori*: Rapid detection of point mutations and assays of macrolide binding to ribosomes. *Antimicrob. Agents Chemother.* **41**:2724–2728.
30. Oldenbreit S., Till M., and Haas R., 1996, Optimized BlaM-transposon shuttle mutagenesis of *Helicobacter pylori* allows identification of novel genetic loci involved in bacterial virulence. *Mol. Microbiol.* **20**:361–373.
31. Sanford J. P., Gilbert D. N., and Sande M. A., 1996, Guide to Antimicrobial Therapy, 26th edn. Antimicrobial Therapy, Inc., Dalls. pp.55.
32. Schnappinger D., and Hillen W., 1996, Tetracyclines: antibiotic action, uptake, and resistance mechanisms. *Arch. Microbiol.* **165**:359–369.
33. Sisson G., Jeong J. Y., Goodwin A., Bryden L., Rossler N., Lim-Morrison S., Raudonikiene A., Berg D. E., and Hoffman P. S., 2000, Metronidazole activation is mutagenic and causes DNA fragmentation in *Helicobacter pylori* and in *Escherichia coli* containing a cloned *H. pylori* RdxA(+) (Nitroreductase) gene. *J. Bacteriol.* **182**:5091–5096.
34. Smeets L. C., Bijlsma J. J., Boomkens S. Y., Vandenbroucke-Grauls C. M., and Kusters J. G., 2000a, *comH*, a novel gene essential for natural transformation of *Helicobacter pylori*. *J. Bacteriol.* **182**:3948–3954.

35. Smeets L. C., Bijlsma J. J., Kuipers E. J., Vandenbroucke-Grauls C. M., and Kusters J. G., 2000b, The *dprA* gene is required for natural transformation of *Helicobacter pylori*. *FEMS Immunol. Med. Microbiol.* **27**:99–102.
36. Smith M. A., and Edwards D. I., 1997, Oxygen scavenging, NADH oxidase and metronidazole resistance in *Helicobacter pylori*. *J. Antimicrob. Chemother.* **39**:347–353.
37. Solca N. M., Bernasconi M. V., and Piffaretti J. C., 2000, Mechanism of metronidazole resistance in *Helicobacter pylori*: comparison of the *rdxA* gene sequences in 30 strains. *Antimicrob. Agents Chemother.* **44**:2207–2210.
38. Stone G. G., Shortridge D., Versalovic J., Beyer J., Flamm R. K., Graham D. Y., Ghoneim A. T., and Tanaka S. K., 1997, A PCR-oligonucleotide ligation assay to determine the prevalence of 23S rRNA gene mutations in clarithromycin-resistant *Helicobacter pylori*. *Antimicrob. Agents Chemother.* **41**:712–714.
39. Tankovic J., Lamarque D., Delchier J. C., Soussy C. J., Labigne A., and Jenks P. J., 2000, Frequent association between alteration of the *rdxA* gene and metronidazole resistance in French and North African isolates of *Helicobacter pylori*. *Antimicrob. Agents Chemother.* **44**:608–613.
40. Taylor D. E., 1997, Antibiotic resistance mechanisms of *Helicobacter pylori*. In: *Pathogenesis and host response in Helicobacter pylori infections* (Moran A. P., and O'Moran C. A. eds), Normed Verlag, Bad Hamburg—Englewood N.J., pp.101–109.
41. Taylor D. E., Ge Z., Purych D., Lo T., and Hiratsuka K., 1997, Cloning and sequence analysis of the two copies of 23S rRNA genes from *Helicobacter pylori* and association of clarithromycin resistance with 23S rRNA mutations. *Antimicrob. Agents Chemother.* **41**:2621–2628.
42. Taylor D. E., Jiang Q., and Fedorak R. N., 1998, Antibiotic susceptibilities of *Helicobacter pylori* strains isolated in the province of Alberta. *Can. J. Gastroenterol.* **12**:295–298.
43. Van der Wouden E. J., de Jong A., Thijs J. C., Kleibeuker J. H., and van Zwet A. A., 1999, Subpopulations of *Helicobacter pylori* are responsible for discrepancies in the outcome of nitroimidazole susceptibility testing. *Antimicrob. Agents Chemother.* **43**:1484–1486.
44. Van Zwet A. A., Vandenbroucke-Grauls C. M., Thijs J. C., van der Wouden E. J., Gerrits M. M., and Kusters J. G., 1998, Stable amoxicillin resistance in *Helicobacter pylori*. *Lancet* **352**:1595.
45. Versalovic J., Shortridge D., Kibler K., Griffy M. V., Beyer J., Flamm R. K., Tanaka S. K., Graham D. Y., and Go M. F., 1996, Mutations in 23S rRNA are associated with clarithromycin resistance in *Helicobacter pylori*. *Antimicrob. Agents Chemother.* **40**:477–480.
46. Wang G., and Taylor D. E., 1998, Site-specific mutations in the 23S rRNA gene of *Helicobacter pylori* confer two types of resistance to macrolide-lincosamide-streptogramin B antibiotics. *Antimicrob. Agents Chemother.* **42**:1952–1958.
47. Wang G., Humayun M. Z., and Taylor D. E., 1999a, Mutation as an origin of genetic variability in *Helicobacter pylori*. *Trends Microbiol.* **7**:488–493.
48. Wang G., Rahman M. S., Humayun M. Z., and Taylor D. E., 1999b, Multiplex sequence analysis demonstrates the competitive growth advantage of the A-to-G mutants of clarithromycin-resistant *Helicobacter pylori*. *Antimicrob. Agents Chemother.* **43**:683–685.
49. Wang G., Wilson T. J. M., Jiang Q., and Taylor D. E., Spontaneous mutations that confer antibiotic resistance in *Helicobacter pylori*. *Antimicrob. Agents Chemother.* (in press).
50. Wang Y., Roos K. P., and Taylor D. E., 1993, Transformation of *Helicobacter pylori* by chromosomal metronidazole resistance and by a plasmid with a selectable chloramphenicol resistance marker. *J. Gen. Microbiol.* **139**:2485–2493.
51. Weisblum B., 1995, Erythromycin resistance by ribosome modification. *Antimicrob. Agents Chemother.* **39**:577–585.

7

Anti-*Helicobacter pylori* Activity of Natural Substances

YOSHIMASA YAMAMOTO

1. INTRODUCTION

Helicobacter pylori is well established as an etiological agent of chronic gastritis and peptic ulcer as well as a risk factor for development of gastric cancer.' Eradication of *H. pylori* by antibiotics is thought to be an essential therapy for such gastric diseases. In early studies, clinical trials with an antibiotic alone have mostly failed to eradicate H. *pylori*.[2,3] However, current triple therapy with antibiotics and a proton pump inhibitor shows a high eradication rate and a low incidence of harmful side effects.[4,5] Although high eradication rates have been achieved in clinical trials, some problems still remain for this therapy, such as non-compliance and development of antibiotic resistance.[6] Furthermore, such treatments with antibiotics are designed for therapy, not for a prophylactic purpose to prevent re-infection with *H. pylori*. Under such circumstances, many natural substances obtained from plants, vegetables and tea have been studied and promoted as alternative or additional strategies for treatment of *H. pylori* infection. Since some of these natural substances are consumed as a part of the daily diet intake, their safety is traditionally established. Furthermore, they have been known to have some beneficial effects against gastric diseases. In this chapter, the effects of such natural products

---

YOSHIMASA YAMAMOTO • Department of Medical Microbiology and Immunology, University of South Florida College of Medicine, Tampa, FL 33612.

Helicobacter pylori Infection and Immunity,
Edited by Yamamoto *et al.*, Kluwer Academic/Plenum Publishers, 2002.

on *H. pylori in vitro and in vivo* are highlighted and the value for *H. pylori* treatment discussed.

2. MEDICINAL PLANTS

Since most medicinal plants have historically been used in certain local areas as an alternative medicine for various diseases, including gastric diseases, and some beneficial effects have been traditionally observed, the potential prophylactic or even therapeutic activity of medicinal plants against *H. pylori* seems possible. In this regard, the anti-*H. pylori* activity of a wide variety of medicinal plants has been studied (see Table 1), but most studies utilized only crude extracts. Therefore, in most cases active components of medicinal plants showing anti-*H. pylori* activity are not yet clear. However, in some cases anti-*H. pylori* agents in medicinal plants have been demonstrated by both *in vitro* and *in vivo* systems. Unfortunately,

TABLE 1
Anti-*H. pylori* activity of medicinal plants

Source	Form	Activity[a] (MIC:μg/ml)	Reference
East African medicinal plants			
Terminalia spinosa	Crude extracts	250	(17,18)
West African medicinal plants			
Pteleopsis suberosa	Methanol extract	31.25–250	(19)
Turkish plants	Crude extracts	1.95–250	(7)
Cistus laurifolius	Chloroform fraction	1.95	
Bearberry, cowberry leaves	Aqueous extracts		(20)
	Tannic acid		
Malagasy medicinal plants	Crude extracts		(21)
Brazilian medicinal plants	Methanol extracts	62.5	(12)
Myroxylon peruiferum	Cabreuvin	7.8	
Korean medicinal plants	Crude extracts		
	Decursinol angelate	6–20	(22)
Chinese medicinal plants			
Rahdosia trichocarpa	Trichorabdal A		(23)
Evodia rutaecarpa	Crude extract	0.31%	(24)
Pistacia lentiscus	Mastic	60 (MBC)[c]	(25)
Rose oil	Geraniol	1.75	(10)
....			
Lichen[d]	Protolichesterinic acid	32	(15)

[a]Determined by agar diffusio or disc method.
[c]minimal bactericidal concentration.
[d]Lichen is not a plant.

as is usual in traditional medicine, *in vitro* anti-*H. pylori* activity was not high as compared with that of antibiotics utilized in eradication therapy.

For example, methanol extracts obtained from West African medicinal plants showed 31–250 μg/ml of MICs values against *H. pylori* strains. In some studies, however, extracts of plants showed a strong MIC against clinical as well as standard strains of *H. pylori* at a relatively low concentration of 1.95 μg/ml.[7] The tested extract was only partially purified and probably contained many components. Therefore, it seems likely that further purification of such extracts may yield more potent active compounds.

A Turkish folk medicine prepared from plants, including flowers, cones, herbs, fruits and flowering herbs, has been used historically for the treatment of gastric ailments. Experimental studies of this traditional medicine extracted from Turkish plants confirmed the anti-ulcerogenic effect on restraint-induced stress ulcers in rat models.[8] In addition, current studies using a variety of extractions with several Turkish medicinal plants showed *in vitro* anti-*H. pylori* activity with MICs as low as 1.95 to 250 μg/ml.[7] In particular, the chloroform fraction of flowers of *Cistus laurifolius,* which seemed to be a polysaccharide,[9] showed the most active MIC of 1.95 μg/ml. However, *in vivo* activity against *H. pylori* has not yet been studied. Therefore, whether the *in vivo* anti-ulcerogenic effect of the extracts from Turkish medicinal plants was due to an anti-*H. pylori* activity or other activity is not known.

The strongest *in vitro* anti-*H. pylori* activity between medicinal plants and other related products has been shown for geraniol, an aliphatic terpene alcohol and the major compound of rose oil, with an 1.75 μg/ml MIC_{90} against 25 *H. pylori* isolates.[10] This compound also showed antibacterial activity against several other bacterial genera such as *Pseudomonas, Staphylococcus* and *Escherichia.* Even though an earlier study showed a beneficial effect of rose oil on gastric ulcers induced experimentally in animals,[11] further investigations are needed to evaluate whether rose oil preparations are useful for prevention and treatment of gastric diseases caused by *H. pylori* infection.

A current study by a Japanese group shows an interesting approach to examine agents in natural substances having selective antibacterial activity against *H. pylori.*[12] The methanol extract of *Myroxylon peruiferum,* a Brazilian medicinal plant, showed mild anti-*H. pylori* activity with a 62.5 μg/ml MIC. The active component of the extract was identified as an isoflavone, cabreuvin (Figure 1), which had a 7.8 μg/ml MIC against *H. pylori.* The antimicrobial activity of this compound was also tested against other microorganisms, such as gram-positive and gram-negative bacteria as well as yeasts. The results showed that cabreuvin did not have any antimicrobial activity against such microorganisms even as high as 625 μg/ml. Even though the antibacterial activity of cabreuvin against *H. pylori* is not markedly high, the selectivity against *H. pylori* is useful because present chemotherapy available sometimes causes development of resistances not only of *H. pylori* but also other bacteria due to their broad antibacterial spectrum. Therefore, selectivity against *H. pylori* is highly desirable for therapy. Even though

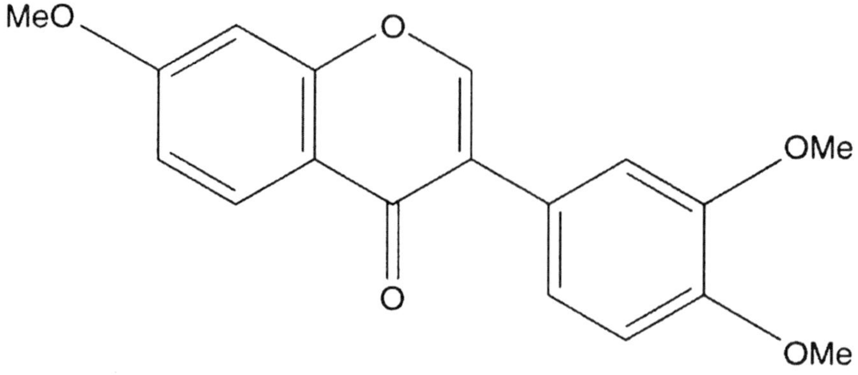

FIGURE 1. Chemical structure of cabreuvin (from ref. 12).

there is not enough data to be conclusive, a possible active substance possessing highly selectivity of natural products against *H. pylori* is very likely. Furthermore, such findings warrant examination of natural products for a new type of anti-*H. pylori* agent.

The lichen *Cetraria islandica,* commonly known as Iceland moss, has been used in European traditional medicine for treatment of minor ailments such as throat irritation and cough, but also for tuberculosis, asthma, and gastrointestinal conditions such as gastritis.[13] Investigations of the biological activity of lichens revealed their antimicrobial activity against a wide variety of microbes including *Mycobacterium, Streptococcus, Staphylococcus, Bacillus* and *Candida.*[14] With reference to the use of Iceland moss to relieve symptoms of gastric and duodenal ulcer, an investigation was undertaken whereby extracts of the lichen were screened for *in vitro* inhibitory activity against *H. pylori.*[15] The MIC_{90} for 34 clinical isolates and a standard strain of *H. pylori* with sodium protolichesterinate, an aliphatic cc-methylene-γ-lactone that is an active component of *C. islandica,* proved to be 32 μg/ml. The protolichesterinic acid has also *in vitro* inhibitory activity against 5-lipoxygenese,[16] which has as a metabolic product leukotriens, which are implicated as mediators of inflammatory responses in the gastrointestinal tract. Therefore, it is likely that the beneficial effects of Iceland moss in cases of gastritis and gastric and duodenal ulcer could be due not only to inhibitory activity of protolichesterinic acid against *H. pylori* but also their pharmacological activity, as is often observed with alternative medicines.

3. NUTRITIONAL AGENTS

The protective effect of certain diets has been implicated in lowering the frequency of peptic ulcers and coincidence of gastric cancer.[26–29] Therefore, it is conjectured that some nutritional agents may have a protective activity due to their anti *H. pylori* activity in peptic ulcers and gastric cancer, since *H. pylori* is a casual factor for peptic ulcers and some gastric cancer.

Capsaicin, the active ingredient in chili peppers, is known to have both detrimental as well as cytoprotective effects on the gastric mucosa. A case-control study evaluating factors responsible for the geographic variation in gastric cancer in Italy correlated ingestion of chili with a decreased risk of gastric cancer.[29] In this regard, a current study showed that capsaicin effectively exerts a time- and concentration-dependent inhibition of the growth of *H. pylori in vitro.*[30] The concentration of capsaicin showing *in vitro* anti-*H. pylori* activity is 50 μg/ml, which corresponds to 1 mg/ml of chili. This concentration can be achieved through diet in populations with a high consumption of chili. For cxample, the per capita consumption of chili in India is 3 g per day.[31] The antimicrobial activity of capsaicin is relatively unique, because this compound does not show any antimicrobial activity *in vitro* to *E. coli,* a bacterium in the same category as *H. pylori.* The *in vivo* protective effect of either capsicin or chili against *H. pylori* infection is not yet clear due to a lack of controlled experimental study, even an epidemiological study with persons having a high dietary intake of chili who may show a lower frequency of ulcer disease compared with controls.[26]

Honey has been used with some beneficial effects as a traditional remedy for dyspepsia including gastritis, duodenitis and ulceration.[32,33] Such traditional experiences stimulated studies to obtain scientific evidence explaining the possible beneficial effects of honey. As a result of such efforts, the possible antibacterial properties of honey have been established.[34] The spectrum of the antibacterial activity of honey was found to be broad, but activity varies markedly and depends on the floral source of the honey. A recent study added *H. pylori* to the list as new susceptible bacterial species.[35] However, the activity of honey against *H. pylori* is not high; complete inhibition of bacterial growth requires the presence of 5% honey in the culture. However, such an effective concentration would be expected in a stomach with a dose of 2.5 ml of honey for 50 ml or less of gastric fluid.[35] Although characterization of active component(s) of honey against *H. pylori* has not been studied, it is conjectured that daily consumption of honey may contribute somewhat to prevention of *H. pylori* infection.

Allium vegetables such as garlic have been used throughout history for their medical properties, especially for their antibacterial and fungicidal properties.[36,37] Several studies also have shown a decreased risk of gastric cancer with an increasing consumption of Allium vegetables, possibly by an effect on *H. pylori.*[38] Therefore, it is likely that Allium vegetables possess an anti-*H. pylori* activity. In fact, the *in vitro* anti*H. pylori* activity of garlic has been demonstrated. For example, oil-macerated garlic constituents could suppress the growth of *H. pylori.*[39] In particular, ajoenes (*E*- and *Z*- 4,5,9-trithiadodeca-1,6,11-triene-9-oxide), which are the main constituents of oil-macerated garlic extract, showed inhibition of *H. pylori* growth at concentrations of 10 to 25 μg/ml. Jonkers *et al.*, also showed an antibacterial effect of a home-made raw garlic extract and commercial garlic tablets alone and in combination with omeprazole against clinical isolates of *H. pylori.*[40] As is usual for other natural products, the MIC values of these garlic products were low, such as 10–17 mg/ml. However, there was an *in vitro* synergistic effect of the combination of garlic and omeprazole. Purified garlic components, such as diallyl sulfide (DAS), showed more impressive *in vitro* antibacterial activity against *H. pylori,* similar to that of ajoenes. That is, anti-*H. pylori* activity with about 50% growth inhibition against 22 clinical isolates at a concentration of 25 μg DAS/ml has been observed.[41] Thus, these findings indicate that garlic may contain at least several anti-*H. pylori* compounds. However, even these *in vitro* findings indicating the effectiveness of garlic on *H. pylori* in regard to a possible therapeutic effect of garlic is controversial due to ineffectiveness on *H. pylori* infection in human trials.[42]

4. TEA

In the field of nutrition and health, many investigations have dealt with foods that are consumed as solids by humans. Many believe it is also important to determine the role of beverages. Worldwide, ever since it was introduced as a beverage in China some 4,000 years ago, tea is the second most common beverage consumed by humans.[43] Green tea, popular in the Far East, differs from the black tea familiar in the West in that an oxidation step occurs in the processing of the black but not green tea. Although this beverage has little nutritional value per se, tea is refreshing, mildly stimulating, and produces a feeling of well-being.[44] The beneficial health effects of tea, besides such refreshing, are also speculated. In one of the earliest reports regarding the beneficial health effects of tea, especially microbiological effects, an army surgeon recommended the use of tea in soldiers' water bottles as a prophylactic against typhoid.[45] Epidemiological findings of possible prophylactic effect of tea consumption against cancer have also been known.[46] Thus, daily consumption of tea beverages may contribute mentally as well as physically to the global health of humans. In addition, recent laboratory studies provided new information about the effect of consumption of tea and various biochemical and physiological parameters associated with tea use.[43]

4.1. Microbiological Effects of Tea

In vitro antimicrobial activity of tea was demonstrated more than 90 years ago.[47] After the first demonstration of antimicrobial activity of tea, a number of reports regarding the microbiological effects of tea and tea components has been published.[44] For example, tea extracts show a strong antimicrobial activity at "cup-of-tea" concentrations against a wide variety of microorganisms, such as

Staphylococcus aureus, S. epidermidis, Salmonella typhi, S. typhimurium, S. enteritidis, Shigella flexneri, S. dysenteriae, Vibrio spp., including *Vibrio cholerae* and others.[48,49] Methicillin-resistant *Staphylococcus aureus* is also susceptible to tea extracts.[50,51] However, the antimicrobial activity of tea is not extended to all microorganisms. For example, tea is active against *Mycoplasma pneumoniae* and *M. orale,* but not against *M. salivarium.*[52] Some yeasts, such as *Candida albicans* and *Cryptococcus neoformans,* are also resistant to the antimicrobial activity of tea, even though *Trichophyton mentagrophytes* and *T. rubrum* are susceptible.[53] The evidence of *in vitro* antimicrobial activities demonstrated by modem laboratory assays support the traditional use of tea as a prophylactic beverage for microbial infections in areas such as Bangladesh.[54] As usual for traditional medicine, most reports of experiences with tea regarding a possible prophylactic effect against infectious diseases have not been analyzed in well-controlled studies. However, current efforts by several groups may contribute to the success of scientific demonstration of *in vivo* antimicrobial effects of tea.[55–58]

The active components of tea extracts responsible for antimicrobial activity have been studied. Even though the chemical composition of tea is complex and not completely understood, detailed investigations indicate that the active antimicrobial components are polyphenolic compounds, which make up some 30% of the dry weight of a tea leaf.[44] The simplest compounds in this class are the catechins, which constitute 7 compounds in tea extracts. As shown in Table 2, epigalocatechin gallate (EGCG) is a major catechin compound in both green and black tea extracts. The biological components EGCG and epicatechin gallate (ECg) show remarkable antimicrobial activity against many bacterial species and also possess anticarcinogenic properties.[59–63] Therefore, it is widely recognized that the active components of tea responsible for antimicrobial activity are catechins.

TABLE 2
Catechin contents of green tea and black tea extract

Component	Green tea	Black tea
Total catechins (g/g tea extract)	0.26	0.10
(+)-Catechin (%)	4	5
(+)-Gallocatechin (%)	4	5
(+)-Gallocateehin gailate (%)	1	0
(−)-Epicatechin (%)	13	1.1
(−)-Epigallocatechin (%)	24	18
(−)-Epicatechin gallate (%)	1.8	20
(−)-Epigallocatechin gailate (%)	36	42

[a]Total catechin content measured by spectrophotometry after complex formation with DMACA, individual catechins measured by HPLC and expressed as percentage of total catechins. (From ref. 73)

It is widely believed in certain areas that drinking tea contributes to good health. Such traditional ideas are supported epidemiologically by the evidence of a low incidence of gastric diseases, including gastric cancer, in certain area, of individuals who drink much tea daily.[64] From such a view point, prevention and treatment of gastric infection with *H. pylori* by tea drinking may be likely.

4.2. Anti-*H. pylori* Activity of Tea Catechins

The *in vitro* anti-*H. pylori* activity of tea catechins has been studied by several groups.[65–67] The MIC of six catechins has been studied using clinical isolates as well as a standard strain of *H. pylori* (ATCC 43504). Only two catechin compounds, EGCG and ECg, show considerable antimicrobial activity against *H. pylori* as determined by the standard agar dilution method.[68] As shown in Table 3, other catechins such as C, EC, GC, and EGC, which do not have gallic acid in their chemical structure (Figure 2), have not shown any significant anti-*H. pylori* activity. Therefore, it seems likely that the anti-*H. pylori* activity of catechins may be related to the gallic acid moiety, similar to the structures with antimicrobial activity to other bacteria.[63] Such a relationship between antimicrobial activity and the chemical structure of catechins is also supported by current work regarding the biological activity of tea catechins on the lipid bilayer.[69] Membrane damage caused by catechins may be one of the mechanisms responsible for the antimicrobial activity of catechins. The MICs of catechins, even though the strongest activity is possessed by EGCG, are much lower as compared with that

TABLE 3
MICs of tea catechins and antibiotics against clinical isolates of *H. pylori*

	MIC (μg/Ml)[a]		
Compound	50.%	90.%	Range
Cathechin	>200	>200	>200
Epicatechin	>200	>200	>200
Gallocatechin	>200	>200	>200
Epigallocatechin	>200	>200	100–>200
Epicatechin gallate	100	100	*50–100*
Epigallocatechin gailate	*50*	100	12.5–100
Metronidazole	8	16	1–>16
Clarithromycin	0.12	2	<0.03–>2
Amoxicillin	0.12	0.25	<0.03–0.5

[a]Thirty eight clinical isolates of *H. pylori* were tested in MIC assay.

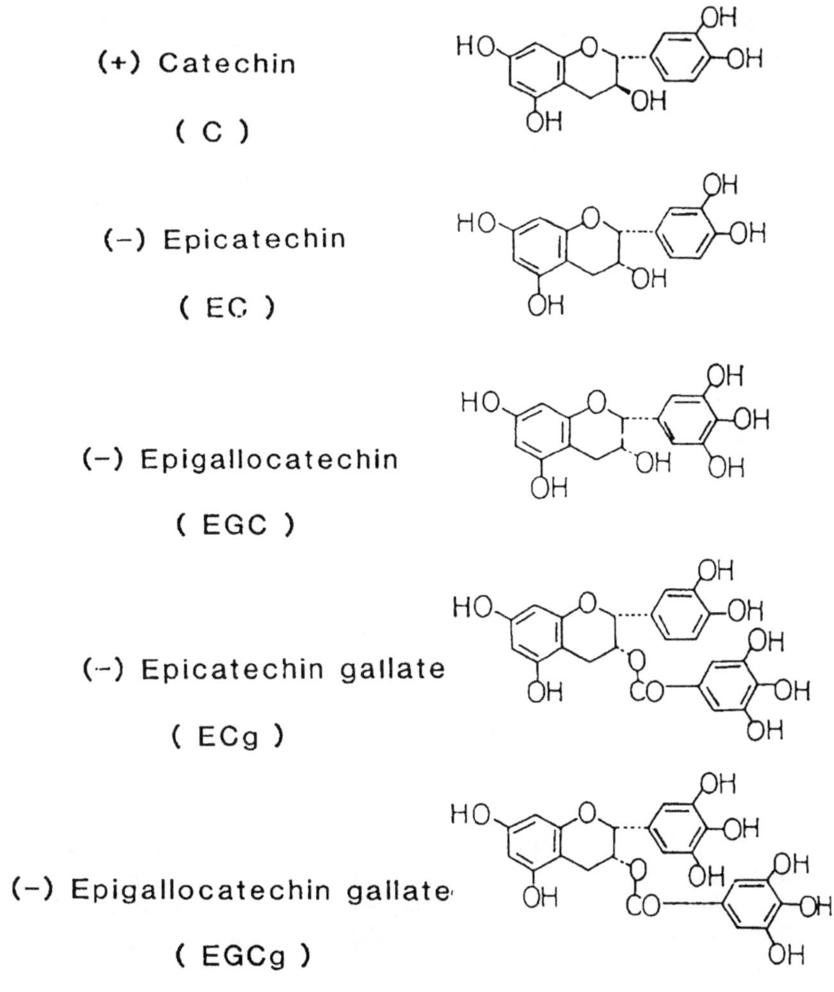

FIGURE 2. Chemical structures of tea catechins.

of antibiotics, such as clarithromycin and amoxicillin widely used for eradication therapy of *H pylori* infection. However, the actual concentrations of tea catechins after drinking a cup of tea may easily increase to the MIC in a stomach. For example, a cup of green tea (200 ml) may contain approximately –160 μg/ml of EGCG, because about 0.94% of the dry weight of green tea extract is EGCG (see Table 2). In a suspension culture of *H. pylori,* EGCG shows more activity against bacteria with a bactericidal activity as low as 50 μg/ml (Figure 3). However,

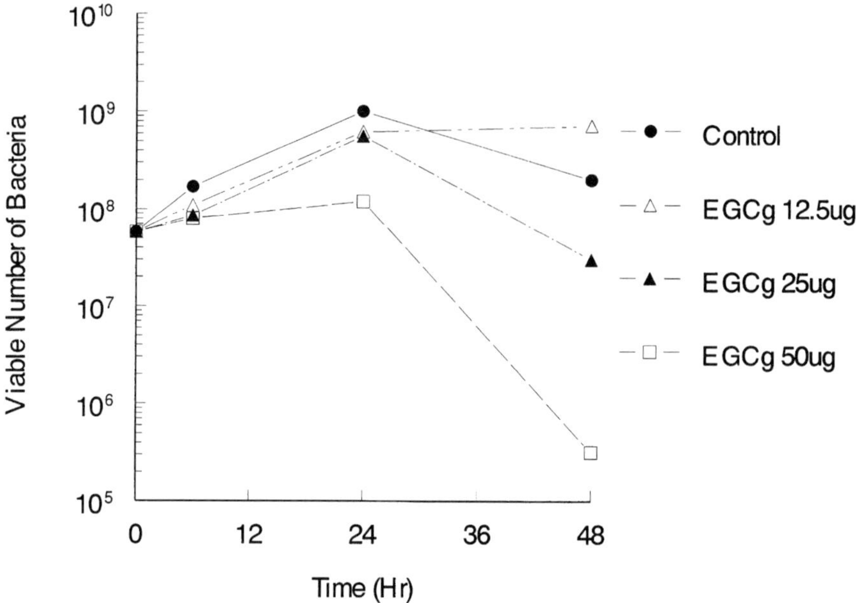

FIGURE 3. Effect of tea catechin EGCG on the growth of *H. pylori*. *H. pylori* cultured in Brucella broth supplemented with 10% fetal calf serum in the presence or absence of indicated concentrations of EGCG for 48 hrs at 37°C in a microaerobic atmosphere. The viable number of bacteria (CFU) was measured on Brucella agar containing 7% horse blood.

the antimicrobial activity of catechins on bacteria is slow and requires more than 24 hrs contact. The reason for a difference of concentration showing anti-*H. pylori* activity between the agar dilution assay and suspension culture assay may be due to the experimental conditions used. Thus, cup-of-tea concentrations may reach the concentrations necessary to inhibit or kill *H. pylori*, even though prolonged time is required.

4.3. *In Vivo* Activity of Tea Catechins

An experimental animal model using Mongolian gerbils has been reported for assessment of effectiveness of tea catechins (Polyphenon 70S, a mixture of catechins) against *H. pylori* infection.[66] The Mongolian gerbil model for *H. pylori* infection provides a stable, reliable infection system and provides relatively comparable pathological features of gastritis to that of human cases.[70] Six weeks after inoculation of bacteria, animals were treated for 2 weeks with a 1% catechin-containing diet plus 0.5% catechin-containing water. After the animals were fasted for 24 hrs, their stomachs were removed for microbiological as well as pathological analysis. The hemorrhage scores and the scores of injury to the gastric mucosa caused by *H. pylori* infection were significantly decreased in all catechin-fed groups, with a 10 to 36% eradication rate. Thus, even a relatively short period of catechin consumption compared with that of humans who drink tea on a daily basis for years showed evidence of improvement, with some eradication of *H. pylori*.

An eradication trial of *H. pylori* from stomachs of human cases with green tea extracts has also been conducted.[67] Thirty-four patients with gastric ulcer, duodenal ulcer, or with chronic gastritis who proved to be *H. pylori* infected took capsules of tea extracts (700 mg/day) orally for one month. Infection was confirmed by serological tests (serum anti-*H. pylori* IgG antibody) and specific culture. No patient received specific treatment for *H. pylori* before or during testing. A ^{13}C-urea breath test was performed to determine the *H. pylori* status of the patient before and after treatment. Eradication of *H. pylori* was assessed as a negative breath test at one month after the end of treatment. More than half of the 34 patients who received tea extracts were found to have a decreased ^{13}C-urea activity one month after treatment. Eradication of *H. pylori* was documented in 6 out of the 34 patients one month after completion of treatment. The results of this *in vivo* clinical trial of tea catechins or tea extracts suggest that tea catechins have, at least, some antimicrobial effects on the presence of *H. pylori* in the stomach and may contribute to improvement of diseases caused by *H. pylori*, even though such studies did not have a sufficient number of patients and were not well controlled in regards to acceptable clinical epidemiological standards.

The *in vivo* effects of tea catechins on gastric diseases caused by *H. pylori* infection may not be derived only from the antimicrobial activity of tea catechins, since tea catechins have a variety of the biological effects including antioxidative[71] and anti-inflammatory effects.[72] The multiple biological effects of tea catechins, even though each activity may not be strong as compared with other agents, may be synergistic or even additive on certain diseases such as gastric diseases caused by *H. pylori* infection. Furthermore, tea catechins are effective against *H. pylori* resistant to certain antibiotics,[65] like metronidazole, which is also widely used as an eradication agent for *H. pylori* infection, and resistance to tea catechins does not occur even with prolonged consumption of tea.

However, tea may not be a good therapeutic agent for gastric diseases caused by *H. pylori* infection, even though tea catechins have anti-*H. pylori* activity, because their antimicrobial activity is not strong bactericidally and requires prolonged contact with the target bacteria. On the other hand, tea may be excellent for prevention of gastric diseases caused by *H. pylori* because of its multifunctional activities, including anti-inflammatory and anti-oxidant activities. Furthermore, tea does not have any side effect, if taken as a beverage, and may not induce bacterial resistance. From such a view point, it seems reasonable why tea has been widely used for more than 4,000 years.

5. CONCLUSION

As reviewed in this chapter, it is obvious there are anti-*H. pylori* agents in natural substances. Some reports are based on well-controlled studies, but some do not provide enough data due to the complexity of the nature of natural products. In some cases, the reports of the efficacy of such natural products are considered controversial, especially the usefulness of such products as a therapeutic agent for gastric diseases caused by *H. pylori* infection. However, it seems reasonable to seek agents specific to *H. pylori* for the therapy or prevention from *H. pylori* infection in natural substances. Further studies concerning the *in vivo* efficacy of natural substances on *H. pylori* infection are warranted.

REFERENCES

1. Marshall B. J., 1994, *Helicobacter pylori. Am. J. Gastroenterol.*, **89**:*S* 1 16.
2. Chiba N., Rano B. V., Rademarker J. W., and Hunt R. H., 1992, Meta-analysis of the efficacy of antibiotic therapy in eradicating *Helicobacter pylori. Am. J. Gastroenterol.*, **87**:1716.
3. Mertens J. C., Dekker W., Lightvoet E. E., and Blok P., 1989, Treatment failure of norfloxacin against *Campylobacter pylori* and chronic gastritis in patients with nonulcer dyspesia. *Antimicrob. Agents Chemother.*, **33**:256.
4. Axon A. T. R., and Moayyedi P., 1996, Eradication of *Helicobacter pylori:* omeprazole in combination with antibiotics. *Scand. J. Gastroenterol.*, *3* **1** (Suppl. 215):82.
5. Misiewicz J. J., Harris A. W., Bardhan K. D., Levi S., O'Morian C., Cooper B. T., Kerr G. D., Dixon M. F., Langworthy H., and Piper D., 1997, One week triple therapy for *Helicobacter pylori:* a multicentre comparative study. *Gut,* **41**:735.
6. Ling T. K. W., Cheng A. F. B., Sung J. J. Y., Yiu P. Y. L., and Chung S. S. C., 1996, AD increase in *Helicobacter-pylori* strains resistance to metronidazole: a five-year study. *Helicobacter* **1**:57.
7. Yesilada E., Giirbiiz L., and Shibata H., 1999, Screening of Turkish anti-ulcerogenic folk remedies for anti-*Helicobacter pylori* activity. *J. Ethanopharmacol,* **66**:289.
8. Yesilada E., Sezik E., Fujita T., Tanaka S., and Tabata M., 1993, Screening of some Turkish medicinal plants for their antiulcerogenic activity. *Phytotherapty Res.*, **7**:263.
9. Yesilada E., Gflrbiiz L., and Ergun E., 1997, Effects of Cistus laurifolius L. flowers on gastric and duodenal lesions. *J. Ethnopharmacol,* **55**:201.
10. Boyanova L., and Neshev G., 1999, Inhibitory effect of rose oil products on *Helicobacter pylori growth in vitro*: preliminary report. *J. Gen. Microbiol.*, **48**:705.
11. Neshev G., 1990, Bulgarian rose oil—pharmacological and clinical studies. Thesis. Medical University, Sofia, Bulgaria.
12. Ohsaki A., Takashima J., Chiba N., and Kawamura M., 1999, Microanalysis of a selective potent anti-*Helicobacter pylori* compound in a Brazilian medicinal plant, *Myroxylon peruiferum* and the activity of analogues. *Bioorg. Med. Chem. Lett.*, **9**:1109.
13. Kartnig T., 1987, Cetraria islandica-lsliindisches Moos. *Z. Phytother.*, **8**:127.
14. Ingolifsdottir K., Bloomfield S. F., and Hylands P. J., 1985, *In vitro* evaluation of the antimi-crobial activity of lichen metabolites as potential preservatives. *Antimicrob. Agents Chemother.*, **28**:289.
15. Ingolfsdottir K., Hjalmarsdottir M. A., Sigurdsson A., Gudjonsdottir G. A., Brynjolfsdottir A., and Steingrimsson O., 1997, *In vitro* susceptibility of *Helicobacter pylori* to protolichesterinic acid from the lichen *Cetraria islandica. Antimicrob. Agents Chemother.*, **41**:215.

16. Ingolifsdottir K., Breu W., Huneck S., Gudjonsdottir G. A., Miiller-Jakic B., and Wagner H., 1994, *In vitro* inhibition of 5-lipoxygenase by protolichesterinic acid from *Cetraria islandica. Phytomedicine,* **1**:187.
17. Fabry W., Okemo P., and Ansorg R., 1996, Activity of east African medicinal plants against *Helicobacter pylori. Chemotherapy*, **42**:315.
18. Fabry W., Okemo P., Mwatha W. E., Chhabra S. C., and Ansorg R., 1996, Susceptibility of *Helicobacter pylori* and Candida spp. to the east African plant *Terminalia spinosa. Arzneimittelforschung,* **46**:539.
19. Germano M. P., Sanogo R., Guglielmo M., De Pasquale R., Crisafi G., and Bisignano G., 1998, Effects of *Pteleopsis suberosa* extracts on experimental gastric ulcers and *Helicobacter pylori* growth. *J. EthnopharmacoL,* **59**:167.
20. Annuk H., Hirmo S., Turi E., Mikelsaar M., Arak E., and Wadstrom T., 1999, Effect on cell surface hydrophobicity and susceptibility of *Helicobacter pylori* to medicinal plant extracts. *FEMS Microbiol. Lett.*, **172**:41.
21. Cassel-Beraud A. M., Le Jan J., Mouden J. C., Andriantsoa M., and Andriantsiferana R., 1991, Preliminary study of the prevalence of *Helicobacter pylori* in Tananarive, Madagascar and the antibacterial activity *in vitro* of 13 Malagasy medicinal plants on this gen-n. *Arch. Inst. Pasteur Madagascar,* **59**:9.
22. Bae E. A., Han M. J., Kim N. J., and Kim D. H., 1998, *Anti-Helicobacter pylori* activity of herbal medicines. *Biol. Pharm. Bull.*, **21**:990.
23. Kadota S., Basnet P., Ishii E., Tamura T., and Namba T., 1997, Antibacterial activity of trichorabdal A from *Rabdosia trichocarpa against Helicobacter pylori. Zentrabl. Bakteriol,* **286**:63.
24. Higuchi K., Arakawa T., Ando K., Fujiwara Y., Uchida T., and Kuroki T., 1999, Eradication of *Helicobacter pylori* with a Chinese herbal medicine without emergence of resistant colonies. *Am. J. Gastroenterol.*, **94**:1419.
25. Huwez F. U., and Thirlwell D., 1998, Mastic gum kills *Helicobacterpylori. N. Engl. J. Med.*, **339**:1946.
26. Kang J. Y., Yeoh K. G., Chia H. P., Lee H. P., Chia Y. W., Guan R., and Yap L., 1995, Chili-protective factor against peptic ulcer? *Dig. Dis. Sci.*, **40**:576.
27. Dorant E., Van Den Brandt P. A., Golbohm R. A., and Sturmans F., 1996, Consumption of onions and a reduced risk of stomach carcinoma. *Gastroenterology, I* **10**:12.
28. You W., Blot W. J., Chang Y., Ershow A. G., Yang Z., An Q., Henderson B., Xu G., Fraumeni J. F., and Wang T., 1989, Allium vegetables and reduced risk of stomach cancer. *J. Natl. Cancer Inst.*, **81**:162.
29. Buiatti E., Paiii D., Decarli A., Amadori D., Avellini C., Bianchi S., Bisemi R., Cipriani F., Cocco P., Giacosa A., Marubini E., Puntoni R., Vindigni C., Fraumeni J., and Blot W., 1989, A case-control study of gastric cancer and diet in Italy. *Int. J. Cancer,* **44**:611.
30. Jones N. L., Shabib S., and Sherman P. M., 1997, Capsaicin as an inhibitor of the growth of the gastric pathogen *Helicobacter pylori. FEMS Microbiol. Lett.*, **146**:223.
31. Desai H. G., Venugopalan K., and Antia F. P., 1973, Effect of red chili powder on DNA content of gastric aspirates. *Gut,* **14**:974.
32. Editorial, 1982, Hospitals using honey as a fast new antibiotic. *Am. Bee J,* **122**:247.
33. Men'shikov F. K., and Feidman S. I., 1949, Curing stomach ulcers with honey. *Sov. Med.*, **10**:13.
34. Molan P. C., 1992, The antibacterial activity of honey. *Bee World,* **73**:5.
35. Somal N. A., Coley K. E., Molan P. C., and Hancock B. M., 1994, Susceptibility of *Helicobacter pylori* to the antibacterial activity of manuka honey. *J. Royal Soc. Med.*, **87**:9.
36. Cavallito C. J., and Bailey J. H., 1944, Allicin, the antibacterial principle of allium sativum. I. Isolation, physical properties and antibacterial action. *J. Am. Chem. Soc.*, **66**:1950.
37. Hughes B. G., and Lawson L. D., 1991, Antimicrobial effects of Allium sativum L. (Garlic), Allium ampeloprasum L. (Elephant garlic), and Allium cepa L. (onion), garlic compounds and commercial garlic supplement products. *Phytother. Res.*, **5**:154.

38. Dorant E., van den Brandt P. A., Goldbohm R. A., and Sturmans F., 1996, Consumption of onions and a reduced risk of stomach carcinoma. *Gastroenterology*, II **0**:12.
39. Ohta R., Yamada N., Kaneko H., Ishikawa K., Fukuda H., Fujino T., and Suzuki A., 1999, *In vitro* inhibition of the growth of *Helicobacter pylori* by oil-marcerated garlic constituents. *Antimicrob. Agents Chemother.*, **43**:1811.
40. Jonkers D., van den Broek E., Thijs C., Dorant E., Hageman G., and Stobberingh E., 1999, Antibacterial effect of garlic and omeprazole on *Helicobacter pylori*. *J. Antimicrob. Chemother.*, **43**:837.
41. Chung J. G., Chen G. W., Wu L. T., Chang H. L., Lin J. G., Yeh C. C., and Wang T. F., 1998, Effects of garlic compounds diallyl sulfide and diallyl disulfide on arylamine N-acetyltransferase activity in strains of *Helicobacter pylori* from peptic ulcer patients. *Am. J. Chinese Med*, **24**:353.
42. Graham D. Y., Anderson S-Y., and Lang T., 1999, Garlic or jalapeño peppers for treatment of *Helicobacter pylori* infection. *Am. J. Gastroenterol.*, **94**:1200.
43. Weisburger J. H., 1999, Second international scientific symposium on tea and human health: an introduction. *Proc. Soc. Exp. Biol. Med.*, **220**:193.
44. Hamilton-Miller J. M. T., 1995, Antimicrobial properties of tea (*Camellia sinensis L.*). *Antimicrob. Agents Chemother.*, **39**:2375.
45. Annon, 1923, Using tea to fight typhoid. *Tea and Coffee Trade J*, July: 129.
46. Kohlmeier L., Weterings K. G. C., Steck S., and Kok F. J., 1997, Tea and cancer prevention: an evaluation of the epidemiologic literature. *Nutr Cancer*, **27**:1.
47. McNaught J. G., 1906, On the action of cold or lukewarm tea on *Bacillus typhosus*. *J. Royal Army Med Corps*, **7**:372.
48. Toda M., Okubo S., Hiyoshi R., and Shimamura T., 1989, The bactericidal activity of tea and coffee. *Lett. Appl. Microbiol.*, **8**:123.
49. Yam T. S., Shah S., and Hamilton-Miller J. M. T., 1997, Microbiological activity of whole and fractionated crude extracts of tea (*Camellia sinensis*), and of tea components. *FEAFS Microbiol. Letters*, **152**:169.
50. Toda M., Okubo S., Hara Y., and Shimamura T., 1991, Antibacterial and bactericidal activities of tea extracts and catechins against methicillin-resistant *Staphylococcus aureus*. *Jpn. J. Bacteriol.*, **46**:839.
51. Yam T. S., Hamilton-Miller J. M. T., and Shah S., 1997, The effect of a component of tea (*Camellia sinesis*) *on* methicillin resistance, PBP2' synthesis, and P-lactamase production in *Staphylococcus aureus*. *J. Antimicrob. Chemother.*, **152**:169.
52. Chosa H., Toda M., Okubo S., Hara Y., and Shimamura T., 1992, Antimicrobial and microbicidal activities of tea and catechins against Mycoplasma. *J. Jpn. Assoc. Infect. Dis.*, **66**:606.
53. Okubo S., Toda M., Hara Y., and Shimamura T., 1991, Antifungal and fungicidal activities of tea extract and catechin. *Jpn. J. Bacteriol.*, **46**:509.
54. ••, 1992, International center for diarrheal disease research: easy way to treat diarrhea. *Babladesh News Letter*, **4**:7.
55. Ryu E., 1980, Prophylactic effect of tea on pathogenic microorganism infection to human and animals. *Int. J. Zoonos.*, **7**:164.
56. Nakayama M., Toda M., and Okubo S., *et al.*, 1994, Inhibition of influenza virus infection by black tea extract: *in vivo* study. *J. Jpn. Assoc. Infect. Dis.*, **68**:824.
57. Nakayama M., Ichikawa H., and Toda M., *et al.*, 1993, Inhibition of pig natural influenza infection by tea catechin. *Jpn. J. Bacteriol.*, **48**:323.
58. Lwata M., Toda M., and Nakayama M., *et al.*, 1997, Prophylactic effect of gargling with black tea extract against influenza infection. *J. Jpn. Assoc. Infect. Dis.*, **71**:487.
59. Ahn Y. J., Kawamura T., Kim M., Yamamoto T., and Mitsuoka T., 1991, Tea polyphenols: selective growth inhibitors of *Clostridium spp. Agric. Biol Chem.*, **55**:1425.
60. Das D. N., 1962, Studies on the antibiotic activity of tea. *J. Ind Chem. Soc.*, **39**:849.

61. Kawamura J., and Takeo T., 1989, Antibacterial activity of tea catechin to *Streptococcus mutans*. *J. Jpn. Soc. Food Sci. Technol.*, **36**:463.
62. Otake S., Makimura M., Kuroki T., Nishihara Y., and Hirasawa M., 1991, Anticaries effects of polyphenolic compounds from Japanese green tea. *Caries Res.*, **25**:43 8.
63. Toda M., and Shimamura T., 1997, Catechin: multifunctional biodefense agent. *Showa Medical J.*, **57**:175.
64. Oguni L., Nasu K., Kanaya S., Ota Y., Yamamoto S., and Nomura T., 1989, Epidemiological and experimental studies on the antitumor activity by green tea extracts. *Jpn. J. Nutr.*, **47**:93.
65. Yamamoto Y., Okubo S., Yanagawa Y., Hara Y., and Shimamura T., 1998, Tea catechins have anti-*Helicobacter pylori* activity and enhance antibacterial activity of antibiotics. 38th ICAAC, San Diego, CA, September 24–27.
66. Mabe K., Yamada M., Oguri T., and Takahashi T., 1999, *In vitro* and *in vivo* activities of tea catechins against *Helicobacter pylori*. *Antimicrob. Agents Chemother.*, **43**:1788.
67. Yamada M., Murohisa B., Kitagawa M., Takehira Y., Tamakoshi K., Mizushima N., Nakamura T., Hirasawa K., Horiuchi T., Oguni I., Harada N., and Hara Y., 1998, Effects of tea polyphenols against *Helicobacter pylori*. *In* Functional Foods for Disease, Prevention 1: Fruits, Vegetable, and Teas. ed., Shibamoto T., Terao J., Osawa T., American Chemical Soc., Washington, DC. p.217.
68. Yamamoto Y., Yanagawa Y., and Shimamura T., ••, Unpublished data.
69. Ikigai H., Nakae T., Hara Y., and Shimamura T., 1993, Bactericidal catechins damage the lipid bilayer. *Biochim. Biophys. Acta*, **1147**:132.
70. Hirayama M., Ikeda T., lwao E., Takagi S., and Yokoyama H., 1996, Establishment of gastric *Helicobacter pyrori* infection in mongolian gerbils. *J. Gastroenterol.*, **31**:24.
71. Nanjo F., Goto K., Seto R., Suzuki M., Sakai M., and Hara Y., 1996, Scavenging effects of tea catechins and their derivatives on 1, 1-diphenyl-2-picrylhydrazyl radical. *Free Radic. Biol. Med*, **21**:895.
72. Suganuma M., Okabe S., Sueoka E., Iida N., Komori A., Kim S., and Fujiki H., 1996, A new process of cancer prevention mediated through inhibition of tumor necrosis factor a expression. *Cancer Res.*, **56**:3711.
73. van het Hof K. H., Wiseman S. A., Yang C. S., and Tijburg L. B. M., 1999, Plasma and lipoprotein levels of tea catechins following repeated tea consumption. *Proc. Soc. Exp. Biol Med*, **220**:203.

8

Adherence of *Helicobacter pylori* to Gastric Cell

SHIGERU KAMIYA and HIROYUKI YAMAGUCHI

1. ADHERENCE PROPERTIES OF *H. pylori* TO GASTRIC CELL

1.1. Specificity of Adherence of *H. pylori*

H. pylori specifically colonizes the surface of the gastric mucosal epithelium in the antrum of the stomach. Adherence of *H. pylori* to the gastric epithelium is a primary and important step for the colonization in gastric mucosa and the induction of gastritis. *H. pylori* infects only gastric type mucosa and gastric metaplasia in the duodenum.[1] In contrast, *H. pylori* is never seen on intestinal epithelium. *In vitro* assay, Dunn *et al.*,[2] reported that *H. pylori* adhered more efficiently to human gastric epithelial (KatoIII) cells than human intestine (Int-407) cells and yolk sac-like epithelial cells. Similarly, the adherence rate of *H. pylori* to gastric cell lines (KatoIII, MKN45) was shown to be significantly higher than that to Int-407 cells.[3] These results indicate that *H. pylori* has specific binding activity to human gastric epithelial cells.

1.2. Adherence of Spiral and Coccoid Forms of *H. pylori*

H. pylori has a spiral morphology in a logarithmic phase under a good nourishment. However, conversion from the spiral to coccoid form can be induced by

---

SHIGERU KAMIYA and HIROYUKI YAMAGUCHI • Department of Microbiology, Kyorin University School of Medicine, 6-20-2 Shinkawa, Mitaka, Tokyo 181-8611, Japan.

Helicobacter pylori Infection and Immunity,
Edited by Yamamoto *et al.*, Kluwer Academic/Plenum Publishers, 2002.

alkaline pH, increased temperature, antibiotic treatment, aerobic or anaerobic conditions, or extended incubation.[4] The coccoid form of *H. pylori* is considered to be viable but non-culturable form. The coccoid form of *H. pylori* adheres to gastric epithelial MKN45 cells as well as spiral form (Figure 1). Although it is unclear whether the coccoid form serves any function in the pathogenesis of infection, Cole *et al.*[5] reported that the coccoid form binds poorly to gastric epithelial cells and induces little interleukin-8 (IL-8) secretion by these cells in comparison to spiral form. On the other hand, the coccoid form was reported to induce cellular changes of pedestal formation more frequently than spiral form of *H. pylori*.[6]

1.3. Attaching and Effacement by Adherence of *H. pylori*

Attaching and effacement is characterized by microvilli effacement, actin rearrangement and pedestal formation following bacterial adhesion to cells as described for enteropathogenic *Escherichia coli* (EPEC).[7] Adhesion of *H. pylori* to gastric cells was reported to induce the attaching and effacement (Figure 2).[6,8] Following attachment of *H. pylori* to gastric epithelial cells, tyrosine phosphorylation of two host cellular proteins (145 kDa and 105 kDa) was reported to be induced.[5] Although the role of tyrosine phosphorylation of host cell proteins in the pathogenesis of gastric diseases associated with *H. pylori* infection, it is speculated that this event is involved in the inflammatory response in gastric mucosa. However, other investigators showed that *H. pylori* attachment does not result in pedestal formation or actin rearrangement.[9]

2. ADHESIN OF *H. pylori* AND ITS RECEPTOR

H. pylori adheres specifically to gastric cells by its adhesin(s) to the receptor on the surface of gastric cell. There have been many reports on the adhesins and their receptors (Tables 1 & 2). As single antibody to one adhesin does not inhibit completely the adhesion of *H. pylori* to cells, adherence of *H. pylori* is considered to be carried out multifactorially through multiple adhesins and their receptors.

2.1. HpaA (Sialyllactose-Binding Adhesin)

Evans *et al.*[10] purified 20 kDa protein as an adhesin of *H. pylori* recognizing N-acetylneuraminyllactose, and cloned its gene, *hpaA*. This protein, HpaA, acts as hemagglutinin and aggregates with the assembly of fibrillar structure. The HpaA was reported to be an intracellular lipoprotein and inactivation of *hpaA* did not affect the adherence of *H. pylori* to gastric cells.[11] Therefore, the significance of HpaA as adhesin of *H. pylori* is controversial.

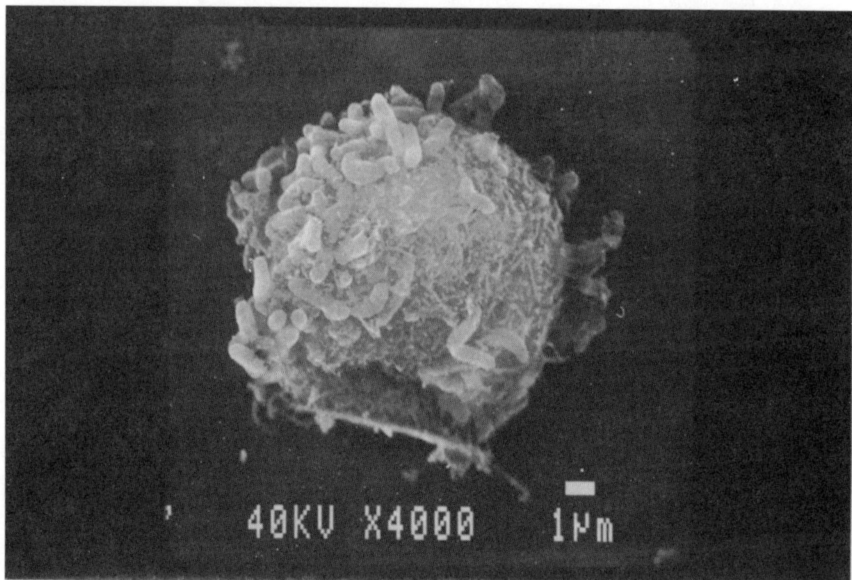

FIGURE 1a.

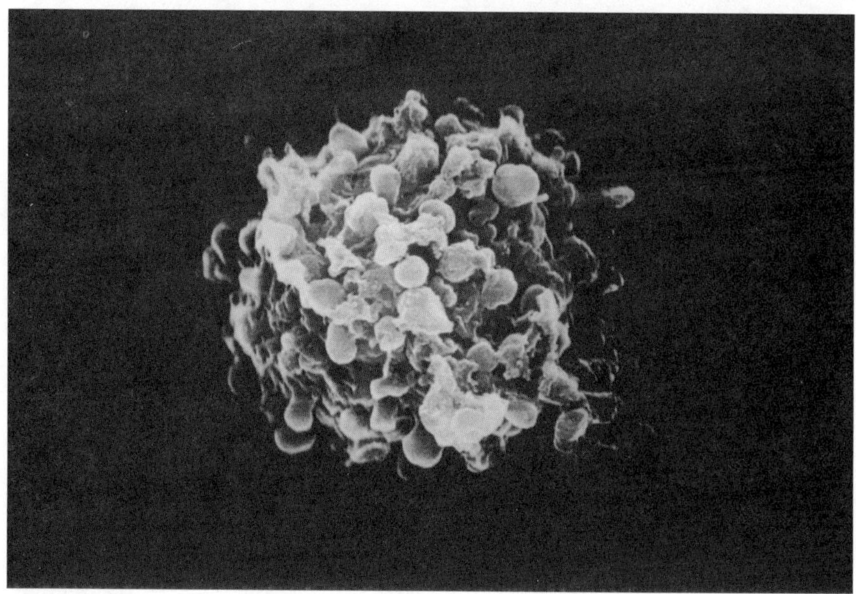

FIGURE 1b. Adherence of spiral (a) and coccoid (b) form of *Helicobacter pylori* to gastric epithelial cells.

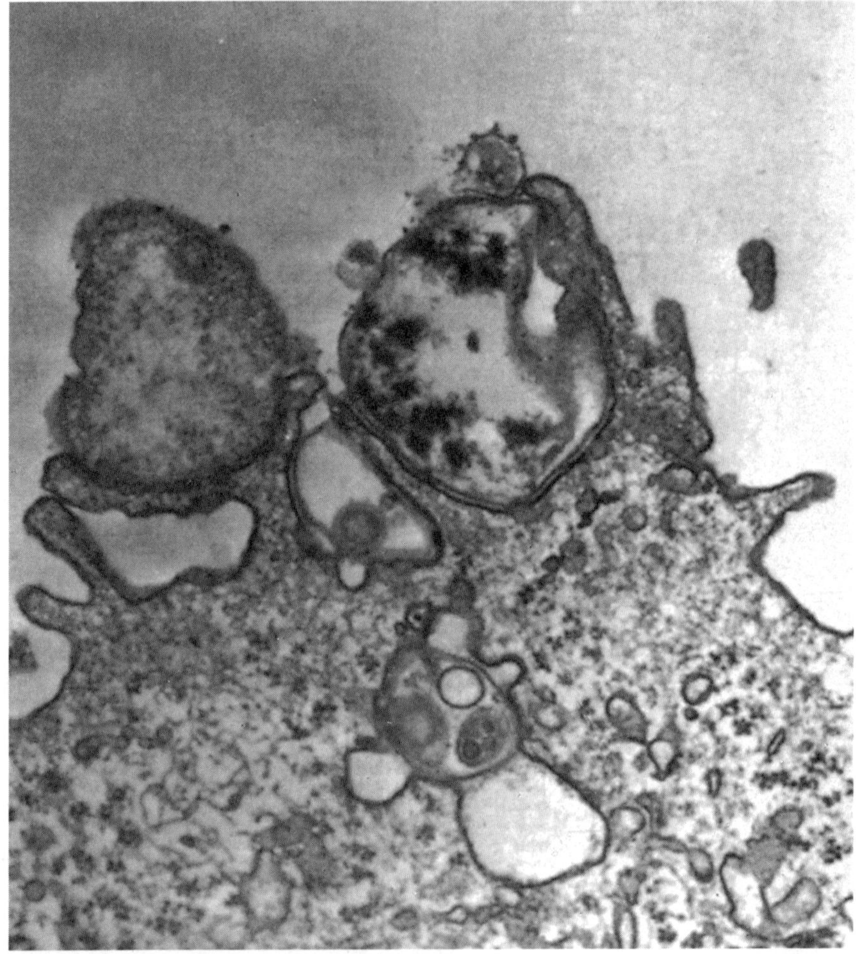

FIGURE 2. Attaching and effacing activity of *Helicobacter pylori*. (Segal *et al.*, *Proc Natl Acad Sci USA* 1996; 93:1259–1264) (ref. 6).

2.2. Adhesin Recognizing Phosphatidylethanolamine

Specific binding of *H. pylori* to a glycerophospholipid species in the antrum of the human stomach was reported.[12] This species was shown to be a form of phosphatidylethanolamine by a thin-layer chromatogram overlay procedure. As similar binding specificity was shown by exoenzyme from *Pseudomonas aeruginosa*, an exoenzyme S-like adhesin was suspected to be responsible for the binding of *H. pylori* to its lipid receptor. Phosphatidylethanol is mainly detected inside

TABLE 1
Putative adhesins of *H. pylori*

Adhesins	Reference
HpaA	10, 11
Adhesin recognizing phosphatidylethanolamine	12
BabA	13, 14
Adhesin recognizing sulfatide	15
Adhesin recognizing extracellular matrix components	16, 17, 18, 19, 20
HSP	21, 22
AlpA, AlpB	23
HopZ	24

of lipid bilayer of cytoplasmic membrane. Detailed analysis on this adhesin is not reported, and the significance of the adhesin recognizing phosphatidylethanolamine in *H. pylori* adherence to gastric cells is not determined.

2.3. BabA Protein Recognizing Lewis^b Antigen

Lewis antigens (Lewis^a, Lewis^b, Lewis^x and Lewis^y) are one of fucosylated blood group antigens, and are expressed on not only erythrocytes but also epithelial cell surface in human. Adherence of *H. pylori* to human gastric epithelial cells was reported to be mediated by Lewis^b antigen that determines blood group O

TABLE 2
Putative receptors for adherence of *H. pylori*

Receptor	Reference
1. Compound lipid	
phospholipid—phosphatidylethanolamine	12
glycerolipid—GM3 ganglioside	25
sulfolipid—sulfatide	15
2. Compound polysaccharide (glycoconjugate)	
glycoprotein—sialylated glycoprotein	26
glycosaminoglycan—heparan sulphate	27
3. Blood group antigen—Lewisb antigen	13, 14
4. Extracellular matrix components	
laminin	17
collagen	18
vitronectin	19
plasminogen	16
lactoferrin	16
fibronectin	20

who are non-secretor.[13] Preferential binding of *H. pylori* to Lewis^b antigen implies a greater risk for developing peptic ulcers in such patients.

Recently, Ilver *et al.*,[14] purified the Lewis^b-binding adhesin (BabA) by receptor activity-directed affinity tagging. The prevalence of *cagA* was associated with BAB (blood group antigen-binding) activity; 73% (54/74) of CagA positive strains were positive for binding to Lewis^b, but only 5% (1/20) of the CagA negative strains were positive for the binding. The sequence of the 20 NH_2-terminal amino acids of the BabA adhesin were used to construct degenerate polymerase chain reaction (PCR) primers for cloning of its gene. Two sets of clones were identified that encode two proteins, BabA (78 kDa) and BabB (75 kDa). The genes corresponding to BabA and BabB were designated as *babA* and *babB*, respectively. By screening an ordered cosmid library, two *babA* genes (*babA1* and *babA2*) and one *babB* gene were mapped (Figure 3). The 10-bp insert with a repeat motif was absent from *babA1*. The *babA* and *babB* sequences were highly similar to the HP1243 gene (91% homology) and HP0896 gene (95% homology) of the published strain 26695,[28] respectively. Inactivation of *babA2* gene abolished BAB activity, but inactivation of *babA1* did not affect BAB activity. The BabA-mediated adherence of *H. pylori* to gastric cells is proposed to play a critical role in efficient delivery of bacterial virulence factors that damage host tissue either directly or through inflammatory or autoimmune reactions, eventually leading to ulcer disease.

2.4. Adhesin Recognizing Sulfatide

Sulfatide (sulfogalactosylceramide) is one of major acidic glycolipid in the human gastric mucosa. Kamisago *et al.*,[15] reported a preferential binding of *H.*

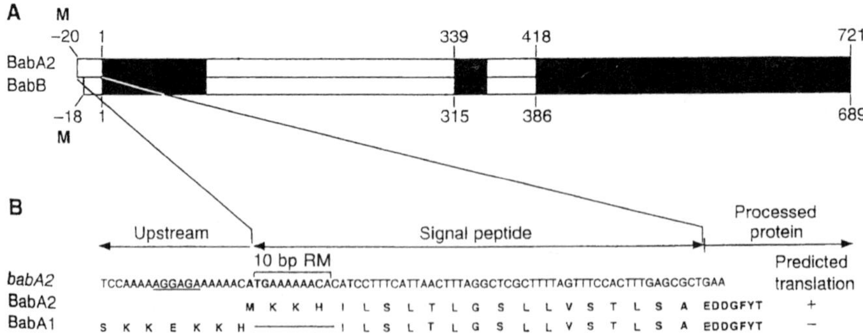

FIGURE 3. (A) The translated *babA* and *babB* sequences showing regions of amino acid sequences similarity and heterogeneity in black and white, respectively. (B) Nucleotide sequence of the upstream and signal peptide regions of the functional adhesin gene *babA2*. (Ilver *et al.*, *Science* 1998; 279:373–377).[14]

pylori to sulphatide on thin-layer chromatography plates. Sulphated glycoconjugates such as heparin and gastric mucin significantly inhibited *H. pylori* adhesion to gastric epithelial KatoIII cells. Anti-sulfatide monoclonal antibody (MAb) also inhibited the adhesion of *H. pylori* to KatoIII cells, but neither anti-GM3 ganglioside, which is another major acidic glycolipid in the gastric mucosa, nor anti-Lewis^b MAb inhibited the adhesion of *H. pylori* to KatoIII cells. In addition, binding of *H. pylori* to only sulfatide in the membrane preparations of KatoIII cells was observed. These results indicate the importance of the sulfatide moiety in the adherence of *H. pylori* to gastric cells. As sulfatide are highly enriched in human gastric mucosa and specifically localized in the epithelial lining of human gastric mucosa, it is speculated that sulfatides can serve as a major receptor for cell adhesion by *H. pylori* in the gastric mucosa.

2.5. Adhesin Recognizing Extracellular Matrix Components

Binding of *H. pylori* to various extracellular matrix components such as vitronectin, heparin sulphate, collagen, fibronectin, lactoferrin, plasminogen and laminin was reported by many investigators.[16–20] Specific attachment of *H. pylori* to extracellular matrix components promotes bacterial colonization.

Plasminogen is a 91 kDa single-chain glycoprotein present in blood and in many tissue fluids. Lactoferrin is an iron-binding glycoprotein both in polymorphonuclear leukocytes and in various body secretions. Khin *et al.*,[16] reported a specific binding of *H. pylori* to plasminogen and lactoferrin. Interestingly, binding of plasminogen and lactoferrin to coccoid form was significantly higher than to spiral form of *H. pylori*. As the ability to acquire iron *in vivo* is an important microbial virulence factor, the iron acquisition system of *H. pylori* by the lactoferrin receptor system may play a major role in the virulence of *H. pylori* infection. Similarly, plasminogen can be converted to an active enzyme (plasmin) by plasminogen activator. The activation could provide a mechanism for bacteria to adopt surface-bound proteolytic activity that allows the microorganism to penetrate into surrounding tissues.

Laminin is a 900 kDa glycoprotein and is important for the structure of the basement membrane by its formation of networks with type IV collagen, entactin and heparin sulphate proteoglycans. Valkonen *et al.*,[17] reported an identification of the N-acetylneuraminllactose-specific laminin-binding protein with molecular weight (MW) of 25 kDa from outer membrane preparations of *H. pylori*. Inhibition experiments with monosaccharides, disaccharides and trisaccharides indicated that the binding was specific for 3-sialyllactose. Similarly, binding of laminin to 25 kDa protein was inhibited when laminin was treated with periodate or sialidase, or laminin was pre-incubated with 3-sialyllactose. These results suggest that glycosylation, particularly sialylation is important for binding by *H. pylori*. In addition, complete inhibition of laminin binding by *H. pylori* strains was achieved only when isolated lipopolysaccharide (LPS) was used as an inhibitor in combination with heat or proteinase treatment of *H. pylori*, suggesting that the 25 kDa outer membrane protein acts in a lectin-like manner with LPS to mediate attachment of *H. pylori* to laminin.

2.6. Heat Shock Protein (HSP)

HSPs are highly conserved proteins found in all prokaryotic and eukaryotic cells, induced by environmental stresses including temperature change, acidic-treatment, inflammation, infection and malignant transformation. HSPs are considered to facilitate folding, unfolding and translocation of polypeptides, as well as the assembly and disassembly of oligomeric protein complexes. Huesca *et al.*,[21] reported that specific binding of HSP70 (DnaK) with MW of 70 kDa of *H. pylori* to sulphatide was increased following brief treatment at low pH. This adhesion was significantly prevented by the inclusion of inhibitors of protein synthesis or by incubation with anti-HSP70. These results suggest that cell surface HSP mediates sulphatide recognition by *H. pylori* under acidic conditions, and they proposed a binary receptor model for the adherence of *H. pylori* to the stomach mucosa. Yamaguchi *et al.*,[22] also reported that HSP60 (GroEL) with MW of 60 kDa was expressed on the surface of *H. pylori* and that the intensity of the surface HSP60 evaluated by flow cytometric analysis correlated with adherence rates of *H. pylori* strains to human gastric MKN45 cells. Moreover, anti-HSP60 MAb was shown to inhibit the adhesion of *H. pylori* to the cells, suggesting that HSP might act as adhesin.

2.7. AlpA and AlpB

Odenbreit *et al.*,[23] screened a library of 135 *H. pylori* in TnMax9 transoposon mutants targeted exclusively in genes encoding exported proteins. Two mutants, P1-140 and P1-179a were defect in adherence to human gastric KatoIII cells. By partial DNA sequencing around the TnMax9 insertion site, the transposon was shown to be inserted exactly 834 bp apart in a single open reading frame (ORF). This ORF designated as *alpA* (adherence-associated lipoprotein A) encodes a putative protein of 518 amino acids, corresponding to a MW of 56.1 kDa. The corresponding ORF in the *H. pylori* 26695 genome sequence was shown to be HP0912 (*omp20*). Exactly 87 nucleotides down stream of the *alpA* stop codon, another ORF was identified. The ORF designated as *alpB* encodes the same number of 518 amino acids with a MW of 55.4 kDa, and corresponded to HP0913 (*omp21*). No transcriptional terminator was found between the two genes, indicating that they might be part of an operon. The C-terminal portion of AlpA and AlpB proteins was predicted to form a porin-like beta-barrel in the outer membrane, consisting of 14 transmembrane amphipathic beta-strands. The isogenic mutant strains of *alpAB* and *alpB* were shown to be defect in the binding to gastric tissue sections. Although the outer membrane prediction for AlpA was supported experimentally by the use of antibodies against AlpA, it is not definitely proved that these Alp proteins are the receptor binding adhesins due to nonspecific binding of the antibodies to other surface proteins of *H. pylori.*

2.8. HopZ

Peck *et al.*,[24] separated 19 proteins from Sarkosyl-insoluble membrane proteins of *H. pylori.* By sequencing of N-terminal peptides, corresponding oligonucleotides were deduced from a lamdaZAP library carrying genomic DNA fragments of *H. pylori.* One of the sequences was shown to hybridize with two different DNA fragments coding for sequences homologous to HopC, a member of the *H. pylori* outer membrane family. One was shown to contain two homologous genes arranged in tandem, and designated as *hopX* and *hopY*. The gene on the second fragment which was designated as *hopZ* encodes a mature protein of 681 amino acid residues of 74.2 kDa, and corresponds to the gene (HP0009) of strain 26695 reported.[28] HopZ was shown to be exposed on the surface of *H. pylori* by immunofluorescence test. The wild type ATCC43505 strain strongly adhered to gastric epithelial cells. but only a few cells of the knockout mutant of *hopZ* strain showed adhesion. These results suggest that the function of HopZ protein is associated with adhesion of *H. pylori* to gastric cells. It was demonstrated that the DNA sequence encoding the signal peptide of the HopZ protein contains stretches of CT dinucleotide repeat. As genotypic variation caused by a slipped-strand mispairing mechanism within these dinucleotide repeats is postulated to switch on or off the expression of the gene, it is possible that the slipped-strand mispairing events within the repetitive sequences of the *hopZ* gene of *H. pylori* would allow the expression of outer membrane protein to be readily switched on or off. Interestingly, HopZ was not able to form pores in bilayer experiment, suggesting that HopZ does not function as a porin.

3. BIOLOGICAL AND PATHOLOGICAL SIGNIFICANCE OF AHDERENCE OF *H. pylori* TO GASTRIC CELL

3.1. Induction of Secretion of Various Cytokines from Gastric Cells

In vivo, gastric infection with *H. pylori* induces the mucosal production of various cytokines in the host, including IL-1beta, IL-6, IL-8 and tumor necrosis factor alpha. Particularly, IL-8 is a small peptide (chemokine) secreted by a variety of cell types, which serves as a potent inflammatory mediator recruiting and activating neutrophils. Stimulation of IL-8 production in gastric epithelial cells by adherence of *H. pylori* was reported.[29] The *cagA* positive strains were shown to induce significantly more IL-8 than *cagA* negative strains. Transposon inactivation of several genes in *cag* pathogenicity island (PAI) showed that various genes (*cagB, C, D, E, G, H, I, L, M*) were responsible for the induction of IL-8 from gastric epithelial cells.[30] Recently, Li *et al.*,[31] reported that multiple genes encoding HP0521, 0525, 0527, 0528 and 0529 ORF in the left half of the *cag* PAI of *H. pylori* are required for tyrosine-kinase dependent transcription of IL-8 in gastric epithelial cells. In addition, Yamaguchi *et al.*,[32] reported the induction of IL-8 by HSP60 of *H. pylori* from gastric epithelial KatoIII cells.

3.2. *iceA* (Induced by Contact with Epithelium)

Adherence of *H. pylori* to gastric epithelium was suggested to provide stimuli that induce expression of some virulence genes. RNAs isolated from *cagA* positive ulcer-derived strain (J166) and *cagA* positive gastritis-derived strain (J178) were used for random arbitrarily primed reverse transcription PCR to identify newly expressed transcribes unique to the ulcer-derived strain following adherence.[33] One of the four primers tested amplified a 900-bp cDNA product from RNA of ulcer strain J166 after adherence to gastric epithelial AGS cells, but not from bacteria that were nonadherent or grown in broth. The DNA sequence of the 900-bp cDNA included an ORF, not previously reported in *H. pylori*, which was designated *iceA*. The *iceA* gene encodes a protein of 178 amino acids with a MW of 20.6 kDa, and demonstrated sequence homology by 60% identity with a gene from *Neisseria lactamica* restriction endonuclease. To investigate *icaA* diversity, the primers for *iceA* were used to amplify genomic DNA from the gastritis strain J178. The longest possible ORF in this region of J178 strain predicted a protein of 59 amino acids, and the sequence in the J178 strain was designated *iceA2*. The published genome sequence of *H. pylori* strain 26695 (28) was shown to contain an *iceA1*, but not *iceA2*. Interestingly, *iceA1* positive strains were significantly associated with peptic ulceration and increased mucosal concentrations of IL-8. Similarly, van Doorn *et al.*,[34] reported that the *iceA* allelic type was independent of the *cagA* and *vacA* status, and there was significant association between the presence of the *iceA1* allele and peptic ulcer disease. In contrast, Yamaoka *et al.*,[34] showed no significant association between *iceA1* and clinical outcome including gastritis, peptic ulcer diseases and gastric cancer. They also demonstrated that *iceA1* and *iceA2* were significantly frequently detected in *H. pylori* strains isolated from east Asia and United States, respectively.

3.3. Attachment-Related Pathology and Induction of Autoantibodies to Lewis^b Carbohydrated Epitope

Guruge *et al.*,[36] used transgenic mice expressing a human receptor, Lewis^b carbohydrate, for *H. pylori* in their gastric epithelium and examined pathological changes following adherence of *H. pylori* to the gastric cells. No significant difference was observed in the colonization rates and the number of *H. pylori* recovered between normal FVB/N mice lacking Lewis^b expression and Lewis^b-transgenic mice. However, *H. pylori* were only seen in the mucus layer in normal mice while in transgenic mice, bacteria were associated with both the mucus layer and pit/surface mucous cells. In Lewis^b-transgenic mice infected with *H. pylori*, severe inflammation distributed over a greater area of the corpus of the stomach and greater fractional representation of macrophages and NK1.1-positive natural killer cells were demonstrated. In addition, after 8 weeks, 21 of 28 transgenic mice (75%) had autoantibodies that reacted with parietal cells compared with only 3 of 23 (13%) nontransgeneic mice. These results indicate that the biological consequences of attachment of *H. pylori* depends on the presence of a putative receptor (Lewis^b) for *H. pylori* adhesins, and that the effect of *H. pylori* attachment was to promote development of autoantibodies to acid-producing epithelial cells, chronic gastritis, and loss of parietal cells.

3.4. Induction of Tyrosine Phosphorylation of Host Cell Proteins

Segal *et al.*,[6] reported that adherence of *H. pylori* to gastric AGS cells resulted in effacement of microvilli, cytoskeletal rearrangement directly beneath the bacterium and cup/pedestal formation at the site of attachment. Binding of *H. pylori* induced tyrosine phosphorylation of two host cell proteins of 145 kDa and 105 kDa, suggesting that *H. pylori* adhesion triggers signal transduction. Cytoskeletal components, responding to transduction signals induced by extracellular signals, can be affected in both structure and function of tyrosine phosphorylation. Su *et al.*,[37] reported a signal transduction-mediated adherence and entry of *H. pylori* into gastric epithelial cells. Tyrosine kinase activity was required for efficient adherence of *H. pylori* to gastric AGS cells, and tyrosine kinase inhibitor, genistein, inhibited the adherence of *H. pylori*. Induction of phosphorylation of 125–130 kDa protein, similar in size to the target protein of *Yersinia* YopH tyrosine phosphatase for protein participating in focal adhesions such as p130cas and FAK (focal adhesion kinase). In addition, adherence of *H. pylori* was inhibited by *Yersinia* organisms expressing enzymatically active YopH but not by inactive YopH. The adherence of *H. pylori* to beta-1 integrin-transfected mouse fibroblast cells was more efficiently observed than to beta1 integrin-deficient cell line GD25. Integrins, E-cadherin and CD66 have been shown to act as ligands for bacteria such as *Yersinia*, *Listeria* and *Neisseria*, allowing both adherence and subsequent internalization.[38] Integrins are known to cluster on the plasma membrane and interact with the cytoskeleton, promoting the assembly of adhesive structures. These results indicate that tyrosine kinase activity and tyrosine phosphorylation of proteins targeted by the YopH tyrosine phosphatase play a role in *H. pylori* adherence. It has been suggested that *H. pylori* enters gastric epithelial cells although *H. pylori* is not intracellular parasitic bacteria. Integrins are normally not expressed on the apical side of polarized epithelial cells. However, the apical membranes of M cells in the intestine were shown to express beta-1-integrin using the gut loop model. Although the presence of M cells in gastric mucosa is not known, the entry mediated by integrin through M cells as reported for *Shigella* and *Yersinia* is speculated for *H. pylori.*

REFERENCES

1. Logan R. P. H., 1996, Adherence of *Helicobacter pylori. Aliment Pharmacol. Ther.* **10**(Suppl. 1): 3–15.
2. Dunn B. E., Altmann M., and Campbell G. P., 1991, Adherence of *Helicobacter pylori* to gastric carcinoma cells: Analysis by flow cytometry. *Rev. Infect. Dis.* **13**(Suppl. 8):S657–S664.
3. Yamamoto-Osaki T., Yamaguchi H., Taguchi H., Ogata S., and Kamiya S., 1995, Adherence of *Helicobacter pylori* to cultured human gastric carcinoma cells. *Eur. J. Gastroenterol. Hepatol.* **7**(Suppl. 1):S89–S92.
4. Catrenich C. E., and Makin K. M., 1991, Characterization of the morphologic conversion of *Helicobacter pylori* from bacillary to coccoid forms. *Scand. J. Gastroenterol.* **181**(Suppl. 1):58–64.
5. Cole S. P., Cirillo D., Kagnoff M. F., Guiney D. G., and Eckmann L., 1997, Coccoid and spiral *Helicobacter pylori* differ in their abilities to adhere to gastric epithelial cells and induce interleukin-8 secretion. *Infect. Immun.* **65**:843–846.
6. Segal E. D., Falkow S., and Tompkins L. S., 1996, *Helicobacter pylori* attachment to gastric cells induces cytoskeletal rearrangements and tyrosine phosphorylation of host cell proteins. *Proc. Natl. Acad. Sci. USA* **93**:1259–1264.
7. Moon H. W., Whipp S. C., Argenzio R. A., Levine M. M., and Giannella R. A., 1983, Attaching and effacing activities of rabbit and human enteropathogenic *Escherichia coli* in pig and rabbit intestines. *Infect. Immun.* **41**:1340–1351.
8. Smoot D. T., Resau J. H., Naab T., *et al.*, 1993, Adherence of *Helicobacter pylori* to cultured human gastric epithelial cells. *Infect. Immun.* **61**:350–355.
9. Dytoc M., Gold B., Louie M., *et al.*, 1993, Comparison of *Helicobacter pylori* and attaching-effacing *Escherichia coli* adhesion to eukaryotic cells. *Infect. Immun.* **61**:448–456.
10. Evans D. G., Karjalainen T. K., Evans D. J. Jr, Graham D. Y., and Lee C. H., 1993, Cloning, nucleotide sequence, and expression of a gene encoding an adhesin subunit protein of *Helicobacter pylori. J. Bacteriol.* **175**:674–683.
11. O'Toole P. W., Janzon L., Doig P., Huang J., Kostrzynska M., and Trust T. J., 1995, The putative neuraminyllactose-binding hemagglutinin HpaA of *Helicobacter pylori* CCUG 17874 is a lipoprotein. *J. Bacteriol.* **177**:6049–6057.
12. Lingwood C. A., Huesca M., and Kuksis A., 1992, The glycerolipid receptor for *Helicobacter pylori* (and exoenzyme S) is phosphatidylethanolamine. *Infect. Immun.* **60**:2470–2474.
13. Boren T., Falk P., Roth K. A., Larson G., and Normark S., 1993, Attachment of *Helicobacter pylori* to human gastric epithelium mediated by blood group antigens. *Science* **262**:1892–1895.
14. Ilver D., Amqvist A., Ogren J., *et al.*, 1998, *Helicobacter pylori* adhesin binding fucosylated histo-blood group antigens revealed by retagging. *Science* **279**:373–377.
15. Kamisago S., Iwamori M., Tai T., Mitamura K., Yazaki Y., and Sugano K., 1996, Role of sulfatides in adhesion of *Helicobacter pylori* to gastric cancer cells. *Infect. Immun.* **64**:624–628.
16. Khin M. M., Ringner M., Aleljung P., Wadstrom T., and Ho B., 1996, Binding of human plasminogen and lactoferrin by *Helicobacter pylori* coccoid forms. *J. Med. Microbiol.* **45**:433–439.

17. Valkonen K. H., Wadstrom T., and Moran A. P., 1997, Identification of the N-acetylneuraminyllactose-specific laminin-binding protein of *Helicobacter pylori*. *Infect. Immun.* **65**:916–923.
18. Trust T. J., Doig P., Emody I., Kienle Z., Wadstrom T., and O'Toole P., 1991, High-affinity binding of the basement membrane proteins collagen type IV and laminin to the gastric pathogen *Helicobacter pylori*. *Infect. Immun.* **59**:4398–4404.
19. Ringneer M., Paulsson M., and Wadstrom T., 1992, Vitronectin binding by *Helicobacter pylori*. *FEMS Microbiol. Immunol.* **105**:219–224.
20. Kondo I., Nagate T., Akashi T., Kaneda Y., Miyachi J., and Yamaguchi M., 1993, Presence of receptors for laminin, collagen, fibronectin and vitronectin on the cell surface of *Helicobacter pylori*. *Eur. J. Gastroenterol. Hepatol.* **5**:S63–S67.
21. Huesca M., Goodwin A., Bhagwansingh A., Hoffman P., and Lingwood C. A., 1998, Characterization of an acidic-pH-inducible stress protein (hsp70), a putatice sulfatide binding adhesin, from *Helicobacter pylori*. *Infect. Immun.* **66**:4061–4067.
22. Yamaguchi H., Osaki T., Kurihara N., *et al.*, 1997, Heat-shock protein 60 homologue of *Helicobacter pylori* is associated with adhesion of *H. pylori* to human gastric epithelial cells. *J. Med. Microbiol.* **46**:825–831.
23. Odenbreit S., Till M., Hofreuter D., Faller G., and Haas R., 1999, Genetic and functional characterization of the *alpAB* gene locus essential for the adhesion of *Helicobacter pylori* to human gastric tissue. *Mol. Microbiol.* **31**:1537–1548.
24. Peck B., Ortkamp M., Diehl K. D., Hundt E., and Knapp B., 1999, Conservation, localization and expression of HopZ, a protein involved in adhesion of *Helicobacter pylori*. *Nucleic. Acids. Res.* **27**:3325–3333.
25. Saitoh T., Natomi H., Zhao W., *et al.*, 1991, Identification of glycolipid receptors for *Helicobacter pylori* by TLC-immunostaining. *FEBS Lett.* **282**:385–387.
26. Lelwala-Guruge J., Ascencio F., Kreger A. S., Ljungh A., and Wadstrom T., 1992, Isolation of a sialic acid-specific surface haemagglutinin of *Helicobacter pylori* strain NCTC 11637. *Zbl. Bact.* **280**:93–106.
27. Ascencio F., Fransson L. A., and Wadstrom T., 1993, Affinity of the gastric pathogen *Helicobacter pylori* for the N-sulphated glycosaminoglycan heparin sulphate. *J. Med. Microbiol.* **38**:240–244.
28. Tomb J.-F., White O., Kerlavage A. R., *et al.*, 1997, The complete genome sequence of the gastric pathogen *Helicobacter pylori*. *Nature* **388**:539–547.
29. Sharma S. A., Tummuru M. K. R., Miller G. G., and Blaser M. J., 1995, Interleukin-8 response of gastric epithelial cell lines to *Helicobacter pylori* stimulation *in vitro*. *Infect. Immun.* **63**:1681–1687.
30. Censini S., Lange C., Xiang Z., *et al.*, 1996, *cag*, a pathogenicity island of *Helicobacter pylori*, encodes type I-specific and disease-associated virulence factors. *Proc. Natl. Acad. Sci. USA* **93**:14648–14653.
31. Li S. D., Kersulyte D., Lindley I. J. D., Neelam B., Berg D. E., and Crabtree J. E., 1999, Multiple genes in the left half of the *cag* pathogenicity island of *Helicobacter pylori* are required for tyrosine kinase-dependent transcription of interleukin-8 in gastric epithelial cells. *Infect. Immun.* **67**: 3893–3899.
32. Yamaguchi H., Osaki T., Kurihara N., *et al.*, 1999, Induction of secretion of interleukin-8 from human gastric epithelial cells by heat-shock protein 60 homologue of *Helicobacter pylori*. *J. Med. Microbiol.* **48**:927–933.
33. Peek R. M. Jr, Tompson S. A., Donahue J. P., *et al.*, 1998, Adherence to gastric epithelial cells induces expression of a *Helicobacter pylori* gene, *iceA*, that is associated with clinical outcome. *Proc. Asso. Am. Phys.* **110**:531–544.
34. van Doorn L.-J., Figueiredo C., Sanna R., *et al.*, 1998, Clinical relevance of the *cagA*, *vacA*, and *iceA* status of *Helicobacter pylori*. *Gastroenterology* **115**:58–66.
35. Yamaoka Y., Kodama T., Gutierrez O., Kim J. G., Kashima K., and Graham D. Y., 1999, Relationship between *Helicobacter pylori iceA*, *cagA*, and *vacA* status and clinical outcome: Studies in four different countries. *J. Clin. Microbiol.* **37**:2274–2279.

36. Guruge J. L., Falk P. G., Lorenz R. G., *et al.*, 1998, Epithelial attachment alters the outcome of *Helicobacter pylori* infection. *Proc. Natl. Acad. Sci. USA* **95**:3925–3930.
37. Su B., Johansson S., Fallman M., Patarroyo M., Granstorom M., and Normark S., 1999, Signal transduction-mediated adherence and entry of *Helicobacter pylori* into cultured cells. *Gastroenterology* **117**:595–604.
38. Lreton K., and Cossart P., 1998, Interaction of invasive bacteria with host signaling pathway. *Curr. Opin. Cell Biol.* **10**:276–283.

9

Helicobacter pylori, Molecular Mimicry and Autoimmunity

BEN J. APPELMELK,[1] GERHARD FALLER,[2] and CHRISTINA M.J.E. VANDENBROUCKE-GRAULS[1]

1. INTRODUCTION

The lipopolysaccharide (LPS) of the Gram-negative human gastric pathogen *H. pylori* expresses Lewis blood group antigens (Tables 1 and 2). Le^x and Le^y are most often expressed,[1,2] but other blood group antigens have also been found.[3,4] Of notice, gastric human epithelial cells also express similar $Le^{x/y}$ blood group antigens. The expression by microorganisms of surface structures similar to those found in the host is called molecular mimicry. Examples of other pathogens displaying molecular mimicry are Campylobacter *jejuni* and *Neisseria spp.* The role of mimicry in pathogenesis may be two-fold. On the one hand mimicry might provide immune escape by preventing the formation of antibodies directed to the epitopes shared by self and microorganism; this might contribute to persistence of infection. On the other hand, infection might break tolerance to the shared epitopes and induces autoantibodies; bound antibodies might fix complement and an autoimmune attack on self might ensue.

In this chapter, we will discuss the structure and biosynthesis of *H. pylori* LPS Lewis antigens as well as their biological significance, in particular the pathogenic

BEN J. APPELMELK and CHRISTINA M.J.E. VANDENBROUCKE-GRAULS • Dept. Medical Microbiology, Vrije Universiteit, Amsterdam, The Netherlands. GERHARD FALLER • Dept. Pathology, University Erlangen, Germany.

Helicobacter pylori Infection and Immunity,
Edited by Yamamoto *et al.*, Kluwer Academic/Plenum Publishers, 2002.

role of Lewis antigen mimicry. Secondly, the pathogenic significance of H. *pylori*-induced anti-gastric autoantibodies will be discussed.

2. STRUCTURE OF *H. pylori* LPS

The structure of LPS of a variety of *H. pylori* strains has been determined chemically. Its overall architecture proved similar to that of LPS of other Gram-negative pathogens: the lipid A part, that is inserted in the outer leaflet of the outer membrane is connected to the oligosaccharide core region that again is connected to the O-antigen (= Lewis antigen). A peculiar feature of *H. pylori* LPS is the occurrence in some strains (e.g., strain MO19) of a polymeric heptose region between O-antigen and core. In many strains, the O-antigen consists of Le^x and/or Le^y (Table 1) but other blood group antigens [H type 1, Le^a, Le^b, non-fucosylated polylactosamine (= i-antigen), blood group A] have been found, too.[1–5]

TABLE 1
Structures of Lewis blood group antigens and glycosyltransferases required

Structure	Antigen	Glycosyltransferases
Fucα1 → 2Galβ1 → 3GlcNAc	H type 1	α2FucT, β3GalT
Fucα1 → 2Galβ1 → 4GlcNAc	H type 2	α2FucT, β4GalT
Galβ1 → 4GlcNAc 3 ↑ Fucα1	Lewis x (Le^x)	α3FucT, β4GalT
Fucα1 → 2Galβ1 → 4GlcNAc 3 ↑ Fucα1	Lewis y (Le^y)	α2FucT, α3FucT, β4GalT
Galβ1 → 3GlcNAc 4 ↑ Fucα1	Lewis a (Le^a)	α4FucT, β3GalT
Fucα1 → 2Galβ1 → 3GlcNAc 4 ↑ Fucα1	Lewis b (Le^b)	α2FucT, α4FucT, β3GalT
→3 (Galβ1 → 4GlcNAcβ1 →)$_n$	i-antigen	β4GalT
NANA2 → 3 Galβ1 → 4GlcNAc 3 ↑ Fucα1	sialyl Lewis x (sLe^x)	α3FucT, β4GalT, sialylT

Gal, D-galactose; Fuc, L-fucose; GlcNAc, *N*-acetyl-D-glucosamine. NANA, N-acetylneuraminic acid (= sialic acid). α2/3/4FucT = α2/3/4 fucosyltransferase; β3/4GalT = β3/4 galactosyltransferase. For all structures a β3-GlcNAcT is also required.

TABLE 2
Structures of *Helicobacter pylori* LPS

Structure	Strain
$(Le^x)_n$-core-lipid A	NCTC 11637[1]
Le^y-$(Le^x)_n$-core-lipid A	P466[2]
Le^y-$(heptose)_n$-core-lipid A	MO19
Polylactosamine-core-lipid A	J233[3]
Le^a-core-lipid A	UA948[4]

[1]NCTC 11637 also expresses Le^y and H type 1.
[2]P466 can express sialyl Le^x.
[3]J223 also expresses H type 1.
[4]UA948 also expresses Le^x.

Strains expressing H type 2 have not been found. Often, strains express more than one Lewis antigen (Table 2). For example, strain NCTC 11637 expresses polymeric Le^x $(Le^x)_n$ with n up to 8 or 9, that is non-stoichiometrically substituted terminally with Le^y or H type 1.

It is also possible to determine *H. pylori* blood group antigen expression by serological methods, e.g., ELISA or immunoblot with specific anti-blood group antigen monoclonal antibodies (Mabs). Epidemiological surveys have shown that at least 80% of the *H. pylori* strains react with anti-Lewis Mabs.[6–8] Possibly, this percentage represents an underestimation: it was demonstrated that some *H. pylori* strains do not react with anti-Le^x Mabs while structurally they were shown to express Lewis x.[9] On the other hand, for at least a few strains it has been shown by structural chemical analysis that Lewis antigens were not present.[10] Thus, Lewis antigen expression in *H. pylori* is highly conserved.

3. LEWIS ANTIGEN BIOSYNTHESIS

The sequencing of the genome of two *H. pylori* strains has been of great value for identifying LPS-related genes.[11,12] For biosynthesis of Lewis antigens, at least two different groups of enzymes are required: the enzymes required for biosynthesis of the nucleotide-activated monosaccharides (the donors), and the glycosyltransferases. Two genes involved in transformation of GDP-mannose into GDP-fucose, the fucose donor for both α3- and α2-fucosyltransferases, have been identified on a homology basis:[13] HP0044 (*rfbD*) and HP0045 (*wbcJ*) code for a dehydratase and epimerase-reductase, respectively. Inactivation of *wbcJ* leads to loss of $Le^{x/y}$ expression.[14] Inactivation of *rfbM* (HP0043, GDP-mannose pyrophosphorylase) that is involved in biosynthesis of GDP-mannose yields a fucose-lacking LPS that expresses the i-antigen;[15] inactivation of *galE* (HP0360, UDP-galactose-4-epimerase) yielded a galactose-lacking, truncated LPS;[15,16] Two similar but non-identical α3-*fucT* genes have been identified: HP0379 and HP0651.[17,18] Functional studies with the cloned and expressed gene products show that both genes are involved in biosynthesis of $Le^{x/y}$, but differ in fine-specificity.[19] The HP0379-coded α3-FucT has a preference for internal GlcNAc residues (i.e., not located at the non-reducing terminus) and yields polymeric Le^{x}, while HP0651 α3FucT has a preference for terminal GlcNAc residues and forms mono/oligomeric Le^{x}.[19] The HP0379 α3-FucT can also function as an α4-FucT, and can therefore also form $Le^{a/b}$.[20]

HP0093/94 is an α2-*fucT*; the gene product is required for biosynthesis of both Le^{y} [21,22] and H type 1 (B. J. Appelmelk, unpublished). H type 2 epitopes do not occur in *H. pylori* LPS, and knocking out both α3-*fucT* genes in a strain that expresses $Le^{x/y}$ yields LPS that expresses i-antigen but no H type 2.[19] We conclude that α3-fucosylation precedes α2-fucosylation. This was confirmed in enzyme assays with cloned α2FucT that forms Le^{y} from synthetic Le^{x} but not H type 2 from Galβ1.4GlcNAc.[22] In contrast, this enzyme is able to form H type 1 with a Galβ1.3GlcNac acceptor.[22] The gene coding for β1.4 GalT has been identified (HP0826) and its recombinant product characterized by in vitro acceptor analysis.[23] Insertional inactivation of this gene in strain SS-1 (which expresses $Le^{x/y}$) yields a mutant that expresses a truncated LPS existing of lipid A and a core substituted with a single fucosylated GlcNAc.[23] At least two transferases that are important for Lewis antigen biosynthesis have not been identified yet: the β3GlcNAcT that together with β1.4 GalT is required for biosynthesis of the polylactosamine backbone. Second, sialylT required for biosynthesis of sialylLe^{x}. The β1.3 GalT that is required for biosynthesis of H type 1 and $Le^{a/b}$ is under investigation (B. J. Appelmelk, unpublished).

It has become clear that biosynthesis of the O-antigen (polymeric Le^{x}) proceeds through sequential transfer of monosaccharides, and not through prior assembly of O-antigen building blocks (i.e., Le^{x}) followed by their polymerization. In this respect LPS biosynthesis in *H. pylori* is different from that in other Gram-negative bacteria that expresses polymeric O-antigens (*Escherichia coli*, *Klebsiella spp.*). This different pathway explains why in *H. pylori* some O-antigen substitutions are not present in stoichiometric amounts: although strain NCTC 11637 expresses polymeric Le^{x}, not all the GlcNAc residues are α3-fucosylated.[2]

4. PHASE VARIATION

Several but not all of the glycosyltransferase genes described above carry long poly-C stretches close to the 5′ end of the gene. These are present in both α2- and α3-*fucT* genes (Figure 1), but not in the β1.4 *galT* gene.

C-tracts are also present in LPS genes of Neisseria *spp.* and are a well characterized cause of LPS phase variation, i.e., the high frequency change in LPS phenotype. Due to DNA slippage, on replication C-tracts may give rise to daughter DNA that is either one C shorter or longer; this can occur at very high

ATGTTCCAACCCCTATTAGACGCCTTTATAGAAAGCGCTTCCATTGAAAAAATGGCCTCTAAATC
TCCCCCCCCCCCCCTAAAAATCGCTGTGGCGAATTGGTGGGGAGATGAAGAAATTAAAGAATT
TAAAAAGAGCGTTCTTTATTTTATCCTAAGCCAACGCTACGCAATCACCCTCCACCAAAACCCCA
ATGAATTTTCAGATCTAGTTTTTAGCAATCCTCTTGGAGCGGCTAGAAAGATTTTATCTTATCAA
AACACTAAACGAGTGTTTTACACCGGTGAAAACGAATCACCTAATTTCAACCTCTTTGATTACGC
CATAGGCTTTGATGAATTGGATTTTAATGATCGTTATTTGAGAATGCCTTTGTATTATGCCCATTT
GCACTATAAAGCCGAGCTTGTTAATGACACCACTGCGCCCTACAAACTCAAAGACAACAGCCTT
TATGCTTTAAAAAAACCCTCTCATCATTTTAAAGAAAACCACCCTAATTTGTGCGCAGTAGTGAA
TGATGAGAGCGATCTTTTAAAAAGAGGGTTTGCCAGTTTTGTAGCGAGCAACGCTAACGCTCCT
ATGAGGAACGCTTTTTATGACGCTCTAAATTCCATAGAGCCAGTTACTGGGGGAGGAAGTGTGA
GAAACACTTTAGGCTATAAGGTTGGAAACAAAAGCGAGTTTTTAAGCCAATACAAGTTCAATCT
CTGTTTTGAAAACTCGCAAGGTTATGGCTATGTAACCGAAAAAATCCTTGATGCGTATTTTAGCC
ATACCATTCCTATTTATTGGGGGAGTCCCAGCGTGGCGAAAGATTTTAACCCTAAAAGTTTTGTG
AATGTGCATGATTTCAACAACTTTGATGAAGCGATTGATTATATCAAATACCTGCACACGCACC
CAAACGCTTATTTAGACATGCTCTATGAAAACCCTTTAAACACCCTTGATGGGAAAGCTTACTTT
TACCAAGATTTGAGTTTTAAAAAAATCCTAGATTTTTTTAAAACGATTTTAGAAAACGATACGAT
TTATCACAAATTCTCAACATCTTTCATGTGGGAGTACGATCTGCATAAGCCGTTAGTATCCATTG
ATGATTTGAGGGTTAATTATGATGATTTGAGGGTTAATTATGACCGGCTTTTACAAAACGCTTCG
CCTTTATTAGAACTCTCTCAAAACACCACTTTTAAAATCTATCGCAAAGCTTATCAAAAATCCTT
GCCTTTGTTGCGCGCGGTGAGAAAGTTGGTTAAAAAATTGGGTTTG

FIGURE 1. Nucleotide sequence of an α3-*fucT*. Note the C13 stretch near the 5′ end of the gene that allows a high frequency phase variation based on DNA slippage during replication. A C13 tract leads to biosynthesis of an active full-length gene product, but C12 will lead to a TAA stop codon right after the tract.

(1%) frequencies. The result is a high-frequency, reversible frame shifting. The consequence is a rapid on-off switching of enzyme activity. When in the parent strain a C-tract is present that leads to a full-length, active gene product, in the C + 1 (or C − 1) daughters, the frame shifting will lead either to the production of nonsense polypeptides that have no or little enzyme activity, or, due to the occurrence of early stop codons, to a truncated inactive gene product.[19] A second mechanism for phase variation was observed in the α2-*fucT* (HP0093/94) gene, namely a sequence (AAAAAAG) that allows mRNA slippage at the translational level.[21] The result of this slippage is a −1 frame shift. This second mechanism may therefore compensate for +1 frame shifting due to C-tracts. These two mechanisms operate in the genome strain 26695. While this strain expresses Le^y,[3] its α2-*fucT* gene is frameshifted due to the C-tract and theoretically would yield an inactive α2FucT. However, presence of the translational −1 frameshift cassette AAAAAAG downstream of a Shine-Dalgarno-like sequence causes a −1 shift in reading frame, an active enzyme to be formed and Le^y synthesis to take place.

Also in non-glycosyltransferase genes relevant to LPS biosynthesis, C-tracts may be present: for instance in *neuB* (HP0178), a gene required for biosynthesis of sialyl-Le^x there is a C6-tract (strains 26695 and J99).

Due to phase variation, within a culture of *H. pylori*, a variety of LPS are expressed depending on the on-off status of the enzymes involved. In colony blot, phase variation shows up through the presence of colonies that do not react with specific Lewis Mabs, others that do react, and still others that are sectored (Figure 2).

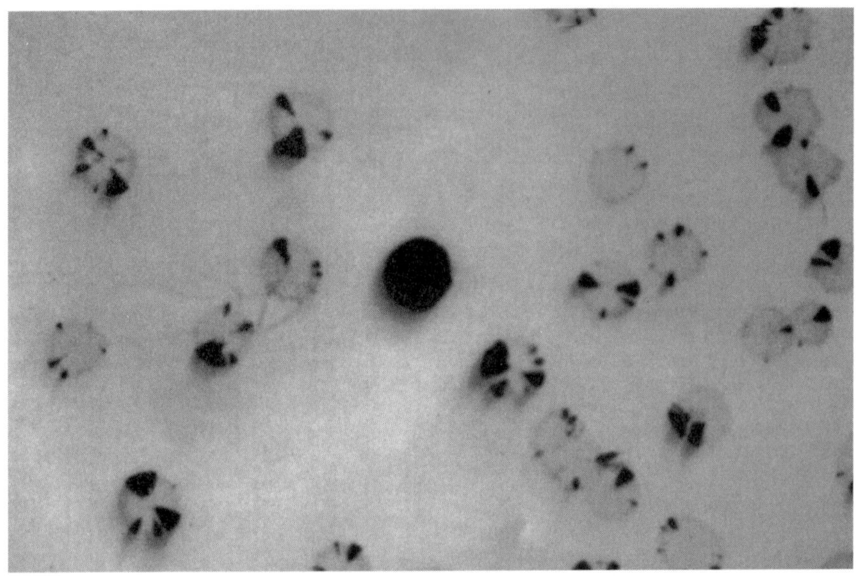

FIGURE 2. LPS phase variation in *H. pylori*.

A list of LPS phase variants isolated from NCTC 11637 is presented in Table 3; these data show that many of the currently known *H. pylori* LPS serotypes described in other strains can be isolated as phase variants from strain NCTC 11637.[24]

The molecular basis of phase variation was determined by sequencing the C-tracts in the α3-*fucT* genes of the parent strain (NCTC 11637) and in the phase variants.[19] In the NCTC 11637 HP0651 is "off" due to the presence of a C9 tract; HP0379 is "on" in this strain (C10). In the phase variant expressing i-Ag plus H type 1 (variant K4.1) both HP0651 (C9) and HP0379 (C11) are off, which explains the lack of Le^x and the biosynthesis of non-fucosylated polylactosamine (= i-Antigen) in strain K4.1. In strain K5.1, the Le^x-positive switch-back variant isolated from K4.1, HP0379 is "on" again (C10). Thus, phase variation from Le^x to i-Ag and back to Le^x can be understood at the molecular level through reversible length changes in the C-tract of α3-*fucT* gene HP0379.

Is phase variation relevant in vivo? We isolated multiple *H. pylori* colonies (n = 30) from a single patient and found that 20% of the colonies expressed $Le^{x/y}$, while 80% express the i-Ag. By molecular typing we demonstrated that they are phase variants of the same strain.[25] Thus, LPS phase variation contributes to strain diversity in vivo. The factor(s) that determine(s) which LPS variant predominates (either in vivo or in vitro) in a particular strain are currently unknown.

TABLE 3
LPS phase variants of strain NCTC 11637

Phase variant	Serotype	Equivalent strain[1]
1b	Le^y	MO19, O6
1c	Le^y, $(Le^x)_n$; see legend[2]	P466
2b	$Le^y \ldots (Le^x)_n$, H type 1	NCTC 11637[3]
3a	Le^a, $(Le^x)_n$	UA948
D1.1	Non-typable	
K4.1[4]	i-Ag, H type 1	J223
K5.1[4]	$Le^y \ldots (Le^x)_n$, H type 1	NCTC 11637
H11	Le^y,$(Le^x)_n$, i-Ag	

[1]Strain with an O-antigen structure identical to that of a particular NCTC 11637 LPS phase variant.
[2]Le^y, $(Le^x)_n$ designates a strong expression of both Le^x and Le^y (variant 1c, strain P466); $Le^y \ldots (Le^x)_n$ designates a weak expression of Le^y and a strong expression of Le^x (variant 2b, strain NCTC 11637).
[3]Variant 2b represents the predominant serotype of strain NCTC 11637.
[4]K4.1 was isolated from NCTC 11637 as a i-Ag positive phase variant, K5.1 was isolated from K4.1 as a Le^x-positive variant and expresses a serotype identical to that of strain NCTC 11637.

5. BIOLOGICAL ROLE OF *H. pylori* LPS LEWIS ANTIGENS

There are various reasons to suspect that *H. pylori* Lewis antigens might fulfill a role in pathogenesis, apart from providing length to the LPS. First of all, almost all *H. pylori* strains express Lewis antigens. This is remarkable as in many other Gram-negative bacteria like *E. coli* and *Klebsiella spp.* many structurally strongly different O-antigens are expressed. Secondly, Lewis antigens are also expressed by the niche in which *H. pylori* is living, i.e., the gastric mucosa. Superficial epithelium predominantly expresses $Le^{a/b}$, while $Le^{x/y}$ predominates at deeper locations. Thus, *H. pylori* displays molecular mimicry with the host, a phenomenon that is also observed in other pathogens and which is thought to be of pathogenic relevance (see below). Thirdly, eukaryotic Lewis antigens interact with various lectins (C-type lectins, selectins) and this might also be the case for Lewis antigens derived from *H. pylori.* Over the years as least three views have been put forward with regard to the biological role of *H. pylori* Lewis antigens and molecular mimicry.

5.1. *H. pylori* Mimicry is Pathogenic

Upon infection, *H. pylori* LPS might induce anti-$Le^{x/y}$ antibodies that bind to the bacteria but also to the gastric epithelial cells; when followed by complement fixation this may lead to tissue injury.[26] Immunization of mice with *H. pylori* indeed induces anti-$Le^{x/y}$ Mabs that cross-react with gastric epithelium, in particular with gastric H$^+$,K$^+$-ATPase, the proton pump that is localized in the parietal cell canaliculi.[26–28] *H. pylori* infection in mice also induce autoantibodies that bind to parietal cells and that can be absorbed with synthetic Lewis antigens.[29] Thus in the murine system *H. pylori* induces autoantibodies through mimicry. Earlier experiments had already shown that high levels of circulating anti-Le^y monoclonal antibodies may damage the host.[30] It was already known that *H. pylori* infection in humans also induces autoantibodies that recognize gastric parietal cells[27,30] and in analogy with the *H. pylori* infection in mice, it was thought that those human autoantibodies also arose through mimicry. Indeed, in patient sera, high titers of antibodies to *H. pylori* LPS are found.[26] However, the epitope-specificity of human anti-*H. pylori* LPS remains enigmatic: in an initial study, anti-Le^x antibodies were found in a few patient sera.[26] However, in a larger survey comprising more than 100 patients, *H. pylori* infection was not found to induce anti-Le$^{x/y}$ antibodies in man.[31] In fact, anti-Le$^{x/y}$ antibodies occur naturally in sera from persons not infected by *H. pylori.* One exception to the rule that anti-Le$^{x/y}$ antibodies are not formed in humans might be non-secretors (persons that do not express Le^b in gastric mucosa) where low affinity, *H. pylori*-associated of anti-Le$^{x/y}$ antibodies were detected in serum.[32] The question remains to what epitopes of *H. pylori* LPS human antibodies are directed. Data have been presented that show that fucose is *not* part of the epitope recognized by human anti-*H. pylori* LPS antibodies but the nature of this epitope remains elusive.[33] Finally, antigastric autoantibodies present n sera of *H. pylori* infected patients are directed to gastric parietal canaliculi but absorption with *H. pylori* does not diminish autoantibody reactivity.[34] This shows that the autoantibodies are not due to mimicry. Thus, current evidence suggests that *H. pylori* Le$^{x/y}$ antigens do not induce autoantibodies in infected human patients. However, the studies discussed above all refer to measurements in serum, and it cannot be excluded that *H. pylori* induce anti-Le$^{x/y}$ antibodies locally that all bind to gastric mucosal epitopes.

5.2. Lewis Antigen Mimicry Provides Immune Escape

In analogy to the AB0 blood group antigens, a host that expresses Le^x would be expected to be able to form anti-Le^y but not anti-Le^x antibodies. Hence, a Le^x-positive *H. pylori* that infects a Le^x-positive host would escape immune attack and be able to persist, while a Le^y-positive strain would not escape and be eradicated. Experimental infection in Rhesus monkeys confirms this concept: an *H. pylori* strain isolated from Le^y-positive (as determined on gastric mucosa) animals expresses more Le^y than Le^x; the same strain expresses more Le^x than Le ^{y} when isolated after colonization of Le^x-positive animals.[35] Thus, the expression of *H. pylori* Le$^{x/y}$ epitopes depends on the host. How adaptation occurs was not investigated, but phase variation between Le^x and Le^y has been reported (see above). It is conceivable that *in vivo* outgrowth of Le^y-expressing *H. pylori* variants is favored because variant expressing Le^x are suppressed in Le^y-positive hosts that form anti-Le^x but not anti-Le^y antibodies.

In analogy with other pathogens, phase variation itself is a random process, and environmental pressure (antibodies, complement etc.) selects the phenotype that survives best. If indeed *H. pylori* infection of Rhesus monkeys induces anti-$Le^{x/y}$ antibodies was not investigated. Studies in humans gave far less consistent results and in two out of three studies no correlation between the Lewis phenotypes of host and pathogen was found.[8,36,37] In addition, strains expressing Le^x, and strains expressing Le^y can be isolated from a single patient, an additional argument against adaptation based on Lewis antigens. Finally, selection and outgrowth of *H. pylori* $Le^{x/y}$ LPS variants would be driven by anti-$Le^{x/y}$ antibodies, and these are not found in infected patients.[31]

5.3. *H. pylori* Lewis Antigens Mediate Adhesion and Colonization

The expression of $Le^{x/y}$ is crucial for *in vivo* colonization of mice: mutants with inactivated β1,4-GalT express a shorter LPS (see above) and do not colonize mice.[23] However, this does not prove that Lewis antigens per se are essential: from other Gram-negative pathogens it is known that shortening of LPS will lead to a decrease in virulence. Therefore a double knockout was created in which both α3-*fucT* genes (HP0379 and HP0651) were inactivated. This mutant expresses a long polylactosamine chain (i-antigen) and H type 1. The parent strain ($Le^{x/y}$ positive) colonized mice well, but the mutant did not (S.L. Martin, submitted) which demonstrates that $Le^{x/y}$ antigens are essential for colonization.

Recent data suggest that Le^x plays a role in adhesion. A Mab specific for *H. pylori* LPS inhibits adhesion of bacteria to gastric epithelial cells;[38] this Mab is specific for Le^x (B.J. Appelmelk and H. Yamaguchi, unpublished). Strains knocked-out in *galE* or *rfbM*, expressing either a truncated nontypable LPS or polymeric i-Ag, respectively, did not adhere to gastric tissue sections, while the parent (strain NCTC 11637, $Le^{x/y}$ positive) adhered well.[15] Infection studies with these two mutants have not yet been performed. In addition, synthetic Le^x coupled to bacterium-sized polystyrene beads bound to human gastric epithelial cells.[15] Clinical studies also suggest a role for $Le^{x/y}$ in adhesion: studies in gastritis patients demonstrated that *H. pylori* strains that expressed $Le^{x/y}$ strongly cause a higher colonization density than strains that express $Le^{x/y}$ weakly.[8] These data suggest that Le^x mediates colonization through adhesion and predicts the existence of gastric Le^x-binding lectins. Preliminary data of experimental studies confirmed this: Le^x-binding polypeptides of 16–29 kDa are found in gastric epithelial cells;[39] the identity of these proteins is unknown but the presence of low MW galactose-binding lectins (galectins) in the stomach has been reported. Other studies have shown that surfactant protein D, a lectin belonging to the innate defense system and expressed in the stomach, is able to bind *H. pylori* LPS;[40] which part of the

LPS is recognized is unknown. Thus, a role for LPS/$Le^{x/y}$ in adherence seems likely but this role is not absolute: $Le^{x/y}$ negative mutants adhered as strongly as their $Le^{x/y}$-positive parents when the strain expresses the Le^{b}-binding lectin BabA and when the host expresses Le^{b} (T. Boren, unpublished). In addition, $Le^{x/y}$-negative strains colonize human hosts well.[41] Thus a $Le^{x/y}$-lectin interaction may contribute to adhesion only for *H. pylori* strains that do not express BabA, or for strains that colonize non-secretors.

6. *Helicobacter pylori* AND AUTOIMMUNITY

In a considerable number of *H. pylori* infected patients serum autoantibodies develop that are directed to gastric parietal cells. As discussed above, molecular mimicry between *H. pylori* and the host is not involved in this autoimmune process. We will now review the present data that suggest a close relationship between classic autoimmune gastritis (AIG, type A gastritis) and *H. pylori* (type B) gastritis. Finally, a mechanism for mimicry-independent, *H. pylori*-induced autoimmunity is proposed.

6.1. From A to B: Autoimmune Gastritis and the Possible Pathogenic Role of *H. pylori* Infection

AIG is characterized histologically by a severe chronic inflammatory infiltration of the gastric corpus with gland destruction, mucosal atrophy and hyperplasia of endocrine cells. In contrast, the mucosa of the antrum is typically devoid of major histopathologic alterations.[42,43] In most cases of AIG, autoantibodies against parietal cells of the gastric mucosa can be found in the patients' serum. Furthermore, many patients develop pernicious anemia, which is accompanied by anti-intrinsic factor autoantibodies.[44]

In contrast to what is seen in patients with AIG, *H. pylori* induces an inflammatory response predominantly in the antrum mucosa.[42,43] Because of the absence of major pathologic alterations in the corpus mucosa, in particular atrophy, gastritis due to *H. pylori* (type B gastritis) was considered until recently a separate entity, clearly distinct from AIG.[45,46] However, in the last few years it has become evident, that many morphological features typical for AIG can also be found in a subset of *H. pylori* gastritis, i.e., body mucosal atrophy,[47,48] hyperplasia of endocrine cells[49] and periglandular infiltrates and gland destruction in the body mucosa.[50,51] Thus, AIG and a subtype of *H. pylori* gastritis show considerable morphological similarities and a clear differentiation between these entities might be difficult. Furthermore, some studies indicate that the development of parietal cell autoantibodies and AIG are preceded or accompanied by *H. pylori* infection.[51-55]

6.2. From B to A: *H. pylori* Gastritis and the Possible Pathogenic Role of Antigastric Autoimmune Reactions

More indications for a relationship between antigastric autoimmunity and *H. pylori* gastritis came from serological analysis in *H. pylori* gastritis. In older patients, the development of antiparietal cell antibodies is associated with *H. pylori* infection.[56] Additionally, some of the *H. pylori* infected patients, observed for 32 years were found to develop anti-parietal cell antibodies as well as chronic atrophic gastritis; finally, these patients became negative for *H. pylori*.[48] Also Negrini *et al.*,[30] reported on autoantibodies against gastric epithelial cells in up to 84% of *H. pylori*-infected subjects.

When sera of *H. pylori*-infected subjects were screened for autoantibodies reacting against human gastric tissue by immunohistochemistry, two different binding sites for these autoantibodies could be demonstrated;[57,58] firstly on the luminal membranes of the foveolar epithelial cells in the antrum and corpus mucosa and secondly on the canalicular membranes of parietal cells in the gastric corpus mucosa. The latter type of autoantibodies was named anticanalicular autoantibodies. The immunohistochemical binding pattern of these anticanalicular autoantibodies is shown in Figure 3.

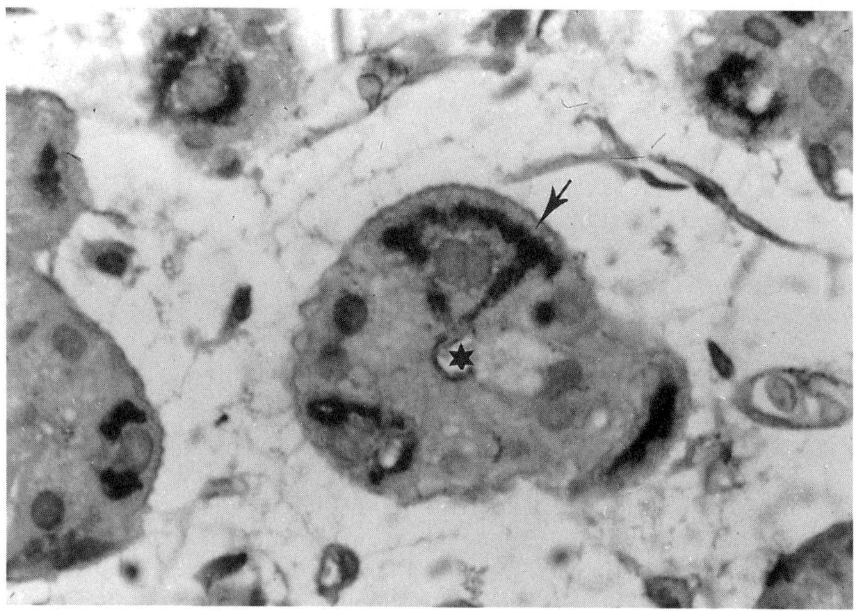

FIGURE 3. Anticanalicular autoantibodies (arrow) in serum of a *H. pylori*-infected patient A microscopic section of the corpus of a non-infected person was incubated with serum from a patient infected with *H. pylori* and stained immunohistochemically. In the middle the lumen of a gland (star) is seen.

Box 1. Evidence for the clinical relevance of antigastric autoimmunity in *H. pylori* gastritis

- severity of body gastritis[27,58]
- increased apoptosis in the corpus mucosa[59]
- body mucosa atrophy[27,31,57,58,60–62]
- higher serum gastrin levels[52,57,58]
- lower pepsinogen levels[58]
- lower gastric acid secretion[63,64]

Both types of antigastric autoantibodies were significantly correlated with *H. pylori* infection. The prevalence of these autoantibodies in *H. pylori*-infected subjects was 30 and 40%, respectively. Anticanalicular autoantibodies showed the strongest association with *H. pylori* gastritis and were analyzed in greater detail.[58]

7. CLINICAL RELEVANCE OF ANTICANALICULAR AUTOANTIBODIES IN *H. pylori* GASTRITIS

In several studies the clinical relevance of antigastric autoimmunity was investigated. Interestingly, the presence of anticanalicular autoantibodies correlates with various histological and clinical parameters of gastric body mucosa atrophy (Box 1). There is no evidence that autoantibodies against the luminal membranes of the foveolar epithelium have any clinical relevance.

8. THE GASTRIC H^+,K^+-ATPASE AS AUTOANTIGEN IN ATROPHIC *H. pylori* GASTRITIS

The close relationship between *H. pylori* gastritis with anticanalicular autoimmunity and AIG is illustrated further by determination of the fine specificity of anticanalicular antibodies. Anticanalicular autoantibodies were detected in 100% of patients with AIG and in about 40% of patients with *H. pylori* gastritis. By immunoprecipitation with the recombinant murine gastric H^+,K^+-ATPase we could show that 50% of *H. pylori* infected patients with anticanalic-ular autoantibodies have autoantibodies against the α and/or β subunits of this enzyme, which is also the key target in classical AIG. In these studies a significant association between anticanalicular/anti-H^+,K^+-ATPase autoantibodies and gastric mucosa atrophy was confirmed. Thus, the anti-H^+,K^+-ATPase reactivity represents not only a marker for classic AIG but also for atrophic *H. pylori* gastritis.[31] It is therefore conceivable that corpus atrophy is autoimmune-mediated, and that at least part of the cases of AIG are due to prior infection with *H. pylori*.[65]

9. A MODEL FOR THE PATHOGENESIS OF *H. pylori* ASSOCIATED ANTIGASTRIC AUTOIMMUNITY

The model is based on the premise that infection with *H. pylori* infection leads to loss of immunological privilege of the gastric mucosa.[31,66,67] It is generally believed that in the uninfected stomach this mucosa is controlled immunologically only by a few scattered intraepithelial lymphocytes. The major alteration in the course of chronic *H. pylori* infection is the influx of B and T cells and the acquisition of a mucosa associated lymphoid tissue. Thus, cells of the immune system can come into close contact with (auto-) antigens, against which no tolerance has been established during the development of the immune system. These autoantigens can be effectively presented to T-cells that subsequently become activated. The autoreactive T cells could provide help for B cell stimulation and autoantibody production. This is a plausible model for the development of mimicry-independent, *H. pylori*-associated antigastric autoimmunity.

Recent data indicate that T-helper 1 (Th1) cells are predominant over Th2 cells in chronic *H. pylori* gastritis.[68–70] This T-cell population could induce MHC class II expression in the gastric epithelium via interferon γ secretion.[71–73] At the same time, interferon γ might give rise to the coexpression of B7-1 (CD80) and B7-2 (CD86) as co-stimulatory factors in gastric mucosa;[74] thus the essential requirements for presentation of autoantigens by gastric epithelium cells are fulfilled, and stimulation and proliferation of autoreactive T is enabled. The loss of glands in the mucosa, i.e., the development of gastric atrophy, could be thus caused by an autoimmune T-cell attack against epithelial cells rather than through autoantibodies. Consequently, antigastric autoantibodies would only serve as marker for ongoing antigastric autoimmunity mainly carried out by autoreactive T cells.

It is interesting that the pathogenic process for the initiation of antigastric autoimmunity in *H. pylori* gastritis needs time. In a twelve year follow-up study a significant increase of anticanalicular autoantibodies in subjects who were chronically infected with *H. pylori* was observed.[60] In addition, the prevalence of this type of autoantibodies is lower in the pediatric population, where the duration of *H. pylori* infection is much shorter.[75–77] Of importance, cure of *H. pylori* infection leads to a rapid decrease of antigastric autoantibodies in the majority of patients.[78]

10. QUESTIONS FOR FUTURE RESEARCH

The severity of gastric inflammation and development of peptic ulcers depend on the presence the cag-pathogenicity island. Future research will show if bacterial factors that contribute to gastric autoimmunity can be identified. It has been shown that certain polymorphisms in the members of Interleukin gene family are associated with development of gastric cancer.[79] Likewise, it is conceivable that host factors will be identified that contribute to development of gastric autoimmunity. Further research should also focus on the role of T-cells in chronic gastritis, particularly in human AIG, atrophic *H. pylori* gastritis and/or in *H. pylori* gastritis with antigastric autoantibodies. One might predict that autoreactive T-cells are present both in AIG and in *H. pylori*-associated gastric autoimmunity but no data are available yet. The characterization of epitope-specificities of human anti-H^+,K^+-ATPase antibodies from *H. pylori*-infected patients and AIG, respectively, might show whether the latter type of antibodies evolve through epitope spreading from the first one. Of clinical importance, it is important whether eradication of *H. pylori* after (early) detection of gastric autoantibodies will reduce the development of AIG and pernicious anemia.

ACKNOWLEDGMENT. We thank A. H. M. Van Vliet for his indispensable help with Reference Manager.

REFERENCES

1. Aspinall G. O., and Monteiro M. A., 1996, Lipopolysaccharides of *Helicobacter pylori* strains P466 and MO19: structures of the O antigen and core oligosaccharide regions, *Biochemistry* **35**:2498.
2. Aspinall G. O., Monteiro M. A., Pang H., Walsh E. J., and Moran A. P., 1996, Lipopolysaccharide of the *Helicobacter pylori* type strain NCTC 11637 (ATCC 43504): Structure of the O antigen chain and core oligosaccharide regions, *Biochemistry* **35**:2489.
3. Monteiro M. A., Appelmelk B. J., Rasko D. A., Moran A. P., Hynes S. O., MacLean L. L., Chan K. H., Michael F. S., Logan S. M., O'Rourke J., Lee A., Taylor D. E., and Perry M. B., 2000, Lipopolysaccharide structures of *Helicobacter pylori* genomic strains 26695 and J99, mouse model *H. pylori* Sydney strain, *H. pylori* P466 carrying sialyl Lewis X, and *H. pylori* UA915 expressing Lewis B Classification of *H. pylori* lipopolysaccharides into glycotype families, *Eur. J. Biochem.* **267**:305.
4. Monteiro M. A., Chan K. H., Rasko D. A., Taylor D. E., Zheng P. Y., Appelmelk B. J., Wirth H. P., Yang M., Blaser M. J., Hynes S. O., Moran A. P., and Perry M. B., 1998, Simultaneous expression of type 1 and type 2 Lewis blood group antigens by *Helicobacter pylori* lipopolysaccharides. Molecular mimicry between *H. pylori* lipopolysaccharides and human gastric epithelial cell surface glycoforms, *J. Biol. Chem.* **273**:11533.
5. Monteiro M. A., Zheng P. Y., Ho B., Yokata S. I., Amano K., Berg D. E., Chan K. H., MacLean L. L., and Perry M. B., 2000, Expression of histo-blood group antigens by lipopolysaccharides of *Helicobacter pylori* strains from Asian hosts: the propensity to express type 1 blood group antigens, *Glycobiology*, in press.
6. Simoons-Smit I. M., Appelmelk B. J., Verboom T., Negrini R., Penner J. L., Aspinall G. O., Moran A. P., Fei S. F., Shi B. S., Rudnica W., Savio A., and de Graaff J., 1996, Typing of *Helicobacter pylori* with monoclonal antibodies against Lewis antigens in lipopolysaccharide, *J. Clin. Microbiol.* **34**:2196.
7. Wirth H. P., Karita M., Yang M., and Blaser M. J., 1996, Expression of Lewis X and Y blood group antigens by *Helicobacter pylori* strains is related to cagA status, *Gastroenterology* **110**:A296.
8. Heneghan M. A., McCarthy C. F., and Moran A. P., 2000, Relationship of blood group determinants on *Helicobacter pylori* lipopolysaccharide with host lewis phenotype and inflammatory response *Infect. Immun.* **68**:937.

9. Knirel Y. A., Kocharova N. A., Hynes S. O., Widmalm G., Andersen L. P., Jansson P. E., and Moran A. P., 1999, Structural studies on lipopolysaccharides of serologically non-typable strains of *Helicobacter pylori*, AF1 and 007, expressing Lewis antigenic determinants, *Eur. J. Biochem.* **266**:123.
10. Kocharova N. A., Knirel Y. A., Widmalm G., Jansson P. E., and Moran A. P., 2000, Structure of an atypical O-antigen polysaccharide of *Helicobacter pylori* containing a novel monosaccharide 3-C-methyl-D-mannose, *Biochemistry* **39**:4755.
11. Tomb J. F., White O., Kerlavage A. R., Clayton R. A., Sutton G. G., Fleischmann R. D., Ketchum K. A., Klenk H. P., Gill S., Dougherty B. A., Nelson K., Quackenbush J., Zhou L., Kirkness E. F., Peterson S., Loftus B., Richardson D., Dodson R., Khalak H. G., Glodek A., McKenney K., Fitzegerald L. M., Lee N., Adams M. D., and Venter J. C., 1997, The complete genome sequence of the gastric pathogen *Helicobacter pylori*, *Nature* **388**:539.
12. Alm R. A., Ling L. S., Moir D. T., King B. L., Brown E. D., Doig P. C., Smith D. R., Noonan B., Guild B. C., deJonge B. L., Carmel G., Tummino P. J., Caruso A., Uria-Nickelsen M., Mills D. M., Ives C., Gibson R., Merberg D., Mills S. D., Jiang Q., Taylor D. E., Vovis G. F., and Trust T. J., 1999, Genomic-sequence comparison of two unrelated isolates of the human gastric pathogen *Helicobacter pylori*, *Nature* **397**:176.
13. Berg D. E., Hoffman P. S., Appelmelk B. J., and Kusters J. G., 1997, The *Helicobacter pylori* genome sequence: genetic factors for long life in the gastric mucosa, *Trends. Microbiol.* **5**:468.
14. McGowan C. C., Necheva A., Thompson S. A., Cover T. L., and Blaser M. J., 1998, Acid-induced expression of an LPS-associated gene in *Helicobacter pylori*, *Mol. Microbiol.* **30**:19.
15. Edwards N. J., Monteiro M. A., Faller G., Walsh E. J., Moran A. P., Roberts I. S., and High N. J., 2000, Lewis X structures in the O antigen side-chain promote adhesion of *Helicobacter pylori* to the gastric epithelium, *Mol. Microbiol.* **35**:1530.
16. Kwon D. H., Woo J. S., Perng C. L., Go M. F., Graham D. Y., and El Zaatari F. A., 1998, The effect of galE gene inactivation on lipopolysaccharide profile of *Helicobacter pylori*, *Curr. Microbiol.* **37**:144.
17. Ge Z. M., Chan N. W. C., Palcic M. M., and Taylor D. E., 1997, Cloning and heterologous expression of an alpha 1,3- fucosyltransferase gene from the gastric pathogen *Helicobacter pylori*, *J. Biol. Chem.* **272**:21357.
18. Martin S. L., Edbrooke M. R., Hodgman T. C., van den Eijnden D. H., and Bird M. I., 1997, Lewis X biosynthesis in *Helicobacter pylori*. Molecular cloning of an alpha(1,3)-fucosyltransferase gene, *J. Biol. Chem.* **272**:21349.
19. Appelmelk B. J., Martin S. L., Monteiro M. A., Clayton C. A., McColm A. A., Zheng P. Y., Verboom T., Maaskant J. J., van den Eijnden D. H., Hokke C. H., Perry M. B., Vandenbroucke-Grauls C. M. J. E., and Kusters J. G., 1999, Phase variation in *Helicobacter pylori* lipopolysaccharide due to changes in the lengths of poly(C) tracts in alpha 3- fucosyltransferase genes, *Infect. Immun.* **67**:5361.
20. Rasko D. A., Wang G., Palcic M. M., and Taylor D. E., 2000, Cloning and characterization of the alpha(1,3/4) fucosyltransferase of *Helicobacter pylori*, *J. Biol. Chem.* **275**:4988.
21. Wang G., Rasko D. A., Sherburne R., and Taylor D. E., 1999, Molecular genetic basis for the variable expression of Lewis Y antigen in *Helicobacter pylori*: analysis of the alpha (1,2) fucosyltransferase gene, *Mol. Microbiol.* **31**:1265.
22. Wang G., Boulton P. G., Chan N. W., Palcic M. M., and Taylor D. E., 1999, Novel *Helicobacter pylori* alpha1,2-fucosyltransferase, a key enzyme in the synthesis of Lewis antigens, *Microbiology* **145**:3245.
23. Logan S. M., Conlan J. W., Monteiro M. A., Wakarchuk W. W., and Altman E., 2000, Functional genomics of *Helicobacter pylori*: identification of a beta-1,4 galactosyltransferase and generation of mutants with altered lipopolysaccharide, *Mol. Microbiol.* **35**:1156.
24. Appelmelk B. J., Shiberu B., Trinks C., Tapsi N., Zheng P. Y., Verboom T., Maaskant J., Hokke C. H., Schiphorst W. E., Blanchard D., Simoons-Smit I. M., van den Eijnden D. H., and

Vandenbroucke-Grauls C. M., 1998, Phase variation in *Helicobacter pylori* lipopolysaccharide, *Infect. Immun.* **66**:70.

25. Appelmelk B. J., Wirth H. P., Lansbergen R., Schilders I., Martin S. L., Verboom T., and Vandenbroucke-Grauls C. M. J. E., 1999, *H. pylori* diversifies in the human host through lipopolysaccharide phase variation, *Gut* **45**:A23.
26. Appelmelk B. J., Simoons-Smit I., Negrini R., Moran A. P., Aspinall G. O., Forte J. G., De Vries T., Quan H., Verboom T., Maaskant J. J., Ghiara P., Kuipers E. J., Bloemena E., Tadema T. M., Townsend R. R., Tyagarajan K., Crothers Jr J. M., Monteiro M. A., Savio A., and de Graaff J., 1996, Potential role of molecular mimicry between *Helicobacter pylori* lipopolysaccharide and host Lewis blood group antigens in autoimmunity, *Infect. Immun.* **64**:2031.
27. Negrini R., Savio A., Poiesi C., Appelmelk B. J., Buffoli F., Paterlini A., Cesari P., Graffeo M., Vaira D., and Franzin G., 1996, Antigenic mimicry between *Helicobacter pylori* and gastric mucosa in the pathogenesis of body atrophic gastritis, *Gastroenterology* **111**:655.
28. Appelmelk B. J., Negrini R., Moran A. P., and Kuipers E. J., 1997, Molecular mimicry between *Helicobacter pylori* and the host, *Trends Microbiol.* **5**:70.
29. Guruge J. L., Falk P. G., Lorenz R. G., Dans M., Wirth H. P., Blaser M. J., Berg D. E., and Gordon J. I., 1998, Epithelial attachment alters the outcome of *Helicobacter pylori* infection, *Proc. Natl. Ac. Sc. USA* **95**:3925.
30. Negrini R., Lisato L., Zanella I., Cavazzini L., Gullini S., Villanacci V., Poiesi C., Albertini A., and Ghielmi S., 1991, *Helicobacter pylori* infection induces antibodies cross-reacting with human gastric mucosa, *Gastroenterology* **101**:437.
31. Claeys D., Faller G., Appelmelk B. J., Negrini R., and Kirchner T., 1998, The gastric H^+,K^+-ATPase is a major autoantigen in chronic *Helicobacter pylori* gastritis with body mucosa atrophy, *Gastroenterology* **115**:340.
32. Kurtenkov O., Klaamas K., Miljukhina L., Shljapnikova L., Ellamaa M., Bovin N., and Wadstrom T., 1999, IgG antibodies to Lewis type 2 antigens in serum of *H. pylori*-infected and noninfected blood donors of different Lewis(a,b) blood-group phenotype, *FEMS Immunol. Med. Microbiol.* **24**:227.
33. Yokota S. I., Amano K. I., Shibata Y., Nakajima M., Suzuki M., Hayashi S., Fujii N., and Yokochi T., 2000, Two distinct antigenic types of the polysaccharide chains of *Helicobacter pylori* lipopolysaccharides characterized by reactivity with sera from humans with natural infection, *Infect. Immun.* **68**:151.
34. Faller G., Steininger H., Appelmelk B., and Kirchner T., 1998, Evidence of novel pathogenic pathways for the formation of antigastric autoantibodies in *Helicobacter pylori* gastritis, *J. Clin. Pathol.* **51**:244.
35. Wirth H. P., Yang M., Dubois A., Berg D. E., and Blaser M. J., 1998, Host Lewis phenotype-dependent selection of H-pylori Lewis expression in rhesus monkeys, *Gut* **43**:A26.
36. Wirth H. P., Yang M., Peek Jr R. M., Tham K. T., and Blaser M. J., 1997, *Helicobacter pylori* Lewis expression is related to the host Lewis phenotype, *Gastroenterology* **113**:1091.
37. Taylor D. E., Rasko D. A., Sherburne R., Ho C., and Jewell L. D., 1998, Lack of correlation between Lewis antigen expression by *Helicobacter pylori* and gastric epithelial cells in infected patients, *Gastroenterology* **115**:1113.
38. Osaki T., Yamaguchi H., Taguchi H., Fukuda M., Kawakami H., Hirano H., Watanabe S., Takagi A., and Kamiya S., 1998, Establishment and characterization of a monoclonal antibody to inhibit adhesion of *Helicobacter pylori* to gastric epithelial cells, *J. Med. Microbiol.* **47**:505.
39. Campbell B. J., Rogerson K. A., and Rhodes J. M., 1999, Adherence of *Helicobacter pylori* to human gastric epithelium mediated by an epithelial cell-surface Lewis(x) carbohydrate- binding protein, *Gastroenterology* **116**:G0565.
40. Eggleton P., Murray E., Dodds A., Worku M., Karim Q., Walker M., Ferris J., Moran A., Appelmelk B., Reid K., and Thursz M., 1999, Surfactant protein D binding to *Helicobacter pylori* lipopolysaccharide, *Gut* **45**:A35.

41. Rasko D. A., Wilson T. J., Zopf D., and Taylor D. E., 2000, Lewis antigen expression and stability in *Helicobacter pylori* isolated from serial gastric biopsies, *J. Infect. Dis.* **181**:1089.
42. Correa P., Chronic gastritis, 1995, in *Gastrointestinal and oesophageal pathology*, R. Whitehead, ed., Churchill Livingstone, New York.
43. Dixon M. F., Genta R. M., Yardley J. H., and Correa P., 1996, Classification and grading of gastritis. The updated Sydney System. International Workshop on the Histopathology of Gastritis, Houston 1994, *Am. J. Surg. Pathol.* **20**:1161.
44. Toh B. H., van Driel I. R., and Gleeson P. A., 1997, Pernicious anemia, *N. Engl. J. Med.* **337**:1441.
45. Price A. B., 1992, The Sydney System: histological division., *J. Gastroenterol. Hepatol.* **6**:209.
46. Wyatt J. I., and Dixon M. F., 1988, Chronic gastritis—a pathogenic approach, *J. Pathol.* **154**:113.
47. Kuipers E. J., Uyterlinde A. M., Pena A. S., Roosendaal R., Pals G., Nelis G. F., Festen H. P., and Meuwissen S. G., 1995, Long-term sequelae of *Helicobacter pylori* gastritis, *Lancet* **345**:1525.
48. Valle J., Kekki M., Sipponen P., Ihamaki T., and Siurala M., 1996, Long-term course and consequences of *Helicobacter pylori* gastritis. Results of a 32-year follow-up study, *Scand. J. Gastroenterol.* **31**:546.
49. Maaroos H. I., Havu N., and Sipponen P., 1998, Follow-up of *Helicobacter pylori* positive gastritis and argyrophil cells pattern during the natural course of gastric ulcer, *Helicobacter* **3**:39.
50. Stolte M., Baumann K., Bethke B., Ritter M., Lauer E., and Eidt H., 1992, Active autoimmune gastritis without total atrophy of the glands, *Z. Gastroenterol.* **30**:729.
51. Eidt S., Oberhuber G., Schneider A., and Stolte M., 1996, The histopathological spectrum of type A gastritis, *Pathol. Res. Pract.* **192**:101.
52. Faisal M. A., Russell R. M., Samloff I. M., and Holt P. R., 1990, *Helicobacter pylori* infection and atrophic gastritis in the elderly, *Gastroenterology* **99**:1543.
53. Cariani G., Bonora G., Vandelli A., Mazzoleni G., and Fontana G., 1991, *Helicobacter pylori* in autoimmune gastritis, *Gastroenterology* **101**:759.
54. Karnes W. J., Samloff I. M., Siurala M., Kekki M., Sipponen P., Kim S. W., and Walsh J. H., 1991, Positive serum antibody and negative tissue staining for *Helicobacter pylori* in subjects with atrophic body gastritis, *Gastroenterology* **101**:167.
55. Ma J. Y., Borch K., Sjostrand S. E., Janzon L., and Mardh S., 1994, Positive correlation between H,K-adenosine triphosphatase autoantibodies and *Helicobacter pylori* antibodies in patients with pernicious anemia, *Scand. J. Gastroenterol.* **29**:961.
56. Uibo R., Vorobjova T., Metskula K., Kisand K., Wadstrom T., and Kivik T., 1995, Association of *Helicobacter pylori* and gastric autoimmunity: a population-based study, *FEMS Immunol. Med. Microbiol.* **11**:65.
57. Faller G., Steininger H., Eck M., Hensen J., Hann E. G., and Kirchner T., 1996, Antigastric autoantibodies in *Helicobacter pylori* gastritis: prevalence, in-situ binding sites and clues for clinical relevance, *Virchows Arch.* **427**:483.
58. Faller G., Steininger H., Kranzlein J., Maul H., Kerkau T., Hensen J., Hahn E. G., and Kirchner T., 1997, Antigastric autoantibodies in *Helicobacter pylori* infection: implications of histological and clinical parameters of gastritis, *Gut* **41**:619.
59. Steininger H., Faller G., Dewald E., Brabletz T., Jung A., and Kirchner T., 1998, Apoptosis in chronic gastritis and its correlation with antigastric autoantibodies, *Virchows Arch.* **433**:13.
60. Vorobjova T., Faller G., Maaroos H. I., Sipponen P., Villako K., Uibo R., and Kirchner T., 2000, Significant increase in antigastric autoantibodies in a long-term follow-up study of *H. pylori* gastritis, *Virchows Arch.* in press.
61. Fixa B., Malfertheiner P., Tuschy P., Komarkova O., and Nozicka Infekce Z., 1995, *Helicobacter pylori* a zaludecni autoimunita—spolecne etiopatogeneticke mechanismy u chronicke gastridy, *Ces. a Slov. Gastroen.* **49**:147.
62. Saxena V., Asante M., Mendall M. A., Neira N., Zaitoun A. M., and Northfield T. C., 1998, Gastric parietal cell antibodies are associated with an altered distribution of *Helicobacter pylori* and increased body atrophy., *Gut* **42** (suppl 1):A79.

63. Faller G., Winter M., Steininger H., Konturek P., Konturek S. J., and Kirchner T., 1998, Antigastric autoantibodies and gastric secretory function in *Helicobacter pylori*-infected patients with duodenal ulcer and non-ulcer dyspepsia, *Scand. J. Gastroenterol.* **33**:276.
64. Parente F., Negrini R., Imbesi V., Maconi G., Cucino C., and Bianchi Porro G., 1999, The presence of gastric autoantibodies impairs gastric secretory function in patients with *H. pylori*-positive duodenal ulcer, *Gut* **45** (suppl 3):A40.
65. Appelmelk B. J., Faller G., Claeys D., Kirchner T., and Vandenbroucke-Grauls C. M., 1998, Bugs on trial: the case of *Helicobacter pylori* and autoimmunity, *Immunol. Today* **19**:296.
66. Fallerand G., and Kirchner T., 2000, Role of antigastric autoantibodies in chronic *Helicobacter pylori* infection, *Microsc. Res. Tech.* **48**:321.
67. Kirchner T., Faller G., and Price A., 1998, The year in *Helicobacter pylori* 1998: Pathology and autoimmunity., *Curr. Opin. Gastroenterol.* **14** (suppl 1):S35–S39.
68. Sommer F., Faller G., Konturek P., Kirchner T., Hahn E. G., Zeus J. R. L. M., and Lohoff M., 1998, Antrum- and Corpus Mucosa-Infiltrating CD4(+) Lymphocytes in *Helicobacter pylori* Gastritis Display a Th1 Phenotype, *Infect. Immun.* **66**:5543.
69. Bamford K. B., Fan X., Crowe S. E., Leary J. F., Gourley W. K., Luthra G. K., Brooks E. G., Graham D. Y., Reyes V. E., and Ernst P. B., 1998, Lymphocytes in the human gastric mucosa during *Helicobacter pylori* have a T helper cell 1 phenotype, *Gastroenterology* **114**:482.
70. D'Elios M. M., Manghetti M., De Carli M., Costa F., Baldari C. T., Burroni D., Telford J. L., Romagnani S., and Del Prete G., 1997, T helper 1 effector cells specific for *Helicobacter pylori* in the gastric antrum of patients with peptic ulcer disease, *J. Immunol.* **158**:962.
71. Engstrand L., Scheynius A., Pahlson C., Grimelius L., Schwan A., and Gustavsson S., 1989, Association of *Campylobacter pylori* with induced expression of class II transplantation antigens on gastric epithelial cells, *Infect. Immun.* **57**:827.
72. Kirchner T., Melber A., Fischbach W., Heilmann K. L., and Müller-Hermelink H. K., Immunohistological patterns of the local immune response in *Helicobacter pylori* gastritis, 1990, in *Helicobacter pylori, gastritis and peptic ulcer*, P. Malfertheiner and H. Ditschuneit, eds., Springer-Verlag, Berlin, Heidelberg.
73. Haeberle H. A., Kubin M., Bamford K. B., Garofalo R., Graham D. Y., El-Zaatari F., Karttunen R., Crowe S. E., Reyes V. E., and Ernst P. B., 1997, Differential stimulation of interleukin-12 (IL-12) and IL-10 by live and killed *Helicobacter pylori in vitro* and association of IL-12 production with gamma interferon-producing T cells in the human gastric mucosa, *Infect. Immun.* **65**:4229.
74. Ye G., Barrera C., Fan X., Gourley W. K., Crowe S. E., Ernst P. B., and Reyes V. E., 1997, Expression of B7-1 and B7-2 costimulatory molecules by human gastric epithelial cells, *J. Clin. Invest.* **99**:1628.
75. Ierardi E., Francavilla R., Balzano T., Negrini R., and Francavilla A., 1998, Autoantibodies reacting with gastric antigens in associated body gastritis of dyspeptic children, *Ital. J. Gastroenterol. Hepatol.* **30**:478.
76. Faller G., Steininger H., Keller K. M., Kühlwein D., and Kirchner T., 1999, *Helicobacter pylori* gastritis and antigastric autoantibodies in children and adolescents, *Pathol. Res. Pract.* **195**:302.
77. Kolho K. L., Jusufovic J., Miettinen A., Savilahti E., and Rautelin H., 2000, Parietal cell antibodies and *Helicobacter pylori* in children, *J. Pediatr. Gastroenterol. Nutr.* **30**:265.
78. Faller G., Winter M., Steininger H., Lehn N., Meining A., Bayerdorffer E., and Kirchner T., 1999, Decrease of antigastric autoantibodies in *Helicobacter pylori* gastritis after cure of infection, *Pathol. Res. Pract.* **195**:243.
79. El Omar E. M., Carrington M., Chow W. H., McColl K. E., Bream J. H., Young H. A., Herrera J., Lissowska J., Yuan C. C., Rothman N., Lanyon G., Martin M., Fraumeni Jr J. F., and Rabkin C. S., 2000, Interleukin-1 polymorphisms associated with increased risk of gastric cancer, *Nature* **404**:398.

10

Apoptosis and the Pathogenesis of *Helicobacter pylori*—Related Disease

EMILIA MIA SORDILLO[1,2] and STEVEN F. MOSS[2]

1. INTRODUCTION

It is an unavoidable, but intriguing, fact that chronic colonization of the stomach by *Helicobacter pylori* has no obvious deleterious consequences in most people. Approximately 10% of all infected individuals will develop a peptic ulcer, and half of those will commence a slow progression of pre-neoplastic changes that will ultimately lead to frank cancer in only a few.[1] Why are certain individuals or populations predisposed to particular clinical outcomes after infection with *H. pylori*? The genetic background of the individual, the timing of first infection, environmental factors, and variations in the degree of bacterial pathogenicity all may contribute to the outcome of infection. One physiologic process that can be influenced by these variables is apoptosis, which when deregulated causes abnormal cell turnover, alterations in epithelial cell subpopulations, and changes in mucosal mass.

Under normal circumstances, apoptosis, sometimes called programmed cell death, is a mechanism by which superfluous or potentially deleterious cells can be

---

EMILIA MIA SORDILLO • Department of Pathology & Laboratory Medicine. STEVEN F. MOSS • Department of Medicine, St. Luke's-Roosevelt Hospital Center/Columbia University New York, NY 10025.

Helicobacter pylori Infection and Immunity,
Edited by Yamamoto *et al.*, Kluwer Academic/Plenum Publishers, 2002.

eliminated. Induction of apoptosis out of the appropriate context is an important factor in the ability of many bacteria to cause disease. There is now consistent and convincing evidence from clinical, animal, and cell culture studies that apoptosis of gastric epithelial cells can be induced by *H. pylori*. Some bacteria, such as *Shigella* and *Listeria*, are well documented to cause apoptosis of neutrophils and macrophages, and this effect on inflammatory cells is a major factor in evasion of host response by those organisms. In contrast, there is little information about the ability of *H. pylori* to induce apoptosis of inflammatory cells. Thus, this review will focus primarily on induction of apoptosis in epithelial cells, and its relationship to the development of disease in *H. pylori*-infected individuals.

As proposed by Zychlinsky and Sansonetti,[2] apoptosis may contribute to pathogenesis in bacterial infections through initiation of inflammation, massive cell deletion, or by inhibition of apoptosis. A role for each of these may be important in the major clinical syndromes that have been linked to *H. pylori* infection. A fairly straightforward connection can be made between ulcer formation or development of atrophy and cell loss. Similarly, a number of studies have evaluated release of inflammatory mediators and the role of inflammatory cells in ulcer development. Inhibition of apoptosis may be a factor in initiation of gastric cancer or lymphoma of the mucosa-associated lymphoid tissue (MALT lymphoma) as a consequence of *H. pylori* infection.

In addition, apoptosis due to *H. pylori* may be important as a stimulus for hyperproliferation and increased cell turnover. It is clear that infection with *H. pylori* is associated with epithelial cell hyperproliferation.[3] Increased numbers of cycling epithelial cells have been noted in *H. pylori*-associated gastritis and in the spectrum of pre-neoplastic histological conditions associated with *H. pylori* infection, as well as in gastric cancer. Although some evidence exists for direct stimulation of proliferation by *H. pylori*, the majority of studies indicate that proliferation is more likely to be a compensatory mechanism, in response to cell deletion. Increased cell turnover is a common feature of many inflammatory, premalignant, and malignant conditions, including chronic gastritis and gastric cancer. In many schema, hyperproliferation caused by inflammation is thought to lead to neoplastic transformation due to the increased chance that a mutant cell will arise during active proliferation. The realization that *H. pylori* is the major cause of chronic gastritis and is closely associated with development of gastric cancer has renewed interest in the effects of *H. pylori* on mucosal epithelial cell kinetics and cell turnover.

2. EVIDENCE OF APOPTOSIS IN HUMAN INFECTION WITH *H. pylori*

Cells carrying degraded DNA, a characteristic feature of apoptosis, can be identified in tissues by terminal deoxynucleotidyl nick end labeling (TUNEL).

Using this method, we and others have demonstrated that the numbers of apoptotic epithelial and inflammatory cells in tissue sections from gastric biopsies are increased in *H. pylori* infection by two to five fold.[4] Eradication of *H. pylori* reduces both apoptosis and proliferation to normal levels. The majority of investigators have shown that the apoptotic epithelial cells found in association with *H. pylori* are located mainly at the gastric lumen, at the site of physiological or "senescent" apoptosis. However, apoptotic epithelial cells have been described throughout the gastric gland, and in *H. pylori* infection they have been observed close to the proliferative zone, where they may represent newly formed mutants which have been eliminated by a self-defensive, altruistic cell death program. Although most studies have examined gastric antral biopsies, we have also found increased epithelial apoptosis in the gastric corpus when *H. pylori* is present.[5] Of note, it has been suggested by two independent groups that apoptosis is increased more by strains of *H. pylori* which did not express CagA, usually considered a marker of more virulent strains,[6,7] but our prospective study failed to confirm this finding.[5]

Although these findings from observational immunohistochemical and epidemiologic studies are highly suggestive, the mechanisms responsible for *H. pylori*—induced apoptosis cannot be determined directly by examination of patient material. Similarly, it is difficult to distinguish among effects caused by bacterial-epithelial cell contact, bacterial products, or components of the associated inflammatory response.

Is apoptosis in *H. pylori* infection a consequence of the inflammatory response? The rapid normalization of increased epithelial apoptosis after the eradication of *H. pylori*, despite the persistence of chronic inflammatory cells, argues against a determining role for the chronic inflammatory infiltrate in the etiology of the increased apoptosis. Attempts to correlate increased apoptosis with parameters of either acute or chronic inflammation have also failed to demonstrate an absolute link between inflammation and apoptosis. However, this should not be construed to mean the inflammatory reaction to *H. pylori* is not important in disease development, especially as the measurement of apoptosis (by TUNEL) and inflammation (by quantitative counting of inflammatory cell numbers) are fairly imprecise. Indeed, increased expression of the CD95 Fas receptor and increased Fas ligand mRNA has been reported in both epithelial cell and inflammatory cell populations in gastric biopsies from infected patients.[8,9] These findings suggest that epithelial cells may be stimulated to undergo apoptosis because of Fas/Fas ligand interactions between the epithelial cell and lymphocytes, or between adjacent epithelial cells—death by "fratricide". A positive relationship between autoantibodies directed against the parietal cell proton pump and apoptosis of these acid-secreting cells was found in one study,[10] and, if corroborated, these findings suggest a link between death of the parietal cell subpopulation and the subsequent development of atrophy. One implication is that autoimmune processes triggered by *H. pylori* may account for the development of gastritis in some individuals.

3. ANIMAL MODELS

The development of animal models has provided new opportunities to study the natural history and long-term sequelae of *H. pylori* infection. Animal models have been used to examine the role of host genetic variability in the pathogenesis of *H. pylori*-related disease. In inbred mice, variations in genetic background determine both the location and extent of the epithelial cell and inflammatory response to gastric *Helicobacter* species. Better understanding of the host's response to *H. pylori* colonization may clarify why only a fraction of *H. pylori*-infected individuals develop active disease, or why disease manifestations differ among those who do.

Host differences in the apoptotic response may be responsible for some of the divergent responses observed, since cell turnover is dependent on both new cell production by proliferation and cell loss by apoptosis. For example, three different, genetically-defined strains of mice had markedly different responses to experimental infection with the *H. pylori*-related animal pathogen, *H.felis.* Both proliferation and apoptosis of the gastric epithelial cells were increased after six weeks in one of the mouse strains (C57BL/6), but not in the two others.[11] The increased cell turnover in the C57BL/6 mice was associated with a loss of highly specialized acid and pepsin-secreting cells and an expansion of an aberrant gastric mucus lineage. A fall in *Helicobacter* colonization density with time was also noted. Since C57BL/6 mice were recently identified as deficient in secretory phospholipase A2, a product of the MOM1 gene (a known modulator of colonic polyp formation in the model of human adenomatous polyposis coli), it has been postulated that secretory phospholipase A2 may be important in determining the change in epithelial turnover associated with *Helicobacter* infection. Other investigators have reported that selective ablation of murine parietal cells increases the extent of gastritis after *H. pylori* infection.[12]

Thus far, there have been few studies of serial changes in parameters of gastric cell turnover associated with *Helicobacter* infection in animals. In both a rat[13] and a Mongolian gerbil model,[14] *H. pylori* infection caused an early rise in the number of apoptotic epithelial cells, followed by a decline over time. In the gerbil, which may be a better model for multistage gastric carcinogenesis, the early rise in epithelial apoptotic activity was followed by hyperproliferation. Increased proliferation unopposed by increased apoptosis may be important in the subsequent development of gastric cancers in this model.

Animal models have also been used to evaluate the role of bacterial or host factors in induction of apoptosis. For example, a possible role for *H. pylori* lipopolysaccharide in induction of apoptosis was suggested from studies with rats. In rats, gastric inoculation with *H. pylori* strains that are VacA- and CagA- are able to increase epithelial apoptosis and delay healing of acetic acid–induced ulcers[15], and administration of *H. pylori* lipopolysaccharide to rats produces apoptosis and gastritis.[16] Although *H. pylori* lipopolysaccharide has not been directly demonstrated to cause epithelial apoptosis in cell culture, Toll-like receptors (for lipopolysaccharides from Gram negative bacteria and some Gram positive bacterial products) recently have been shown to mediate cell activation and apoptosis in mononuclear cells and potentially in epithelial cells.[17] Variations in susceptibility to endotoxin (LPS) are well-recognized in mice, and have been linked in part with variability in Toll-like receptors and associated signaling pathways. Parallel heterogeneity in humans is another possible mechanism for variability in response to *H. pylori.*

Helicobacter infection of mice with specific gene deletions has been used to elucidate the role of these genes in epithelial cell apoptosis. For example, deletion of the cyclo-oxygenase 2 (cox-2) gene has been associated with increased gastritis and apoptosis after *H. pylori* infection, suggesting that cox-2 may protect against excessive apoptosis.[18] Cox-2 is an inducible form of cyclo-oxygenase, which catalyzes the rate-limiting step in the synthesis of prostaglandins from arachidonic acid. Increased expression of cox-2 has been found in several human tumors and in animal models of carcinogenesis. One mechanism by which increased cox-2 is thought to promote cancer is through inhibition of apoptosis.

Experimental *H. pylori* infection of mice lacking one functional p53 allele resulted in increased numbers of proliferating epithelial cells, but whether there was an associated change in apoptosis was not examined in that study.[19] Since p53 has a central role in determining if the apoptotic pathway is activated in response to stress, p53 heterozygous animals may well display an altered apoptotic and pathological response to *Helicobacter* infection. Investigations of the effects of *H. pylori* infection in transgenic animals with alterations in other important oncogenes, tumor suppressor genes and apoptosis-regulatory genes are likely to further our understanding of the determinants of the host response to infection, and particularly to gastric carcinogenesis.

Very recently, an animal model that has the potential to reproduce more closely the pathological changes found in human infection has been described. In this model, intact human fetal stomach is implanted into nude mice.[20] Because these mice potentially can also be implanted with other human tissues, such as lymph node tissue, the effects of *H. pylori* on human gastric cells with or without concurrent human inflammatory cell response potentially can be studied. It remains to be seen whether this model can also be used to study development of gastric cancer or MALT lymphoma, since survival of these mice and the time required for neoplastic transformation have not been determined.

4. MECHANISMS OF APOPTOSIS ASSOCIATED WITH *H. pylori* INFECTION

4.1. Inflammation, IL-8 and Epithelial Cell Apoptosis

IL-8 is a cytokine important for neutrophil chemotaxis and macrophage activation, and is a possible mediator of mucosal damage. Of note, coculture with CagA+VacA+ clinical strains increases IL-8 mRNA expression and protein secretion in many cell lines,[21,22] including the AGS, Kato III, and MKN28 gastric cancer epithelial cell lines that are frequently used to study apoptosis *in vitro*, and in primary gastric epithelial cells[23]. Increased IL-8 secretion has also been tied to intracellular signaling events. A number of studies have linked *H. pylori*-stimulated IL-8 production in AGS cells[24] and in MKN45 cells[25] to signaling through tyrosine kinase, through a tyrosine phosphorylation-independent pathway involving the ser/thr kinase protein kinase G,[26] and to NF-kB activation.[27] However, while apoptosis of the K562 human leukemia cell line in response to IL-8 has recently been demonstrated,[30] this cytokine has not been shown directly to cause apoptosis of epithelial cells. Thus, although this does not preclude involvement of IL-8 in the epithelial cell apoptotic response, increased secretion of IL-8 by epithelial cells may reflect a parallel response to stimuli that also cause apoptosis. Subsequent activation of macrophages by IL-8 to produce TNFα and interferonγ may then promote or enhance *H. pylori*-induced apoptosis.

4.2. Are Intact, Viable Bacteria Required for Induction of Apoptosis?

Studies in our laboratory[29] suggest there is more apoptosis when AGS gastric epithelial cells are inoculated with viable *H. pylori*, than if formalin-treated (killed bacteria) are added in the same bacteria: AGS cell ratio. A possible confounder in these experiments is the potential for continued division of the viable bacteria, which could result in a higher bacterial: AGS cell ratio compared to the experiments using killed bacteria when incubation is prolonged. However, the apoptotic response was also decreased when the inoculum was separated from the epithelial cells by a Transwell membrane, suggesting contact between bacteria and the host cell is a major factor in stimulation of apoptosis.

4.3. The Type IV Secretion System in *H. pylori* Encoded by the *cag* Pathogenicity Island

Genes within the *cag* pathogenicity island encode a type IV secretion system with homology to secretion systems initially found in *Agrobacterium tumefaciens*, and now also described for *Bordetella pertussis*, some *E. coli*, and Brucella suis. *PicB/cagE*, a part of the type IV secretion system in *H. pylori*, has been noted to have a profound effect on the ability of this organism to induce IL-8 secretion and NF-κB activation.[23,27,30-32] Mutant *cag*$^-$ and *picB*$^-$ strains are less potent than *cag*$^+$ strains in induction of MAP kinase activity.[33] Similarly, clinical strains lacking the *cag* pathogenicity island have a decreased ability to induce apoptosis in gastric epithelial cells in some studies[34] but not in others.[35]

In *Agrobacterium*, a plant pathogen that causes the equivalent of neoplastic tumors, the type IV secretion system allows T-DNA transfer to plant cells. It is intriguing to speculate that *cag*$^+$ *H. pylori* might use this system to deliver potentially transforming signals or signals that regulate apoptosis to the host cell.

4.4. VacA Cytotoxin and Apoptosis

VacA cytotoxin was perhaps the first *H. pylori* virulence factor to be clearly associated with cell death, although not necessarily death by apoptosis. Early experiments demonstrated that VacA causes vacuolation of epithelial cells by interference with movement and fusion of late endosomes with the Golgi and lysosomal apparatus, resulting in cytoplasmic swelling and cell death.

Addition of culture supernatants from cytotoxic *H. pylori* to AGS or Kato III cells induces apoptosis in up to 50% of the treated cells.[8] *In vitro* studies with fast protein–liquid chromatography (FPLC) fractions of conditioned media from toxigenic strains suggest that more purified VacA toxin can also induce apoptosis in gastric epithelial cells *in vitro*,[36] and isogenic *vacA*$^-$ *H. pylori* have been shown to cause less apoptosis than the parent wild type strain.[34] Kimura *et al.* have found that VacA toxin causes mitochondrial damage, a known stimulus for caspase activation.[36] VacA toxin also can interfere with actin stress fiber formation and microtubule organization, tyrosine phosphorylation of focal adhesion kinase, and signal transduction.[37,40] Although addition of VacA is able to cause decreased transepithelial resistance in monolayers of T84 human gut epithelium, MDCK1 canine kidney, and epH4 murine mammary gland cells, it did not appear to affect epithelial tight junctions by microscopy.[38] However, the lack of a suitable polarized gastric epithelium-derived cell line limits the degree to which these changes in transepithelial resistance can be extrapolated to the situation *in vivo*. In addition, those cells studied displayed only minimal vacuolation, perhaps indicating the absence of specific receptors.[38] Although both toxigenic and non-toxigenic *H. pylori* make a VacA-like product, only strains with the s1m1 subtype were initially believed to induce vacuolization. Recently, the vacuolization of epithelial cells in response to s1m2 toxin has been shown to depend on the presence of a receptor for the m2 subunit. Thus, yet another host-dependent factor has been demonstrated to be a potential variable in determining the outcome of response to infection. Decreases in transepithelial resistance also were noted after coculture of epithelial cells with toxigenic strains, and even m2 toxin-producing strains without vacuolating ability.[39]

Formaldehyde treatment of VacA results in loss of vacuolating activity and ability of the toxin to induce epithelial damage.[40] Inactivation of preformed toxin could contribute to the decreased apoptotic response of epithelial cells to formalin-treated bacteria.[29]

4.5. Signaling Molecules and Signal Transduction and Apoptosis

Apoptosis caused by addition of *H. pylori* to gastric cancer cells can be enhanced by treatment with TNFα, or by an activating antibody against CD95/Apo-1/Fas receptor, or by gamma-interferon.[35,41] Furthermore, expression of CD95 by AGS or Kato III cells is upregulated by addition of live cytotoxic *H. pylori* or culture supernatants from these bacteria.[8] Jones *et al.*[42] have demonstrated that infection of gastric epithelial cells by a *cagA*$^+$, *cagE*$^+$, VacA$^+$ clinical isolate results in increased Fas receptor expression, and increased sensitivity to Fas-mediated death, as demonstrated by treatment with an agonist monoclonal anti-Fas receptor antibody. However, the gastric epithelial cell also has the potential to protect itself against TNF-induced apoptosis stimulated by *H. pylori* since infection of gastric epithelial cells in culture and in gastric biopsies was associated with the shedding of two types of cell surface TNF-receptors.[41] Other cell surface molecules, which have been implicated in the induction of apoptosis by *H. pylori* infection, are the MHC class II antigens. These molecules are upregulated in *H. pylori* infection, at least partly through the secretion of interferon gamma, and in cell culture act as adhesins for *H. pylori* to attach and stimulate apoptosis.[43]

Studies in our laboratory[29] have indicated that apoptosis in *H. pylori*-treated AGS cells, which have wild-type p53, is preceded by markedly increased expression of the pro-apoptotic protein Bak, apparent by 4h after inoculation. Expression of other members of the Bcl-2 family, including Bax, and Bcl-X_L and Bcl-2 itself, are moderately decreased. The expression of Bak in epithelial cells in gastric biopsies from patients infected with *H. pylori* was also increased, although others have suggested that an imbalance between mucosal Bcl-2 and Bax accompanies apoptosis in ulcer patients.[44] Examining events further downstream in the apoptosis pathway, Wagner *et al* have demonstrated that the induction of apoptosis in *H. pylori*-treated AGS cells can be correlated with 3-5 fold increases in the activity of caspases 3 and 8.[45]

There is mounting evidence for a central role of the phosphorylation cascades in the epithelial cell response to *H. pylori* infection (as mentioned elsewhere in this volume). Several lines of evidence suggest the influence of *H. pylori* on these host signaling pathways may be particularly relevant to induction of apoptosis and the effects of *H. pylori* on the cell cycle. In studies of the mechanism of increased IL-8 secretion in *H. pylori*-infected epithelial cells, Aihara *et al.*[25] used a luciferase reporter construct to demonstrate evidence of activation of the transcription factor NF-κB and the early response transcription factor activator protein—1 (AP-1). Recently, Keates *et al.*[33] have shown that *cag*$^+$ *H. pylori* strains induce activity of the ERK (extracellular signal-regulated kinases), p38, and JNK (c-Jun N-terminal kinase) MAP kinases in *H. pylori*-infected epithelial cells in culture. Activation of AP-1 and generation of NF-κB was also reported after epithelial cell attachment of *cagA*$^+$ *H. pylori* by Naumann and colleagues.[46] These authors describe activation of a stress-activated protein kinase cascade that includes JNK, MAP kinase kinase 4, and p21-activated kinase, as well as the Rho-GTPases Rac1 and Cdc42. The c-Jun pathway may be particularly important in determining the response of a given host cell to infection with *H. pylori*. Studies in fibroblasts[47] suggest that c-Jun plays an essential role, both in progression through the G1 phase of the cell cycle and in protection from UV-induced apoptosis. The potential to influence the specificity of the c-Jun effect by different biochemical mechanisms, possibly related to specific serine phosphorylation, suggests a mechanism by which the ultimate outcome for the host cell in response to a stimulus such as *H. pylori* infection could be modulated by other influences. The requirement for coordination of multiple signal transduction pathways to achieve maximal IL-8 gene expression has recently been demonstrated.[48]

5. ALTERATIONS IN THE CELL CYCLE AND APOPTOSIS RESISTANCE

Many bacteria, including *E. coli*, *Actinobacillus actinomycetemcommitans*, and cytolethal distending toxin producing strains of *Haemophilus ducreyi*, *Campylobacter*, and *Shigella dysenteriae*, appear able to block the cell cycle in G2, as may *H. pylori*.[34] By contrast, data from our laboratory[49] using AGS gastric epithelial cells, and others, using the gastric cell line AZ-521 cells,[36] indicate that *H. pylori* inhibits the cell cycle predominantly at the G1/S transition (Figure1).

We have demonstrated this G1/S block is paradoxically associated with a marked decrease in expression of the cyclin-dependent kinase inhibitor p27^{kip1}, that controls passage from G1 into S (Figure 2). Under normal circumstance, a decrease in p27^{kip1} accompanies entry into the S phase of the cell cycle. Whether passage into S phase is necessary for apoptosis induced by *H. pylori* to occur is not known. In our studies, there was also increased expression of cyclin D, as well as moderately decreased expression of PCNA and cyclin A, without altered expression of p53, cyclin E, and pRb. In these experiments, expression of another cyclin-dependent kinase inhibitor p21^{cip1} decreased at 6 h, but then increased in comparison with controls by 12 h after addition of live *H. pylori*. *H. pylori* has been reported to produce a 100 kd antiproliferative protein with reversible effects,[50] but its effects on the cell cycle are not known. Of interest, the anaerobic bacterium *Fusobacterium nucleatum* produces a 95 kd heterodimeric protein which blocks cells in mid G1 phase.[51]

We have found that expression of p27^{kip1} is stably decreased in cells that have been chronically exposed to *H. pylori*.[52] These chronically-exposed cells become

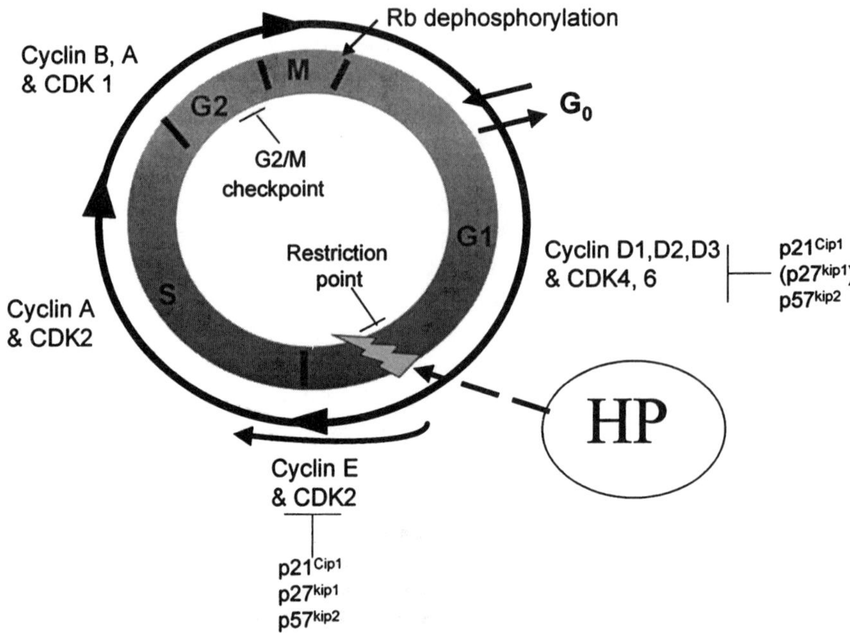

FIGURE 1. In addition to inducing apoptosis, *H. pylori* (HP) affects the growth of AGS cells in culture through inhibition of the transition from G1-S phases of the cell cycle.

resistant to apoptosis induced by *H. pylori* and also by many other agents commonly used to treat gastrointestinal cancers, such as 5-fluorouracil and irradiation. We have found a similar decrease in $p27^{kip1}$ expression in tissue biopsies from *H. pylori*-infected patients. The sustained decrease in $p27^{kip1}$, both in AGS cells chronically exposed *in vitro* to *H. pylori* and in biopsies from infected patients, is particularly noteworthy in light of the correlation between decreased $p27^{kip1}$ expression and aggressive behavior in a variety of tumors.[53] Additionally, increased susceptibility to tumor development has been demonstrated in mice either heterozygous or homozygous for deletion of the $p27^{kip1}$ gene,[54] suggesting that the decrease in $p27^{kip1}$ associated with *H. pylori* infection is responsible for apoptosis-resistance and tumorigenesis.

6. ADHERENCE AND APOPTOSIS

Although direct adherence of *H. pylori* may not be required for demonstration of all the organism's pathogenic effects *in vitro*, it remains a critical characteristic to enable infection to be established *in vivo*. Perhaps more important in the

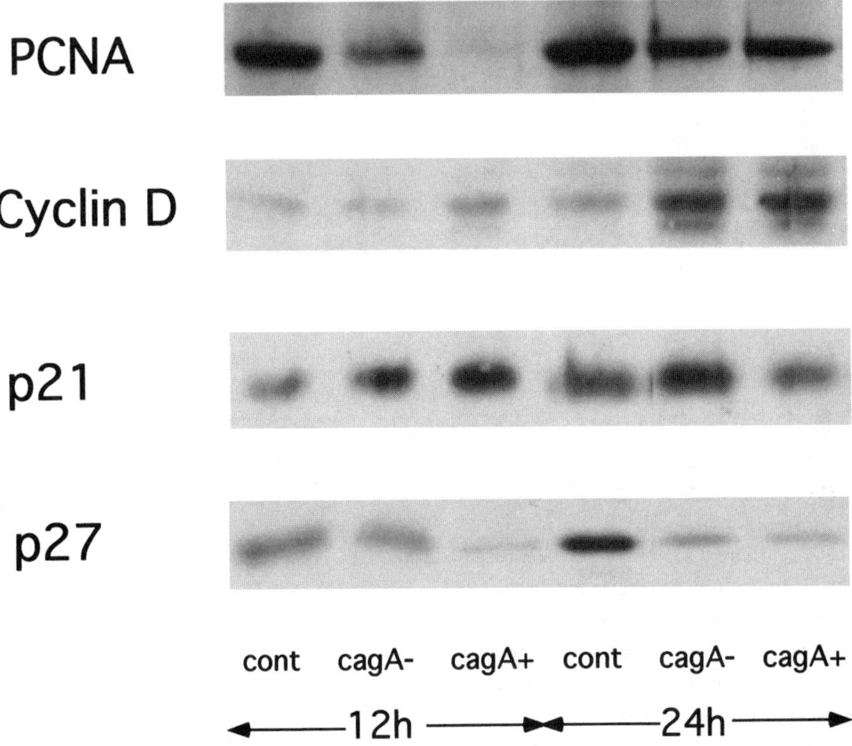

FIGURE 2. Effects of *H. pylori* on the expression of PCNA, cyclin D, $p21^{cip1}$ and $p27^{kip1}$. Wild type *cagA*+ *H. pylori* and an isogenic *cagA*– mutant were added to AGS cells, and the cells subsequently harvested for Western blotting at the time intervals specified. Uninfected AGS cells served as controls ("Con"). From reference 49, with permission.

intact animal, the presence of the type IV secretion system can theoretically potentiate virulence by enhanced or directed transfer of VacA toxin or other bacterial products.

Many adhesins and receptors have been proposed to mediate *H. pylori* binding to gastric epithelial cells, including hemagglutinin, sialic acid-binding adhesins, the N-acetylneuramininyllactose-binding adhesin HpaA, fucose-binding adhesins such as the Lewis blood group antigens, various basement membrane components, lipid binding adhesins, fimbriae-like adhesins, and mucin.[55] The *H. pylori* adhesin, called BabA, responsible for binding to the Lewis b antigen on human erythrocytes and epithelial cells, recently has been characterized, localized on the bacterial outer membrane, and the coding sequence for the *bab* genes identified.[56] Bacterial binding through the Lewis blood group antigens may explain in

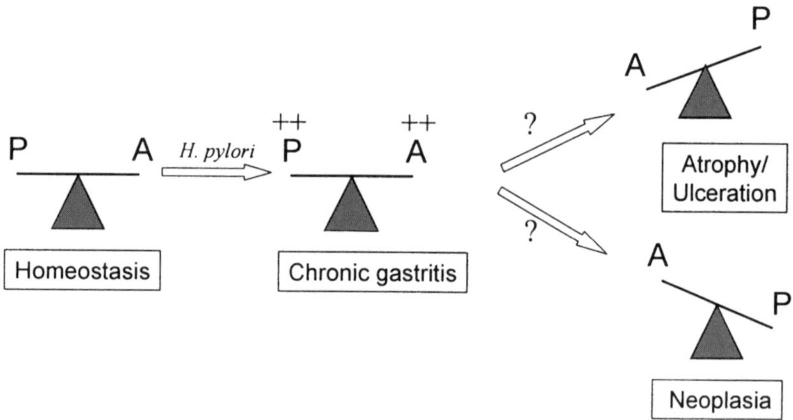

FIGURE 3. *H. pylori* is associated with a state of balanced increased cell turnover. Both proliferation and apoptosis are increased in chronic gastritis. Subsequently some patients develop an imbalanced state, associated with disease.

part variations in host susceptibility to infection by *H. pylori* infection and its sequelae, including apoptosis.

7. APOPTOSIS AND PATHOGENESIS OF ULCERS AND CANCER

In the stomach, excessive epithelial apoptosis may result in mucosal ulceration, whereas insufficient cell death could explain hypertrophic and neoplastic mucosal growth. In fact, this area has not previously been well studied, and there is little hard and consistent data. It is unknown whether excessive apoptosis leads to gastric ulcers and atrophy. In chronic gastritis, cell turnover is increased, and there are increased numbers of both apoptotic and proliferating cells. Hypothetically, this state of "balanced" increased cell turnover may become unbalanced, with excessive apoptosis relative to proliferation leading to ulceration and atrophy (Figure 3).

Although there have been no good studies of apoptotic and proliferating cells in ulcers to test this hypothesis, increased numbers of apoptotic cells have been described in the base of the gastric gland in patients with atrophic gastritis.[10,57] In the report by Steininger and Colleagues,[10] increased apoptosis at the base of the

FIGURE 4. Proliferation, apoptosis and the proliferation to apoptosis ratio in a cohort of patients with chronic gastritis followed for over 30 years. Some patients developed atrophic gastritis (cases) whereas most did not (controls). From reference 58, with permission.

A

PROLIFERATION
PROLERATING CELLS/GLAND
6
5
4
3
2
1
0
p=0.48

B

APOPTOSIS
APOPTOTIC CELLS/GLAND
12
11
10
9
8
7
6
5
4
3
2
1
0
p=0.27

C

PROLIFERATION/APOPTOSIS
P/A RATIO
0.6
0.4
0.2
0
p=0.32
CASES
CONTROLS

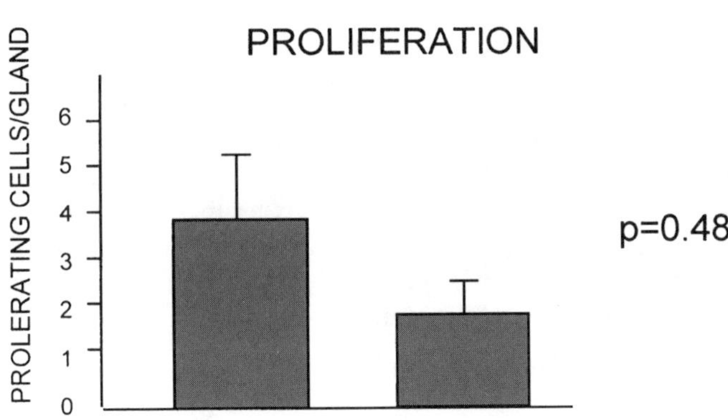

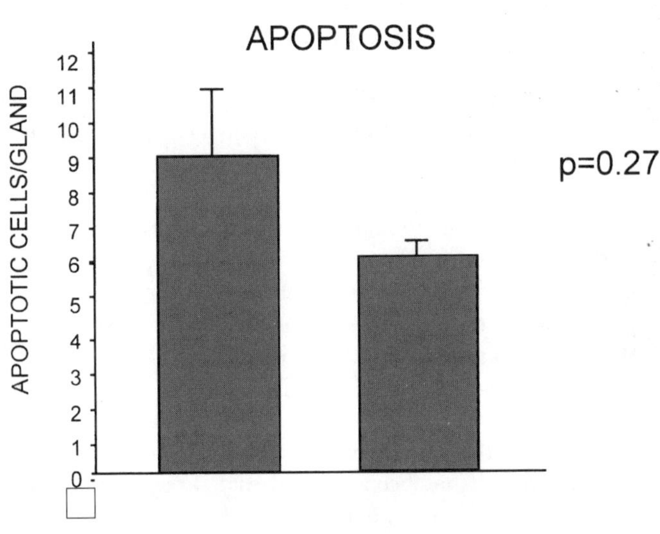

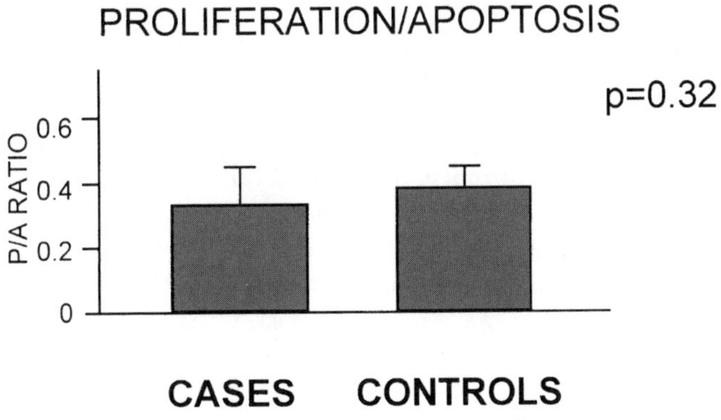

gastric gland (where the specialized acid-secreting parietal cells are normally located) was found to be associated with anti-canalicular gastric autoantibodies, suggesting that glandular apoptosis may result from an autoimmune mechanism. In a prospective study, we studied whether the ratio of apoptotic to proliferating epithelial cells in gastric biopsies from patients with chronic gastritis is predictive of the later development of atrophy.[58] We found no significant difference in this ratio between the atrophy patients (cases) and those in whom there were still no changes of atrophic gastritis (controls) after over 30 years, although the atrophy patients did have moderately higher scores for both proliferation and apoptosis at onset (Figure 4).

8. IS A DEFICIENCY IN APOPTOSIS RESPONSIBLE FOR THE DEVELOPMENT OF CANCER?

Atrophic gastritis, characterized by a loss in specialized acid-secreting cells at the gland base, is an early step in the sequence of changes driven by *H. pylori* that may ultimately result in the common, intestinal, type of gastric cancer. Following atrophy, the gland base becomes repopulated by epithelial cells that appear similar to those found in the intestine (intestinal metaplasia). It is from cells in this lineage that dysplastic and frankly neoplastic cells arise. Although it is well known that this sequence of changes is accompanied by progressively increased proliferation, the contribution of altered or dysregulated apoptosis to the development of gastric carcinogenesis has not been defined.

In the incomplete (type III) form of intestinal metaplasia, which is the type most closely associated with gastric cancer, increased numbers of apoptotic cells are found near the base of the gland, close to the proliferative zone from where new cells arise. It has been inferred that these apoptotic cells have undergone appropriate "altruistic" apoptosis soon after they have been generated, presumably because they carry potentially harmful mutations.[57,59] Theoretically, failure of apoptosis in these circumstances would have dangerous consequences, and may be enhanced by acquisition of mutations in key apoptosis-regulatory genes such as p53 or the type II transforming growth factor beta receptor (often associated with microsatellite instability). Such mutations commonly occur during gastric carcinogenesis.

Members of the Bcl-2 protein family play a central role in the regulation of apoptosis, and accordingly there have been several studies to evaluate expression of these molecules during carcinogenesis. Some have reported increased expression of the anti-apoptotic Bcl-2 protein in cancer,[60,61] whereas other authors have found changes in other members of this family, such as Bcl-X_L, Bax and Bak, to be more important markers of neoplasia.[61,62] Survivin, a member of a completely unrelated of apoptosis inhibitory group of proteins, is overexpressed in gastric cancer.[63] Whether *H. pylori* can alter expression of survivin has not been evaluated. The demonstration of the Fas ligand on the cancer cell membrane provides further evidence to support a relative inhibition of apoptosis in gastric cancer. According to the "Fas counterattack" model of tumorigenesis, expression of Fas ligand by epithelial cells leads to the death of lymphocytes that conduct immune surveillance - a function normally essential for control of cancer formation.[64]

9. CONCLUSIONS AND SPECULATIONS

H. pylori infection hastens the death of epithelial cells lining the stomach, which is likely to contribute to the damage caused by this bacterium. The precise mechanisms used by *H. pylori* to induce apoptosis are not understood, nor is it known why, despite infection over decades, most individuals colonized by *H. pylori* do not develop clinically relevant consequences. It is possible that in some infected people, deregulation of apoptosis contributes to the development of gastric malignancy.

Why does *H. pylori* induce apoptosis? According to Syder and colleagues,[11] selective loss of specialized acid-secreting cells within the gastric gland leads to a shift in the organism's ecological niche, and ultimately results in decreased bacterial adherence. It is difficult to argue that this is advantageous for the bacterium. A speculative and unproven housekeeping function for the organism, is that apoptosis-enhanced elimination of unwanted cells is advantageous to the host, and thus ultimately to the colonizing bacterium. Another possibility is that apoptosis is an inadvertent outcome of infection, occurring only in certain hosts primed for an apoptotic response either genetically, or because of other environmental signals. Improved understanding of the relationships among proliferation, apoptosis and transformation and how they are modulated by *H. pylori* may provide answers to these questions in the next few years.

REFERENCES

1. Blaser M. J., and Parsonnet J. *et al.*, 1994, Parasitism by the "slow" bacterium *Helicobacter pylori* leads to altered gastric homeostasis and neoplasia. *J. Clin. Invest.* 94:4–8
2. Zychlinsky A., and Sansonetti P. J. *et al.*, 1997, Apoptosis as a proinflammatory event: What can we learn from bacteria-induced cell death? *Trends in Microbiology* 5:201–204
3. Anti M., Armuzzi A., Gasbarrini A., and Gasbarrini G. *et al.*, 1998, Importance of changes in epithelial cell turnover during *Helicobacter pylori* infection in gastric carcinogenesis. *Gut.* 43 (suppl 1):S27–32
4. Shirin H., and Moss S. F. *et al.*, 1998, Leading article: *Helicobacter pylori*-induced apoptosis. *Gut.* 43:592–594

5. Abdalla A. M., Krivosheyev V., Hanzely Z., Holt P. R., Perez-Perez G. I., Blaser M. J., and Moss S. F. *et al.*, 1998, Increased epithelial cell turnover in antrum and corpus of *H. pylori*-infected stomach, irrespective of CagA status. *Gastroenterology* 114:A50
6. Peek R. M., Moss S. F., Tham K. T., Perez-Perez G. I., Miller G. G., Atherton J. C., Holt P. R., and Blaser M. J. *et al.*, 1997, *Helicobacter pylori* cagA+ strains and dissociation of gastric epithelial proliferation from apoptosis. *J. Natl. Cancer Inst.* 89:863–868
7. Rokkas T., Ladas S., Liatsos C., Petridou E., Papatheodorou G., Theocharis S., Karameris A., and Raptis S. *et al.*, 1999, Relationship of *Helicobacter pylori* CagA status to gastric cell proliferation and apoptosis. *Dig. Dis. Sci.* 44: 487–493
8. Rudi J., Kuck D., Strand S., von Herbay A., Mariani S. M., Krammer P. H., Galle P. R., and Stremmel W. *et al.*, 1998, Involvement of the CD95 (APO-1/Fas) receptor and ligand system in *Helicobacter pylori*-induced gastric epithelial apoptosis. *J. Clin. Invest.* 102:1506–1514
9. Houghton J., Korah R. M., Condon M. R., and Kim K. H. *et al.*, 1999, Apoptosis in *Helicobacter pylori*-associated gastric and duodenal ulcer disease is mediated via the Fas antigen pathway. *Dig. Dis. Sci.* 44:465–478
10. Steininger H., Faller G., Dewald E., Brabletz T., Jung A., and Kirchner T. *et al.*, 1998, Apoptosis in chronic gastritis and its correlation with antigastric autoantibodies. only *Virchows. Arch.* 433:13–18
11. Wang T. C., Goldenring J. R., Dangler C., Ito S., Mueller A., Jeon W. K., Koh T. J., and Fox J. G. *et al.*, 1998, Mice lacking secretory phospholipase A2 show altered apoptosis and differentiation with *Helicobacter felis* infection. *Gastroenterology* 114:675–689
12. Syder A. J., Guruge J. L., Li Q., Hu Y., Oleksiewicz C. M., Lorenz R. G., Karam S. M., Falk P. G., and Gordon J. I. *et al.*, 1999, *Helicobacter pylori* attaches to NeuAc alpha 2,3Gal beta 1,4 glycoconjugates produced in the stomach of transgenic mice lacking parietal cells. *Mol. Cell* 3:263–274
13. Li H., Andersson E.-M., and Helander H. F. *et al.*, 1999, Reactions from rat gastric mucosa during one year of *Helicobacter pylori* infection. *Dig. Dis. Sci.* 44:116–124
14. Peek R. M., Wirth H. P., Moss S. F., Yang M., Abdalla A. M., Tham K. T., Zhang T., Tang L. H., Modlin I. M., and Blaser M. J. *et al.*, Helicobacter *pylori* alters gastric epithelial cell cycle events and gastrin secretion in Mongolian gerbils. *Gastroenterology* (in press).
15. Li M., Mellgard B., and Helander H. F. *et al.*, 1997, Inoculation of VacA- and CagA-*Helicobacter pylori* delays gastric ulcer healing in the rat. *Scand. J. Gastroenterol.* 32:439–444
16. Piotrowski J., Piotrowski E., Skrodzka D., Slomiany A., and Slomiany B. L. *et al.*, 1997, Induction of acute gastritis and epithelial cell apoptosis by *Helicobacter pylori* lipopolysaccharide. *Scand. J. Gastroenterol.* 32:203–211
17. Aliprantis A. O., Yang R.-B., Mark M. R., Suggett S., Devaux B., Radolf J. D., Klimpel G. R., Godowski P., and Zychlinsky A. *et al.*, 1999, Cell activation and apoptosis by bacterial lipoproteins through Toll-like receptor-2. *Science* 285:736–739
18. Luo X.-L., Ramanujam K. S., Zhao H.-M., Moss S. F., Russell R. G., Drachenberg C. B., and Wilson K. T. *et al.*, 1999, Protective role of COX-2 in *H. pylori* gastritis. *Gastroenterology* 116:A767
19. Fox J. G., Li X., Cahill R. J., Andrutis K., Rustgi A. K., Odze R., and Wang T. C. *et al.*, 1996, Hypertrophic gastropathy in *Helicobacter felis*-infected wild-type C57BL/6 mice and p53 hemizygous transgenic mice. *Gastroenterology* 110:155–166
20. Lozniewski A., Muhale F., Hatier R., Marais A., Conroy M. C., Edert D., le Faou A., Weber M., and Duprez A. *et al.*, 1999, Human embryonic gastric xenografts in nude mice: a new model of *Helicobacter pylori* infection. *Infect. Immun.* 67:1798–1805
21. Crabtree J. E., Farmery S. M., Lindley I. J., Peichl P., and Tompkins D. S. *et al.*, 1994, CagA/cytotoxic strains of *Helicobacter pylori* and interleukin-8 in gastric epithelial cell lines. *J. Clin. Pathol.* 47:945–950
22. Sharma S. A., Tummuru M. K. R., Miller G. G., and Blaser M. J. *et al.*, 1995, Interleukin-8 response of gastric epithelial cell lines to *Helicobacter pylori* stimulation *in vitro*. *Infect. Immun.* 63:1681–1687

23. Ogura K., Takahashi M., Maeda S., Ikenoue T., Kanai F., Yoshida H.; Shiratori Y., Mori K., Mafune K. I., and Ogata M. *et al.*, 1998, Interleukin-8 production in primary cultures of human gastric epithelial cells induced by *Helicobacter pylori. Dig. Dis. Sci.* 43:2738–2743
24. Beales I. L., and Calam J. *et al.*, 1997, Stimulation of IL-8 production in human gastric epithelial cells by *Helicobacter pylori*, IL-1 beta and TNF-alpha requires tyrosine kinase activity, but not protein kinase C. *Cytokine* 9:514–520
25. Aihara M., Tsuchimoto D., Takizawa H., Azuma A., Wakebe H., Ohmoto Y., Imagawa K., Kikuchi M., Mukaida N., and Matsushima K. *et al.*, 1997, Mechanisms involved in *Helicobacter pylori*-induced interleukin-8 production by a gastric cancer cell line, MKN45. *Infect. Immun.* 65:3218–3224
26. Segal E. D., Lange C., Covacci A., Tompkins L. S., and Falkow S. *et al.*, 1997, Induction of host signal transduction pathways by *Helicobacter pylori. Proc. Natl. Acad. Sci. USA* 94:7595–7599
27. Sharma S. A., Tummuru M. K., Blaser M. J., and Kerr L. D. *et al.*, 1998, Activation of IL-8 gene expression by *Helicobacter pylori* is regulated by transcription factor nuclear kappa B in gastric epithelial cells. *J. Immunol.* 160:2401–2407
28. Terui Y., Tomizuka H., Mishima Y., Ikeda M., Kasahara T., Uwai M., Mori M., Itoh T., Tanaka M., Yamada M., Shimamura S., Ishizaka Y., Ozawa K., and Hatake K. *et al.*, 1999, *Cancer Res.* 59:5651–5655
29. Chen G., Sordillo E. M., Ramey W. G., Reidy J., Holt P., Krajewski S., Reed J. C., Blaser M. J., and Moss S. F. *et al.*, 1997, Apoptosis in gastric epithelial cells is induced by *Helicobacter pylori* and accompanied by increased expression of BAK. *Biochem. Biophys. Res. Commun.* 239:626–632
30. Tummuru M. K., Sharma S. A., and Blaser M. J. *et al.*, 1995, *Helicobacter pylori* picB, a homologue of the *Bordetella pertussis* toxin secretion protein, is required for the induction of IL-8 in gastric epithelial cells. *Mol. Microbiol.* 18:867–876
31. Censini S., Lange C., Xiang Z., Crabtree J. E., Ghiara P., Borodovsky M., Rappuoli R., and Covacci A. *et al.*, 1996, *cag*, a pathogenicity island of *Helicobacter pylori*, encodes type I-specific and disease-associated virulence factors. *Proc. Natl. Acad. Sci. USA* 93:14648–14653
32. Munzenmaier A., Lange C., Glocker E., Covacci A., Moran A., Bereswill S., Baeuerle P. A., Kist M., and Pahl H. L. *et al.*, 1997, A secreted/shed product of *Helicobacter pylori* activates transcription factor nuclear factor kappa B. *J. Immunol.* 159:6140–6147
33. Keates S., Keates A. C., Warney M., Peek R. M., Murray P. G., and Kelly C. P. *et al.*, 1999, Differential activation of mitogen-activated protein–kinases in AGS epithelial cells by *cag+* and *cag– Helicobacter pylori. J. Immunol.* 163:5552–5559
34. Peek R. M., Blaser M. J., Mays D. J., Forsyth M. H., Cover T. L., Song S. Y., Krishnan U., and Pietenpol J. A. *et al.*, *Helicobacter pylori* strain-specific genotypes and modulation of the gastric epithelial cell cycle. *Cancer Res.* (in press)
35. Wagner S., Beil W., Westermann J., Logan R. P., Bock C. T., Trautwein C., Bleck J. S., and Manns M. P. *et al.*, 1997, Regulation of gastric epithelial cell growth by *Helicobacter pylori*: evidence for a major role of apoptosis. *Gastroenterology* 113:1836–1847
36. Kimura M., Gotot S., Wada A., Yahiro K., Niidome T., Hatakeyama T., Aoyagi H., Hirayama T.,and Kondo T. *et al.*, 1999, Vacuolating cytotoxin purified from *Helicobacter pylori* causes mitochondrial damage in human gastric cells. *Microb. Pathog.* 26:45–52
37. Pai R., Cover T. L., and Tarnawski A. S. *et al.*, 1999, *Helicobacter pylori* vacuolating cytotoxin (VacA) disorganizes the cytoskeletal architecture of gastric epithelial cells. *Biochem. Biophys. Res. Commun.* 19:245–250
38. Papini E., Satin B., Norais N., deBernard M., Telford J. L., Rappuoli R., and Montecucco C. *et al.*, 1998, Selective increase of the permeability of polarized epithelial cell monolayers by *Helicobacter pylori* vacuolating toxin. *J. Clin. Invest.* 102:813–820
39. Pellici V., Reyrat J. M., Sartori L., Pagliaccia C., Rappuoli R., Telford J. L., Montecucco C., and Papini E. *et al.*, 1999, *Helicobacter pylori* VacA cytotoxin associated with the bacteria increases epithelial permeability independently of its vacuolating activity. *Microbiology* 145:2043–2050

40. Manetti R., Massari P., Marchetti M., Magagnoli C., Nuti S., Lupetti P., Ghiara P., Rappuoli R., and Telford J. L. *et al.*, 1997, Detoxification of the *Helicobacter pylori* cytotoxin. *Infect. Immun.* 65:4615–4619
41. Shibata J., Goto H., Arisawa T., Niwa Y., Hayakawa T., Nakayama A., and Mori N. *et al.*, 1999, Regulation of tumour necrosis factor (TNF) induced apoptosis by soluble TNF receptors in *Helicobacter pylori* infection. *Gut.* 45:24–31
42. Jones N. L., Day A. S., Jennings H. A., and Shernman P. M. *et al.*, 1999, *Helicobacter pylori* induces gastric epithelial cell apoptosis in association with increased Fas receptor expression. *Infect. Immun.* 67:4237–4242
43. Fan X., Crowe S. F., Behar S., Gunasena H., Ye G., Haeberle H., Van Houten N., Gourley W. K., Ernst P. B., and Reyes V. E. *et al.*, 1998, The effect of class II major histocompatibility complex expression on adherence of *Helicobacter pylori* and induction of apoptosis in gastric epithelial cells: A mechanism for T helper cell type-I mediated damage. *J. Exp. Med.* 187: 1659–1669
44. Konturek P. C., Pierzchalski P., Konturek S. J., Meixner H., Faller G., Kirchner T., and Hahn E. G. *et al.*, 1999, *Helicobacter pylori* induces apoptosis in gastric mucosa through an upregulation of Bax expression in humans. *Scand. J. Gastroenterol.* 34:375–383
45. Wagner S., Mix H., Sobek-Koocked I., Obst B., Schmidt H., Bleck J., Kirchner G., Gokeb M., Manns M. P., and Beil W. *et al.*, 1999, Activation of caspase-8 and -3 mediates apoptosis in gastric epithelial cells induced by *Helicobacter pylori. Gastroenterology* 116:347
46. Naumann M. Wessler S., Bartsch C., Wielans B., Covacci A., Haas R., and Meyer T. F. *et al.*, 1999, Activation of activator protein-1 and stress response kinases in epithelial cells colonized by *Helicobacter pylori* encoding the *cag* pathogenicity island. *J. Biol. Chem.* 274:31655–31662
47. Wisdom R., Johnson R. S., and Moore C. *et al.*, 1999, c-Jun regulates cell cycle progression and apoptosis by distinct mechanisms. *EMBO J.* 18:188–197
48. Holtmann H., Winzen R., Holland P., Eickemeier S., Hoffman E., Wallack D., Malinin N. L., Cooper J. A., Resch K., and Kracht M. *et al.*, 1999, Induction of Interleukin-8 synthesis integrates effects on transcription and mRNA degradation from at least three different cytokine- or stress-activated signal transduction pathways. *Mol. Cell Biol.* 19:6742–6753
49. Shirin H., Sordillo E. M., Oh S. H., Yamamoto H., Delohery T., Weinstein I. B., and Moss S. F. *et al.*, 1999, *Helicobacter pylori* inhibits the G1 to S transition in AGS gastric epithelial cells. *Cancer Res.* 59:2277–2281
50. Knipp U., Birkholz S., Kaup W., and Opferkuch W. *et al.*, 1996, Partial characterization of a cell proliferation inhibiting protein produced by *Helicobacter pylori. Infect. Immun.* 64:3491–3496
51. Shenker B. J., and Datar S. *et al.*, 1995, *Fusobacterium nucleatum* inihibits T cell activation by arresting cells in the mid G1 phase of the cell cycle. *Infect. Immun.* 63:4830–4836
52. Shirin H., Sordillo E. M., Delohery T., Weinstein I. B., and Moss S. F. *et al.*, 1999, Reduced expression of the cyclin-dependent kinase inhibitor, $p27^{kip1}$ in subclones of AGS gastric epithelial cells resistant to *H. pylori*-induced apoptosis. *Gastroenterology* 116:A503
53. Lloyd R. V., Erikson L. A., Jin L., Kulig E., Qian X., Cheville J. C., and Scheithauer B. W. *et al.*, 1999, $p27^{kip1}$: A multifunctional cyclin-dependent kinase inhibitor with prognostic significance in human cancer. *Am. J. Pathology* 154:313–323
54. Fero M. L., Randel E., Gurley K. E., Roberts J. M., and Kemp C. J. *et al.*, 1998, The murine gene $p27^{kip1}$ is haplo-insufficient for tumour suppression. *Nature* 396:177–180
55. Doig P., and Trust T. J. *et al.*, 1997, The molecular basis for *H. pylori* adherence and colonization, in: *The Immunobiology of H. pylori: From Pathogenesis to Prevention*, PB Ernst, P Michetti, PD Smith, eds., Lippincott-Raven, Philadelphia
56. Ilver D., Arnqvist A., Ogren J., Frick I.-M., Kersulyte D., Incecik E. T., Berg D. E., Covacci A., Engstrand L., and Borens T. *et al.*, 1998, *Helicobacter pylori* adhesin binding fucosylated histo-blood group antigens revealed by retagging. *Science* 279:373–377

57. Ishida M., Gomyo Y., Ttaebe S., Ohfuji S., and Ito H. *et al.*, 1996, Apoptosis in human gastric mucosa, chronic gastritis, dysplasia and carcinoma: analysis by terminal deoxynucleotidyl transferase-mediated dUTP-biotin nick end labeling. *Virchows. Arch.* 428:229–235
58. Moss S. F., Valle J., Abdalla A. M., Wang S., Siurala M., and Sipponen P. *et al.*, 1999, Gastric cellular turnover and the development of atrophy after 31 years of follow up: a case-control study. *Am. J. Gastroenterology* 94:2109–2114
59. Yabuki N., Sasano H., Tobita M., Imatani A., Hoshi T., Kato K., Ohara S., Asaki S., Toyota T., and Nagura H. *et al.*, 1997, Analysis of cell damage and proliferation in *Helicobacter pylori*-infected human gastric mucosa from patients with gastric adenocarcinoma. *Am. J. Pathol.* 151:821–829
60. Lauwers G. Y., Scott G. V., and Karpeh M. S. *et al.*, 1995, Immunohistochemical evaluation of bcl-2 protein expression in gastric adenocarcinomas. *Cancer* 75:2209–2213
61. Kondo Shinomura Y., Kanayama S., Higashimoto Y., Miyagawa J. I., Minami T., Kiyohara T., Zushi S., Kitamura S., Isozaki K., and Matsuzawa Y. *et al.*, 1996, Over-expression of Bcl-X_L gene in human gastric adenomas and carcinomas. *Int. J. Cancer* 68:727–730
62. Krajewska M., Fenoglio-Preiser C. M., Song K., Macdonald J. S., Stemmerman G., and Reed J. C. *et al.*, 1996, Immunohistochemical analysis of the Bcl-2 family proteins in adenocarcinoma of the stomach. *Am. J. Pathol.* 149:1449–1457
63. Lu C.-D., Altieri D. C., and Tanigawa N. *et al.*, 1998, Expression of a novel antiapoptosis gene, *survivin*, correlated with tumor cell apoptosis and p53 accumulation in gastric carcinomas. *Cancer Res.* 58:1808–1812
64. Bennett M. W., O'Connell J., O'Sullivan G. C., Roche D., Brady C., Kelly J., Collins J. K., and Shanahan F. *et al.*, 1999, Expression of Fas ligand by human gastric adenocarcinomas: a potential mechanism of immune escape in stomach cancer. *Gut.* 44:156–162

11

Toxins, Travels and Tropisms: *H. pylori* and Host Cells

NINA R. SALAMA, STANLEY FALKOW, and KAREN M. OTTEMANN

1. INTRODUCTION

In this chapter we will discuss the ways in which *H. pylori* interacts with and manipulates host cells. Studies with *H. pylori* reveal a number of effects on host cells including attachment-induced membrane and cytoskeletal changes, disruption of endocytic traffic and vacuolation, alteration of transepithelial conductance, induction of proinflamatory cytokines, alteration of antigen processing, induction of cell migration, loss of mucus granules, arrest of cell cycle progression and induction of apoptosis. Molecular identification of bacterial factors responsible for a few of these effects has been achieved, but most remain *H. pylori*-associated phenotypes.

We first review what is known about the interaction of *H. pylori* with the human stomach epithelium and mucus, including adherence to gastric epithelial cells. Next we explore the effects of VacA, the major toxin expressed by *H. pylori* and the best studied *H. pylori* virulence factor. Finally we discuss some of the other cellular changes induced by *H. pylori*, many of which depend on the *cag* pathogenicity island (*Cag* PAI).

NINA R. SALAMA and STANLEY FALKOW • Department of Microbiology and Immunology, Stanford University, Stanford, CA. Karen M. OTTEMANN • Departments of Biology and Environmental Toxicology, University of California at Santa Cruz, Santa Cruz, CA.

Helicobacter pylori Infection and Immunity,
Edited by Yamamoto *et al.*, Kluwer Academic/Plenum Publishers, 2002.

2. ADHERENCE

2.1. In the Real Stomach World

A great deal has been garnered of how *H. pylori* interacts with the gastric mucosa by examining human gastric biopsies. In these fixed samples, most of the bacteria are located in the antral region of the stomach. Numerous assessments have found that about 20% of the bacteria adhere to the epithelial cells, but most are located in the mucus layer over the epithelium.[1–5]

Adherent bacteria are most often attached to certain cell types. Additional foci of adherence are found *in vivo* at intercellular junctions.[1–8] Several reports have noted that *H. pylori* is attached predominantly to the mucus neck cells that line the luminal-proximal portion of the gastric pits.[5,8,9] This pattern of attachment is very similar in appearance to *H. pylori* adherence *in situ* to fixed gastrointestinal epithelium.[10]

In vivo, bacterial-host cell attachment takes several forms. Most frequently (70%), bacteria are seen abutting the cells, with no change in the shape of the cell membrane.[2,4] Less frequently, bacteria are on raised cell membrane pedestals (8–16%),[2,4] or at depressions in the cell membrane (11–17%).[2,4,5,7,9] Rarely (3–10%), bacteria are seen inside cells.[4,5] Attachment can be at either bacterial pole or along the side. Several groups have observed fibril strands between the bacterium and the host,[3,4,11] but the identity of these structures remains unknown.

In the presence of *H. pylori*, the gastric epithelium undergoes degenerative changes. These include loss of microvilli,[2–5,7–9] loss of mucus granules,[2–4,7–9,12,13] and cytoplasm.[2,7] By examining patients with different bacterial loads, the severity of degenerative changes were found to increase with bacterial numbers. These degenerative changes, included loss of epithelial cells and formation of erosions.[12,14,15] Cellular vacuolization is also viable in gastric biopsy specimen[4,13] and can occur in cells that neighbor cells with adherent *H. pylori*, but do not directly contact the bacteria.

3. THE MOLECULAR BASIS FOR *H. pylori* ADHERENCE

There are many studies describing molecules that adhere to *H. pylori* (Table 1). There are, however, few studies that examine how and if *H. pylori* uses these abilities during infection. So while it is clear that *H. pylori* is able to specifically bind many molecules, it is not clear if *H. pylori* requires these abilities, or even encounters these molecule *in vivo*. Two reviews offer further insights into this matter.[16,17] One exceptionally well-studied adherence system is binding of the Lewis B antigen, mediated by the *H. pylori* molecule BabA2.

TABLE 1
Molecules bound by *H. pylori*

Molecule Bound	Affinity	*H. pylori* Receptor	Reference
Lewis Antigens (fucosylated)			
Lewis B	0.1 nM	BabA	19, 20, 24
H1	Nd	BabA	24
H2	Nd	n.d.	113
Lipids			
Phosphatidlyethanolamine	Nd	Unknown; previously hypothesized to be KatA	35, 36
Glycosphingolipids			
lactosylceramide (Galβ4Glcβ1Cer) with sphingosine and 2-D hydroxy fatty acids	Nd	unknown	114
Sulfatide (I^3SO_3-GalCer) See below in sulfated	Nd	unknown	115, 116
GM_3 gangliosides (II^3NeuAc-LacCer)	Nd	Unknown	17, 115
Sialylated Compounds	Nd		
3′siallylactose (NeuAc-alpha2-3Gal-beta1-4Glc) (also called N-acetylneuraminyllactose) which is part of laminin	Nd	An unknown protein[a]	43, 117
Extracellular Matrix Components			
Collagens (Type IV, V)	16 nM	Unknown, probably protein (treatments)	17, 39, 118
Plasminogen (inhibited by sialic acid-rich glycoproteins)	Nd	Unknown	118
Vitronectin (inhibited by sialic acid-rich glycoproteins)	Nd	Unknown	118
Laminin (see 3′siallylactose)	8.5 pM–7.9 nM (partially irreversible)	LPS An unknown protein[a]	39–42
Sulfated molecules			
Sulfatide (sulfoglycolipid) (SO_3-3Galβ1Cer	Nd	Unknown	33, 115, 116
Heparan sulfate	9 nM	Unkown	116, 119
Mucin	Nd	Unkown	26 116
Cell Surface Proteins			
MHC class II (Cell Surf Prot)	nd	Unknown	120

nd = not determined.
[a]originally called HpaA, but subsequently this was shown not to bind to 3′siallylactose.

4. ADHERENCE TO THE LEWIS B ANTIGEN

Lewis B (Le^b) was first suspected as an adherence target when it was noticed, in tissue slices, that the pattern of *H. pylori* binding to mucus neck cells displayed the same pattern as the spatial positioning of the Le^b and H1 blood group antigens.[10] Blood group antigens are a collection of carbohydrates molecules covalently linked to protein and lipid moieties of cells. These antigens share a common core, and are formed by sequential addition of fucose or galactose-derived saccharide residues to carbohydrate precursor structures.[18] In human gastric sections *in situ*, *H. pylori* binding was inhibited by pretreating the sections with compounds that contained fucose or that bound to fucosylated blood group antigens (monoclonal antibodies to H, B or Le^b antigens), but not by those that contained sialic acid.[10,19] This strongly suggested that a fucosylated sugar was required for adherence in this system. Additionally, treatment with proteinase K abolished binding, suggesting that the adherence target contained protein. By using defined carbohydrates, it was found that *H. pylori* bound primarily to Le^b, but also to the related H1 antigen.[20] Most studies focused on the Le^b as the adherence determinant because soluble Le^b could inhibit 100% of *H. pylori* binding, while H1 could inhibit only 50% of binding.[20] Next, in order to test if binding to the Le^b antigen mediated bacterial attachment *in vivo*, transgenic mice that expressed this antigen in the gastric mucus cells were created.[21] Using *in situ* binding assays with either Le^b-minus or Le^b-positive transgenic mouse gastric tissue, the authors demonstrated that *H. pylori* adhered appreciably only when the Le^b antigen was present. To date, however, the gastric tissue Le^b-containing molecule has not been identified. Interestingly, in the transgenic mouse, several epithelial tissues (pit and surface mucus cells of the stomach, jejunal, ileal and colonic enterocytes) were Le^b-positive by immunocytochemical studies. *H. pylori* adhered, however, only to gastric tissue and only gastric tissue was recognized in western blots by a Le^b monoclonal antibody.[21] Thus, while Le^b seems to be present in more than one tissue type, both *H. pylori* and a monoclonal Le^b antibody could recognize only Le^b expressed in gastric tissue. One possible explanation is that there are conformational differences between the Le^b epitope found in gastric tissue and those found elsewhere. This hypothesis may underlie the lack of binding of *H. pylori* to other Le^b-positive tissues.

Le^b is not the only molecule bound by *H. pylori in vivo*. In primary gastric cells and cultured epithelial cells, adherence occurs regardless of Le^b expression or accessibility.[22,23] In fixed gastric tissues, however, Le^b is required for adherence.[10,23] Le^b is expressed in non-gastric human tissues such as the duodenum. *H. pylori* adheres, surprisingly, only to the gastric Le^b-positive tissues. This suggests that there are unique conformations or additional factors, found only in gastric tissues required for adherence, or there are factors in the non-gastric tissues that obscure the Le^b epitope for *H. pylori* binding.[23] This situation is similar to that in the Le^b transgenic mice described above, in which Le^b is expressed in several tissues, but only gastric tissue Le^b is recognized by *H. pylori* and monoclonal antibodies to Le^b. Interestingly, 95% of type II *H. pylori* strains (which do not contain the *Cag* PAI) do not bind Le^b.[24] The Lewis blood group antigens are also attached to gastric mucin.[25] Although *H. pylori* is capable of binding mucus,[26] it has been shown in vitro (http://www.micro.unsw.edu.au/!THEHELI.COP/movie.html) and presumed in vivo, to be swimming unattached in the mucus layer. Thus *H. pylori* would need to migrate through a sea of Le^b carbohydrates in the mucus, and then attach specifically to the Le^b epitopes on the cells. Navigating this conundrum may explain why the context of the Le^b epitope seems to be important to enable *H. pylori* to differentiate mucus Le^b versus Le^b on different cell types.

Using an affinity tagging technique, Ilver *et al.*[24] identified a *H. pylori* surface molecule that binds Le^b. Amino-terminal sequencing of the Le^b-bound protein led to the identification of three genes whose products contained this sequence: *babA1*, *babA2* and *babB* (*B*lood group *A*ntigen *B*inding). The *babA1* gene lacks a start codon, and inactivation of this open reading frame by insertional mutagenesis did not alter Le^b binding. In contrast, insertional inactivation of *babA2* resulted in a decrease in Le^b binding activity. There is no information about how *babB* effects Le^b binding, because large scale affinity tagging, purification and subsequent protein sequencing suggested that BabA contributed most to the binding of Le^b. The *bab* genes belong to a family whose products have amino acid homology in both the amino- and carboxy-terminal domains, and are predicted to reside in the *H. pylori* outer membrane.[27] The functions of the 30 members of this family are still mostly unknown.[28] There are about 500 Le^b-binding molecules per bacterium that bind Le^b with a dissociation constant of 0.1 nM.[24] Although there is no direct information on the control of the expression of BabA, earlier work suggested that Le^b-binding activity was greatest in stationary phase.[10,19] Epidemiologic data also supports that BabA is an important molecule for gastric disease. *H. pylori* strains that contain the *babA2* gene are more likely to be associated with duodenal ulcer and adenocarcinoma, although not with gastritis or mucosa-associated lymphoid tissue (MALT) lymphoma.[29] Further epidemiological studies reveal a dominant genotype among strains from patients with active disease. These strains are triple positive for the *babA2* gene (and the associated ability to adhere to Le^b), the *vacAs1* allele of the vacuolating cytotoxin, and *cagA*, suggesting there is an advantage to carrying all three of these loci. To date, full characterization of the effect of inactivation of the *babA2* gene on both *in vitro* and *in vivo* Le^b binding has not been presented. Thus it is difficult to conclude too much about the role of this activity during infection.

5. BEYOND Le^b TO SEVERAL ALLEGED ADHESINS

Several putative *H. pylori* adhesins, in addition to BabA, have been identified. None of these have been tested for their effect on virulence in animals. *alpA* and *alpB* were originally identified as transposon mutants with reduced binding to KatoIII cells[30] and are now known to encode outer membrane proteins that are also required for binding human gastric tissue in situ.[31] Neither the role(s) of these proteins in pathogenesis, nor the molecules they bind, have been established. Monoclonal antibodies to heat shock protein 60 (Hsp60) block *H. pylori* adherence to human cells, suggesting that an antigenically-related protein may be involved in adherence.[32] Interestingly, the protein recognized by the Hsp60-antibody localizes to the bacterial cell surface.[33]

It has been suggested that *H. pylori* binds phosphatidylethanolamine (PE) via a 63 kilodalton protein.[34–36] The N-terminal sequence of a purified PE-binding protein facilitated cloning of the respective gene, which turned out to be highly homologous to the cytoplasmic enzyme catalase (encoded by *katA*).[36–38] Construction of *katA*-deficient mutants abolished catalase activity, but apparently did not affect adherence to epithelial cells.[38] There is no information regarding the PE–binding ability of the catalase-deficient mutants, so it is unclear if the ability to bind PE is mediated by catalase or required for epithelial cell binding.

H. pylori binds to laminin with very high affinity (kd = 8.5 pM) in a saturable and partially non-reversible manner.[39,40] Binding of laminin has been attributed to both LPS [17,39,41] and a 25 kD protein.[40,42] N-acetylneuraminyllactose (3 sialyllactose) is an oligosaccharide that is found in laminin.[42] The 26–29 kD HpaA protein was cloned as an N-acetylneuraminyllactose-binding protein.[43] This protein was sufficient to allow *E. coli* to bind human gastric epithelial biopsy sections *in situ*.[43] The ability to bind N-acetylneuraminyllactose correlates with the ability to agglutinate red blood cells.[43] Mutants deficient in *hpaA*, however, adhered to cultured gastric cells, human gastric slices and caused hemagglutination as well as the wild-type parent.[44,45] Interestingly, two groups found that HpaA was not involved in binding to cells, they found different subcellular localizations of HpaA: in the cytoplasm[45] or on the flagellar sheath.[44] There is some evidence that freshly isolated *H. pylori* are more likely to bind sialic acid-containing molecules than lab-passaged strains, suggesting that the *hpaA*-minus phenotype should be carefully evaluated in clinical isolates.[46] The relative roles that HpaA and LPS play in N-acetylneuraminyllactose binding remains to be teased apart.

6. WHAT DOES ADHERENCE DO FOR *H. pylori* ANYWAY?

The Le^b-transgenic mice, as well as other studies, strongly suggest that adherence is not required for colonization or persistence in the stomach.[47,48] This observation is consistent with the finding that administration of various anti-adhesion compounds such as 3′-sialyllactose to monkeys or humans had modest or no effect on colonization levels.[49,50] The transgenic mice were tested by comparison of transgenic mice expressing molecules *H. pylori* bound with non-transgenic littermates. Regardless of how many *H. pylori* adhered to the epithelial cells, all the mice were colonized with the same numbers of bacteria, and also retained this level of colonization for extended periods of time. The level of immune response, however, was different between the two groups. In mice with adherent *H. pylori*, there was an increased humoral and cellular immune response.[47,48] This phenomenon may act in human infection as well: in gastric biopsies, elevated numbers of adherent *H. pylori* correlate with increased epithelial damage.[12,14,15] This finding suggests that adherent bacteria lead to an elevated immune response, which in turn leads to host cell damage, as has been suggested with the Le^b-expressing mice. The molecular basis for this is still not known, as immune effector molecules such as NF-kB and IL-8 can be induced by culture supernatants.[51] Adherence could also directly facilitate epithelial cell damage by the delivery of bacterial molecules into host cells. The *Cag*A protein, which affects the host cell cytoskeleton,[52] is delivered directly into host cells by adherent *H. pylori*.[52–55] Toxins such as VacA, however, can be delivered without adherence.[56] Mathematical modeling supports a hypothesis that damage to the epithelial cells provides nutrients to the *H. pylori*.[57,58] In summary, it seems that adherence is not needed by *H. pylori* for colonization, but may lead to increased cellular damage, either directly or indirectly, and this may result in a more favorable environment for the growth of *H. pylori*.

7. THE VACUOLATING CYTOTOXIN, VacA

Shortly after the discovery of *H. pylori*, Leunk *et al.*[59] observed that broth culture supernatants induced noncytotoxic cytopathic effects on a number of mammalian cell lines. These cell lines accumulated large intracellular vacuoles. This activity was found in 110/201 strains (55%) and dubbed vacuolating cytotoxin, or VacA. Later VacA was shown to cause vacuolation of primary human mucosal epithelial cells as well.[60]

8. PRIMARY SEQUENCE AND SEQUENCE VARIABILITY OF *vacA*

Three separate groups sequenced the *vacA* gene from two different strains of *H. pylori* (Figure 1).[61–63] Cover *et al.* purified the 87 kDa VacA protein from strain 60190 (ATCC 49503). Peptide sequencing allowed the use of degenerate primers to screen a genomic library. The identified genomic clone encoded a 139 kDa precursor with a classical signal sequence and a C-terminal transmembrane domain with structural similarities to the amphipathic core domain of other bacterial proteins including the IgA proteases of *Haemophilus influenzae* and *Neisseria gonorrhoeae*. In a fashion similar to the cleavage seen in the IgA proteases, cleavage of the

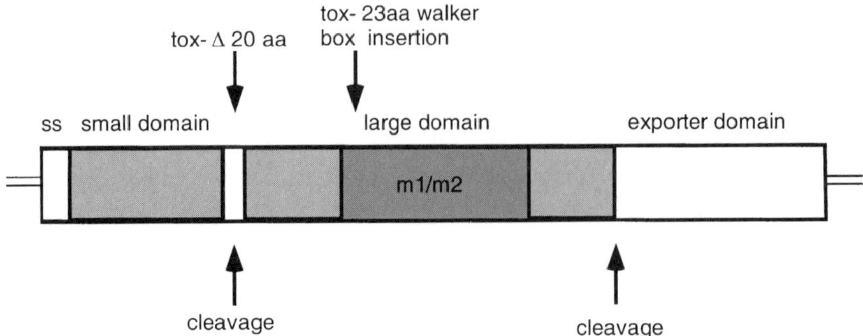

FIGURE 1. Schematic diagram of VacA showing the signal sequence (ss), small domain, large domain containing the variable sequence m1/m2 and the C terminal exporter domain. The sites of proteolytic cleavage are indicated as well as the deletion and insertion observed in the tox– strains.

C-terminal transmembrane domain would leave an 87 kDa polypeptide that corresponds to the observed size of the VacA protein on western blots of whole cell extracts. Antibodies against different portions of VacA revealed that, in addition to the cleavage upon export to release the N-terminal 94 kD piece, a second cleavage event occurred resulting in 37 kD and 58 kD polypeptides (Figure 1).[63] From strain to strain, the size of the full-length and cleaved polypeptides varies. We will refer to the cleavage products of the mature toxin as the small (N-terminal, p37 or p33) and large (C-terminal, p58 or p70) domains.

Disruption of the *vacA* gene confirmed that it was responsible for encoding both protein and vacuolating activity.[61] DNA probes from various parts of the gene were used to check for the presence of the *vacA* gene in a variety of strains, including those that do not express active toxin (tox^-). The *vacA* gene was found in all strains, but there were differences in how well different strains hybridized to probes from different portions of the gene. This was the first indication of the variability between strains in the primary sequence of the *vacA* gene.

As noted, only 50% of strains showed vacuolating toxin activity (tox^+) on cultured HeLa cells. The *vacA* gene, however, appeared to be present in all strains.[64] Possible explanations for this anomaly include non-functional alleles, poor expression, or poor export of the *vacA* gene product in the tox^- strains. Garner *et al.* postulated that there was sequence variability between tox^+ and tox^- strains as manifested by the variable hybridization by some *vacA* probes to tox^- strains.[65] To explore the sequence diversity issue further, they cloned and sequenced different genomic fragments from 3 tox^+ and 3 tox^- strains of *H. pylori*. They found more variability within these *vacA* coding regions than between the non-coding intergenic region just upstream.

Atherton *et al.* further analyzed the vacA sequence variability by sequencing the entire *vacA* gene from the tox$^-$ strain Tx30a.[66] The VacA protein encoded by this gene underwent the same C terminal cleavage as VacA from tox$^+$ strains. Analysis of the DNA sequence revealed three major differences between the Tx30a *vacA* and the three other existing tox$^+$ *vacA* sequences. One difference was in the signal sequence. The first 25 amino acid residues were identical in all strains, while the remainder of the signal sequence of the Tx30a *vacA* gene was completely different. The second major difference was a 20 amino acid deletion spanning a repeat region where the cleavage between the small and large domains occurs. Thirdly, the Tx30a *vacA* gene contained an insertion of 23 amino acids at residue 501. This insertion encoded a potential ATP/GTP binding site motif (GNIYLGKS), corresponding to the Walker A consensus. By sequencing1.5 kb from the middle of one more tox$^+$ and one more tox$^-$ strain, they were able to define a 0.73 kb region where tox$^+$ and tox$^-$ strains were on average only 70.4% identical at the nucleotide level and 58.7% identical at the amino acid level. They called this region m1 in tox$^+$ or m2 in tox$^-$ strains.

An analysis of the m and signal sequence (s) regions of the *vacA* genes of 59 clinical isolates revealed that 22 contained m1 and 37 contained m2 sequences. They found three classes of s regions: s1a corresponds to the signal sequence found in the previously published tox$^+$ strains, s1b which differed from s1a by 12 nucleotide changes that resulted in 6 amino acid changes, and s2 corresponding to the signal sequence in Tx30a. In the 59 clinical isolates, 20 contained s1a, 20 s1b, and 19 s2. Interestingly, though m2 could be associated with all three signal sequence classes, the s2-m1 combination was not represented in the 59 strains examined. They also used the HeLa cell vacuolation assay and an ELISA assay to quantify VacA activity and protein levels in broth culture supernatants of these strains. They found that the s1/m1 combination correlated best with highest activity and protein amount and the s2/m2 combination with lower values for both these parameters. Additionally, using the patient history for these strains, they found a significant correlation between the s1 alleles and gastric ulcer disease.

In most cases, tox$^-$ strains produced very little VacA protein in immunoblots of culture supernatants. Primer extension analysis of 8 tox$^+$ and 9 tox$^-$ strains revealed that tox$^+$ strains often had more mRNA, but this was not always the case.[67] To determine if the *vacA* promoter region dictated this variability, *xylE* gene fusions were used. Using one a high expressing tox$^+$ *vacA* gene promoters and a low expressing *vacA* gene promoter, they ascertained that the XylE activity levels were consistent with the primer extension data in the corresponding strain background. By moving the high expressing promoter to the low expressing strain, and vice versa, they found that strain background determined expression level. This suggests that the expression of other proteins such as transcriptional activators or repressors probably plays a substantial role in determining the transcriptional level of the *vacA* gene.

Paglieaccia *et al.*, shed more light on the mystery of non-functional alleles of *vacA* in an elegant study in which the group characterized the VacA protein from strain 95–54.[68] DNA sequencing of this *vacA* gene revealed it belonged to the s1-m2 group, and immunoblotting demonstrated that the protein was produced and secreted. VacA from this strain did not induce vacuolation when administered exogenously to HeLa cells. However, when HeLa cells were transfected with a plasmid that expressed both the large and small domains, vacuolation was observed. This indicated that the protein was capable of vacuolation, from inside the cell, but was defective for getting into HeLa cells. In fact, they found that the vacuolation defect of 95–54 VacA was specific to HeLa cells because exogenously added 95–54 VacA could vacuolate both a rabbit kidney epithelial cell line (RK13) and primary human epithelial cells. Further binding studies revealed that the m2 allele is defective in binding HeLa cells while the m1 and m2 alleles bind to RK13 cells equally well.

In summary, the *vacA* gene is highly variable. Variability within the signal sequence, as well as difference in strain background, lead to different levels of VacA expression. Differences in the middle region determine cell-type binding.

9. TERTIARY STRUCTURE OF THE VacA PROTEIN

Initial observations suggested that purified VacA exists as an oligomeric complex.[64] Analytical size exclusion chromatography revealed that the VacA complex fractionates at a molecular weight of 660 kD.[69] Quick-freeze, deep-etching electron microscopy revealed that VacA formed both heptamers (70%) and hexamers (30%) with a flower-petal-type radially symmetric structure. On average, the diameter of the flower was 30 nm and contained a central hole of ~12 nm. Interestingly, examination of preparations that had undergone cleavage to the small and large domains revealed a similar structure. However, in these preparations, a small percentage of the flowers had lost their central core. The authors postulated that either the small or large domain comprised the central raised structure while the other made the petal. A second structural study[70] focused on the three dimensional structure of acid-activated VacA. Acid activation had previously been shown to increase the specific activity of purified VacA.[71] Under acidic conditions, VacA sediments at 5S, the size predicted to be monomeric, in contrast to the 22S oligomer seen previously. Using similar electron microscopy techniques as described above, the monomeric VacA appeared as individual petals. Since the acidified protein is more active, dissociation of the oligomer may be important for activity.

One additional study of tertiary structure focused on the large domain of VacA. The large domain, purified from *H. pylori*, could bind to HeLa cells with similar saturation kinetics as the full-length protein, but was not internalized.[72]

This protein was unable to vacuolate cells when administered exogenously or when transfected into HeLa cells. Crosslinking studies showed that the protein forms dimers and quick-freeze, deep-etch electron microscopy revealed a similar structure as that of the individual petals seen in the hexamers of the whole molecule. These results support a model in which the central core consists of the small domain of the protein, while the large domain composes the petals. A paradox remains in that acid activation, which increases activity, results in a structure that looks like individual petals, while the structure of the large domain alone appears as individual petals but is not active.

10. THE RELATIONSHIP BETWEEN STRUCTURE AND FUNCTION

A lot of research has focused on the functions of the two domains and delineation of required residues.[73,74] These studies were done by transfecting HeLa cells with constructs that fused the small and large domains into a single molecule. N-terminal and C-terminal and in frame internal deletions, revealed that well over half of the large domain, including the variable m portion, can be deleted and the protein retained vacuolating activity. However, as described above, the large domain, particularly the m portion, appears to be important for binding and entry into cells. Deletion of more than the first 6 amino acids of the small N-terminal domain abolishes activity. Toxin purified from *H. pylori* containing an in-frame deletion from residues 6 to 27 acts as a dominant negative inhibitor of the wild-type protein.[75] One possible explanation of this behavior is that this protein binds nonproductively to the cellular target of VacA and blocks access of the wild-type toxin. This allele may thus be a very useful reagent for further elucidation of VacA's mechanisms of action.

11. CHARACTERIZATION OF VACUOLES

11.1. The Role of ATPases

The role of vacuolar ATPases (vATPase) in VacA-induced vacuole formation was tested. Specific inhibitors of vATPases including bafilomycin, N-ethylmaleimide, NBD-Cl and DCCD all inhibited vacuolation, suggesting that vacuole formation requires a vATPase. In contrast, inhibiters of P-type, gastric and F_1F_0 ATPases did not alter vacuolation, suggesting these ATPases did not play a role in vacuolation.[76] Pretreatment of the bacterial extract with bafilomycin established that the required ATPase activity was not of bacterial origin.[77] Thus these studies suggested the accumulation of large swollen vacuoles in VacA-intoxicated cells resulted from an osmotic imbalance that depended on the cellular vATPase function.

11.2. From Where Do the Vacuole Membranes Originate?

A number of studies characterized the composition of the induced vacuoles and attempted to identify the source of the membranes that composed them. The normal flow of membranes within the cell, as shown in Figure 2, includes both the biosynthetic pathway and the endocytic pathway. The biosynthetic pathway begins at the Endoplasmic Reticulum (ER) and proceeds to the Golgi apparatus via vesicular intermediates. From the Golgi some vesicles proceed directly to the plasma membrane, while others travel to the endosome and from there to lysosomes. At the same time, endocytosis at the plasma membrane results in the formation of early endosomes. These early endosomes can fuse with each other as well as with vesicles coming from the trans-Golgi network to form late endosomes that can then mature into lysosomes. The first clues to the composition of VacA vacuoles came from the observation that the vacuoles contained rab7, a marker of late endosomes, but not the other rabs.[78] Rab proteins are part of the ras super family of small GTPases and regulate membrane fusion events in the exo- and endocytic pathways of eukaryotic cells. Rab7 accumulated over time in VacA-induced vacuoles.[78] These vacuoles did not contain transferrin receptor, a marker of early endosomes. Both colcicine and nocodazole, which inhibit the transitions from early to late endosome, inhibited vacuolization. This indicated that the VacA-induced vacuoles derive from the endocytic pathway and more likely the late endosome since they contain a marker of late endosomes (rab7) and require early endosome-late endosome fusion for their formation.

Further evidence implicating the late endosome as the source of the VacA vacuoles came from examining the effects of various mutant rab proteins on vacuole formation.[79] Rab5 appears to regulate steps early in the endocytic pathway leading to early endosomes, while rab7 affects early endosome-late endosome fusion, and rab9 functions in membrane cycling between late endosomes and the trans-Golgi network. Dominant negative rab mutations were tested for their effect on vacuolation and EGF receptor degradation. The EGF receptor normally proceeds from the early endosome to late endosomes and ultimately is degraded in lysosomes. Dominant-negative alleles of both rab5 and rab7 inhibited vacuole formation as well as EGF receptor degradation, while no rab9 alleles had any effect. Thus, formation of VacA-induced vacuoles requires rab5 and rab7, but not rab9. The membranes probably derive from the endocytic pathway, since they require two rab proteins that function in the endocytic pathway, and EGF receptor degradation is altered during VacA intoxication. The ability of VacA to stimulate endosome fusion in vitro was tested. Addition of purified VacA to a homotypic endosome-fusion assay had no effect, suggesting that VacA does not directly stimulate membrane fusion.

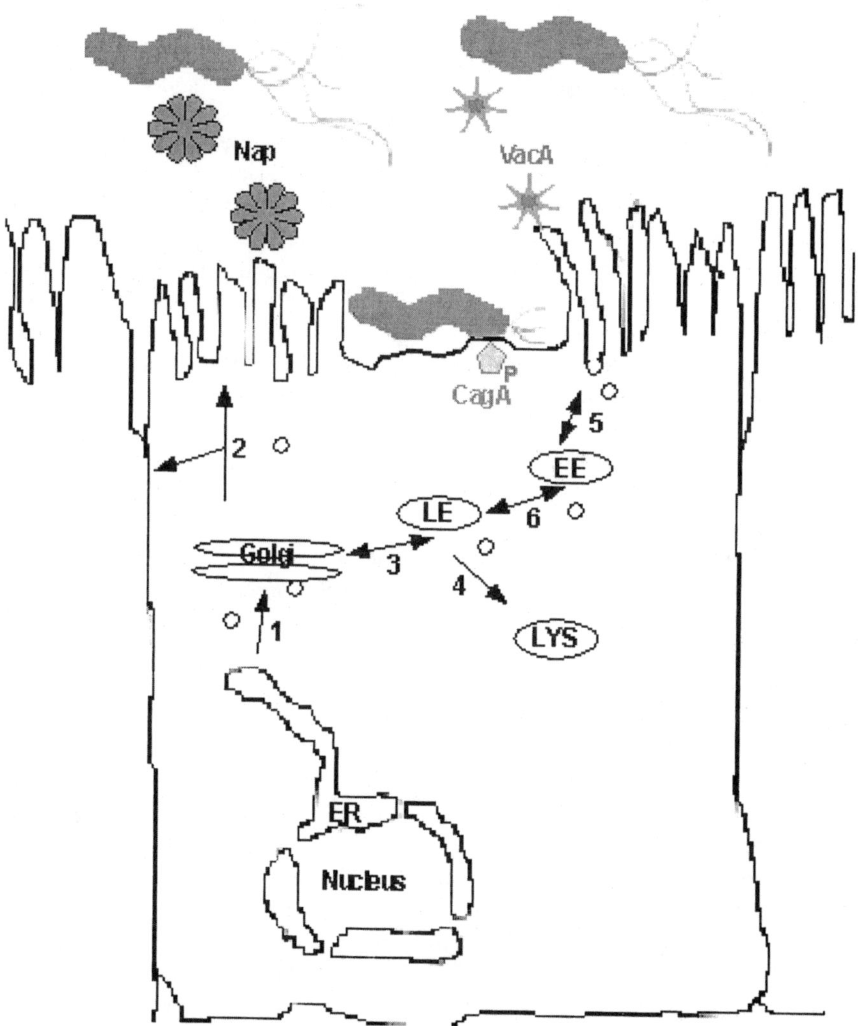

FIGURE 2. The normal biosynthetic pathway in epithelial cells and some known *H. pylori* products that interact with this cell type. Secretory proteins synthesized in the endoplasmic reticulum (ER) can move via vesicular intermediates to the Golgi apparatus (1). From the Golgi, protein-laden vesicles can proceed to the basal lateral or apical plasma membrane (2), or to the late endosome (LE, 3), which can then mature into lysosomes (LYS, 4). At the same time, proteins internalized into vesicles from the plasma membrane by endocytosis can fuse with early endosomes (EE, 5). Some proteins then recycle back to the plasma membrane (5) or proceed to late endosomes. From the late endosome, proteins can go to the lysosome for degradation (4). As indicated by the arrows, many steps in this pathway are reversible. *H. pylori* secretes at least 2 proteins into the medium that can alter host cells: NapA, which activates neutrophils, and VacA, which leads to the accumulation of vacuoles inside cells that have features of late endosomes. When *H. pylori* forms a tight association with the host cell, bacteria which contain the *Cag* PAI inject the *Cag*A protein into the host cell where it becomes phosphorylated and causes alterations in the actin cytoskeleton that ultimately lead to cell migration. A separate activity of the *Cag* PAI leads to activation of the $NF_{\kappa}B$ pathway and induction of expression of pro-inflammatory cytokines.

11.3. What's on and Inside VacA Vacuoles?

Fractionation of membrane compartments of baby hamster kidney (BHK) cells, using isopycnic gradient ultra centrifugation, with and without VacA revealed that the late endosome fractions of VacA-treated cells had additional proteins as compared to untreated cells.[80] After examining a variety of markers, they found that rab7 and the cation-independent mannose 6-P (CI-M6P) receptor showed the same distribution in these gradients +/− VacA, but lgp110, a lysosomal protein, shifted in the gradient to the late endosomal peak position (containing rab7 and CI-M6P) in cells incubated with VacA. Interestingly, CI-M6P receptor immunoreactivity showed the same distribution in cells +/− VacA and did not decorate VacA-induced vesicles. This shows that VacA-induced vacuoles have a similar density to late endosomes, but contain only a subset of late endosomal markers and contain some additional markers that normally are restricted to lysosomes.

Further characterization of VacA vacuoles focused on the effect of VacA on normal intracellular traffic. Satin *et al.* looked at the processing of Cathepsin D and the degradation of EGF receptor in HeLa cells.[81] Cathepsin D maturation was inhibited by VacA with a concomitant release of cathepsin D into the extracellular medium. EGF receptor degradation was also inhibited. Both of these effects could be due to an inhibition of late endosome-lysosome fusion. If this were true, one would expect that both cathepsin D and EGF receptor would be trapped in an endosome that never fused with a lysosome, but this was not the case. However, VacA increased the endosomal-lysosomal pH, which could explain both observations of the impairment of the degradative function of the VacA-intoxicated late endosomes and lysosomes and the mistargetting of cathepsin D and other acidic hydrolases. These authors postulated that the enhanced secretion of hydrolases caused by this defect might assist in degrading the host extracellular matrix and mucus, and thus provide more nutrients for the bacteria. Additionally, impairment of lysosomal degradation could effectively starve cells by limiting nutrient acquisition.[81]

In summary, VacA vacuoles contain membranes derived from the endocytic pathway by a rab7-dependent mechanism. The density of the vesicles is most similar to late endosomes, though they contain a unique mixture of markers, some from endosomes, and some from lysosomes. VacA intoxication disrupts the maturation of the late endosome and lysosome, compromising normal receptor turnover from the plasma membrane and targeting of lysosomal enzymes.

11.4. Mechanisms of VacA Action

Although there have been many studies with the purified toxin, the exact mechanism of action, particularly inside the animal host, is still unclear. There has, however, been considerable progress in understanding the kinetics of internalization of the toxin and its localization inside tissue culture cells. Additionally, a number of potential biochemical activities have been identified.

11.5. How Does VacA Get Inside Cells and Where Does It Localize?

To understand where VacA acts, Garner *et al.* used immunohistochemistry to look at binding and internalization of both the whole protein and the individual domains. Both recombinant subunits bound to AGS cells (gastric adenocarcinoma) at 4°C. If incubation was shifted to 37°C the proteins appeared in the cytosol. There was some punctate perinuclear staining, but no co-localization with vacuoles. This result suggests that the protein was cyotosolic and not membrane bound.

Quantitative assessment of binding showed saturable high affinity binding of VacA to HeLa cells with a Kd of ~1.4 nM.[82] Acid-activated VacA bound slightly less well. Inactivation of the toxin by fixation with formaldehyde resulted in a protein with a higher affinity for HeLa cells, and one that competitively inhibited binding of the native molecule. VacA also bound to Kato III and NIH3T3 cell lines, but not a human T lymphocyte (Jurkat) cell line, implying there is a cell-type specific receptor for VacA.[82]

In order to search for a cellular receptor for VacA, Yahiro *et al.* biotinylated the cell surface of AZ521, AGS, COS-7 and HL-60 cells, added purified VacA and immunoprecipitated with anti-VacA antibodies.[83] Using this technique they found that VacA bound a 140 kD protein in the two gastric cell lines but not the non-gastric cell lines (COS-7 and HL-60). In a subsequent study, further co-immunopreciptations from AZ521 cells with anti-VacA antisera identified a 250 kDa glycosylated protein antibody.[84] The relationship of this protein to the 140 kDa proteins is unclear. Peptide sequencing of the 250 kDa protein revealed it to be a receptor protein-tyrosine phosphatase (RPTPbeta/PTPzeta). Furthermore, p250 reacted with an anti-human RPTPbeta monoclonal antibody.[84] Interestingly, induction of RPTPbeta mRNA in HL-60 cells with phorbol 12-myristate 13-acetate (PMA) also caused this normally resistant cell line to be sensitive to VacA intoxication.[85] Since PMA causes a variety of cellular changes, it is not conclusive that RPTPbeta is the receptor for VacA. Transfection of this receptor into a non-responsive cell line to assess gain of vacuolation would firmly establish the role of this protein as the VacA receptor.

11.6. Pore Forming Activity

H. pylori can be detected in stool samples and can cause diarrhea in malnourished children and AIDS patients.[86] This could indicate an ability of *H. pylori* to compromise the integrity of epithelial monolayers or alter the water homeostasis of the cells. Additionally, VacA has been postulated to be a member of the super family of bacterial AB toxins based solely on its oligomeric two domain structure.[87] In these types of toxins, the B subunit is responsible for target cell binding and pore formation to allow translocation of the catalytic A subunit. Neither the small domain or the large domain share homology with B domains of other toxins, but several groups set out to test whether purified VacA has channel forming activity. The first indication that VacA has channel forming activity came from the observation that it increased the short circuit current in Caco2 cells.[88]

Subsequently, two groups went on to show that purified acid-activated VacA forms anion-selective, voltage-dependent pores in artificial membranes and HeLa cells.[89,90] They defined the permeability sequence of these pores as Cl^-, $HCO_3 \rightarrow$ pyruvate > d-gluconate > K^+, Li^+, Ba^{2+} > NH_4^+. Pore activity was not appreciably affected by membrane composition or by varying the pH between 4.8 and 12. The large domain alone showed no channel forming activity.[90] In HeLa cells, this current formed independent of ATP levels, but did not occur in the presence of anti-VacA antiserum.[89] To rule out the possibility that VacA was affecting endogenous channels, a variety of channel-specific inhibitors were tested for their effects on VacA channel formation.[89] These experiments established that VacA can induce a Cl^- conducting activity in HeLa cells whose properties differs from all the endogenous Cl^- channels.

Further work was done to characterize how the VacA-induced channels affected cells. Opening of Cl^- channels is expected to cause depolarization. Szabo *et al.* showed this was indeed the case using a membrane potential-indicating probe and a voltage sensitive Probe.[89] Another voltage probe that accumulates almost exclusively inside mitochondria was not modified by VacA, indicating the VacA channels do not affect the mitochondria. VacA also caused increased transepithelial conductance to molecules <340 kDa in Madin-Darby canine kidney (MDCK) cell epithelial monolayers.[89] In order to try and separate vacuolating activity from pore activity, seven Cl^- channel inhibitors were examined to see how they altered channel forming activity by VacA in planar lipid bilayers and vacuolation activity in HeLa cells. All inhibited channel formation to varying degrees, while simultaneously inhibiting vacuolation with the same order of severity. Thus, to date, the two activities cannot be uncoupled.[91]

Whether VacA exerts its effects by interacting directly with cellular membranes to form pores or whether it does this through a second cellular protein remains unknown. De Bernard *et al.* attempted to search for a possible cellular target of VacA using a yeast two hybrid system.[92] They identified a single VacA-interacting protein from HeLa cells called VIP54 for Vacuolating toxin Interacting Protein. A glutathione S tranferase-VIP54 fusion protein could bind purified VacA. Antibodies raised to VIP54 were used to demonstrate that VIP54 localized to the cytoplasm and to intermediate filaments, and that it co-precipitated with the intermediate filament protein vimentin. Unfortunately, they could not detect VIP54 staining in VacA-intoxicated cells, or show VIP54 localization to late endosomes in untreated cells. Thus a biologically relevant interaction between VacA and VIP54 remains to be shown.

11.7. Antigen Processing

The vacuoles that accumulate in VacA-intoxicated cells have features of both early endosomes and late endosomes (see above). They contain rab7 and lysosomal membrane glycoproteins but do not contain the cation-independent mannose 6-P receptor. These features are shared by compartments of antigen presenting cells (APCs) in which antigen proteolytic processing takes place. Because of these similarities, Molinari *et al.*[93] checked whether VacA had an effect on antigen presentation. They used a model consisting of tetanus toxoid-specific human ($CD4^{+}$) T cells stimulated by B cells that had been pulsed with the autologous antigen. In this model the B cells process the antigen, via proteolysis and present it on their surfaces to the T cells. VacA inhibited degradation of I^{125}-labeled tetanus toxin in B cells. Similarly, VacA inhibited processing of a variety of antigens in several different B cell clones. Antigen presentation can occur by two pathways. In one, newly synthesized MHCII molecules associate with the invariant chain peptide (Ii) in the endoplasmic reticulum. This peptide is then displaced by the peptide to be presented in the antigen-processing compartment. In the other, mature receptors associate with the peptides to be presented directly in an early endocytic compartment. Using T cell clones specific to epitopes generated by these two different pathways, they showed that VacA inhibited Ii-dependent antigen processing, but not Ii-independent antigen processing. VacA did not inhibit peptide loading or presentation to T cells per se as T cell stimulation was restored by the addition of the appropriate peptide instead of whole protein to the antigen presenting cells.[93]

11.8. Role of VacA in Virulence

The role of VacA in virulence has been tested in several animal models of infection. Ghiara *et al.* administered VacA in broth culture supernatants to BALB/c Mice.[56] They found epithelial cell damage, mono- and polynuclear cell infiltration into the gastric mucosa, and a reduction in the thickness of the mucus layer. Broth culture supernatants from isogenic *vacA* mutants were diminished in their ability to induce epithelial damage. Using *H. pylori* instead of broth culture supernatants in a gnotobiotic piglet model, isogenic *vacA* mutant strains colonized just as well as wild type did, and elicited the same amount of gastritis.[94] In a gerbil model of infection, isogenic *vacA* mutants were slightly reduced in their ability to colonize (25/29 animal infected with *vacA* mutant vs 25/25 with wild type), though the number of organisms recovered from infected animals was unchanged.[95] Thus,

VacA, when administered exogenously to mice can cause damage to the gastric epithelium, but its role in colonization and disease in other models is unclear.

12. *H. pylori* ALTERS CELL PROLIFERATION

In *H. pylori*-infected stomachs, there are occasional changes in the epithelial cell equilibrium: increased cell death and cell proliferation. These phenomena lead, respectively, to ulcerous erosions and gastric cancer. Several studies have examined these aspects in human biopsy specimens and in *in vitro* cell culture systems. Below we summarize the proliferation aspect of this literature; more detail is provided elsewhere in this book which covers *H. pylori* and apoptosis.

Numerous studies have examined the effect of *H. pylori* on proliferation of gastric epithelial cells *in vivo*. Immunohistochemistry of gastric biopsies can be used to detect Proliferating Cell Nuclear Antigen (PCNA), a protein that is present only in dividing cells. Brenes and coworkers used this technique to show that when an *H. pylori* infection was cured (using antibiotic treatment), the number of cells that reacted with PCNA antibodies decreased significantly.[96] These results suggested that *H. pylori* increased the number of proliferating epithelial cells, and that elimination of it rapidly abrogated this proliferation. A similar phenomenon was found using different markers of proliferation (immunohistochemistry with anti-Ki-67 as well as anti-PCNA antibodies, or visual identification of the numbers of cells undergoing mitosis).[97] Furthermore, the decrease in cell proliferation due to *H. pylori* elimination persisted for at least 6 months.[97] The proliferating cells localized mostly to the normal region of gastric epithelial cell proliferation, the gland neck in the middle third of the gland, but also extended deeper into the gland.[96–99] This suggests that *H. pylori* mostly accelerates normal proliferation but can also lead to proliferation of normally non-dividing cells.

In most cases, the number of proliferating cells dropped only when *H. pylori* was eliminated.[96,97] However, in at least some cases the number of proliferating epithelial cells decreased simply with antibiotic treatment, regardless of whether *H. pylori* was eliminated.[99] In this study the authors noted a correlation between the amount of neutrophil inflammation and the numbers of proliferating epithelial cells, suggesting that inflammation increased the numbers of the proliferating cells. In this hypothesis, the inflammatory response and increased neutrophils were caused by the *H. pylori*, but the numbers of neutrophils could be reduced by antibiotic treatment itself. These results suggest that *H. pylori* may not directly cause the increase in cell proliferation, but instead may lead to inflammation which in turn leads to increased proliferation. In support of this idea, Nardone and coworkers used two measures to determine that the amount of proliferation increased in any person with gastritis, whether or not *H. pylori* was present.[98] Antibiotic treatment of the *H. pylori*-positive patients resulted in a concomitant decrease in numbers of proliferating cells and extent of inflammatory infiltrate, measurable up to one year later. Patients who had gastritis but not *H. pylori* were not examined to see if antibiotic treatment affected cell proliferation. Thus whether proliferation is a direct effect of the bacteria, or an effect of the infiltrating immune cells has not been resolved.

Another way to assess proliferation is to culture gastric biopsies with brdU, a DNA analog. The more cell division, the more brdU is incorporated. Similar to the results above, biopsies from patients infected with *H. pylori*, incorporated more brdU, indicating an increased degree of cell proliferation.[100] The amount of incorporated brdU decreased in patients treated with antibiotics who eliminated the *H. pylori*, and remained constant if the *H. pylori* persisted. Using the same approach, Lynch *et al.* compared biopsies from uninfected, *H. pylori*-positive and gastritis-negative, and *H. pylori*-positive and gastritis-positive people.[101] The *H. pylori*-positive gastritis-positive biopsy samples showed increases in brdU incorporation compared to normal or gastritis negative patients. Antibiotic treatment of these gastritis-positive patients decreased the quantity of proliferating cells. At 4 weeks post treatment, this decrease occurred regardless of *H. pylori* eradication. At 12 months post treatment, however, the amount of proliferation in samples that retained the *H. pylori* had climbed to the pretreatment levels. Taken together, these results suggest that antibiotics can have short term effects on cell proliferation directly, but long term increases depend on the presence of *H. pylori*.

In order to further probe how *H. pylori* alters the cell cycle, researchers have attempted to identify the bacterial molecule(s) responsible. Cell-free extracts from several *H. pylori* strains inhibited DNA synthesis, and therefore cell proliferation, of multiple cell lines.[102] This activity inhibited cellular protein synthesis, was reversible and did not kill the cells. Physical and chemical treatment of the soluble extract indicated that the active molecule was a protein with a molecular mass of about 100 kD. The active protein was not urease, CagA or VacA, but its identity is still not known.

Bacteria-free broth culture supernatants were shown to contain factors that impaired cell proliferation.[103] Culture supernatant was found to contain two active components: VacA (or something that depended on *vacA*), and a second smaller molecule that was less than 12 kilodaltons in size. Treatment of the supernatants with anti-VacA antibodies partially eliminated the cell proliferation effect, supporting the idea that one of the active molecules is VacA. The identity of the smaller molecule remains to be determined. From these studies it seems likely that *H. pylori* inhibits cell proliferation of cultured cells. Furthermore, preliminary work has suggested that individual molecules, including VacA, can mediate this response, but the identity of most of these molecules remains to be determined.

13. HOW *H. pylori* AFFECTS CELL SHAPE AND MOTILITY

During the course of infection, *H. pylori* are found primarily in the gastric mucus with a significant number of organisms in close association with gastric epithelial cells within the gastric pits. Based on examination of human biopsy specimens, the microvilli of these cells appear damaged and often missing. This alteration in microvilli may involve a reorganization of the cytoskeletal network. Segal *et al.* examined cytoskeletal rearrangements directly using infection of AGS cells, a gastric epithelial cell line, with *H. pylori*. Using transmission electron microscopy, *H. pylori* were observed on cup-like projections, often with electron-dense material at the base. Immunofluorescence revealed actin polymerization at these sites of bacterial attachment.[104] This phenotype appears related, at a visual level, to the massive actin polymerization and pedestal formation observed during the association of Enteropathogenic *E. coli* (EPEC) with intestinal epithelial cells, although it is less dramatic. EPEC contains a large pathogenicity island encoding a type III secretion system. This system injects a number of proteins into the host cell that facilitate tight binding of the bacteria, and instructs host cell signaling pathways to rearrange the cytoskeleton.

Censini *et al.* and Akopyants *et al.* discovered a pathogenicity island in a subset of *H. pylori* strains upstream of the gene encoding the immunodominant antigen CagA.[105,106] This pathogenicity island, called *Cag* PAI, does not encode a type III secretion system and does not contain homologues of any of the EPEC effector proteins. Many of the genes in this 40 kb island have some homology to genes from type IV secretion systems. Type IV secretion systems are involved in the transfer of large molecules such as DNA by *Agrobacterium tumefaciens* and a protein toxin by *Bordetella* species. The details of the *Cag* PAI are discussed in elsewhere in this volume. The sequence of two pathogenic *H. pylori* strains have been published and both strains contain the *Cag* PAI, and no other large insertions of genes indicative of another pathogenicity island.[27,107] Recently, four groups have shown that the CagA protein is injected into eukaryotic host cells and phosphorylated on tyrosine residues when *H. pylori* are in tight association with host cells.[52–55] The Tir protein of EPEC also is translocated into host cells and phosphorylated, pointing to further similarities between *H. pylori*-gastric cell interactions and EPEC-intestinal cell interactions.[108] Mutations in several other genes in the *Cag* PAI abolish the ability of CagA to fractionate with host cells, suggesting that *H. pylori* may use these proteins to build a secretion system that pumps CagA, and possibly other molecules, into host cells.[53,54] This finding supports the idea that *H. pylori* shares strategies with EPEC to manipulate host cells.

The role of the pathogenicity island in directing host cell cytoskeleton changes are beginning to be fleshed out. Strains that lack the *Cag* PAI show less pronounced actin condensation around the bacteria than strains containing the full *Cag* PAI.[109] However, isogenic mutants that eliminate specific genes of the pathogenicity island and result in loss of other activities of the *Cag* PAI, such as proinflammatory cytokine induction or *Cag*A translocation and phosphorylation, retain high levels of actin polymerization. This observation could mean that there are additional differences between *H. pylori* strains outside of the pathogenicity island, or that elimination of the full *Cag* PAI removes a necessary gene that the smaller mutations don't. A direct relationship between the presence of the pathogenicity island and cytoskeletal alterations has been supported by a detailed study of *H. pylori*-induced cell shape changes.[52] Co-culture of *H. pylori* with AGS cells for long periods (30 hr) in the absence of serum revealed that *H. pylori* can induce dramatic cell shape changes suggestive of cell migration. This phenotype was best seen in an isogenic *vacA*-mutant background in which there is no cell vacuolation. Mutations that eliminate *CagA*, or in the *Cag* PAI genes that block *Cag*A delivery into host cells, block this phenotype. Interestingly, this study uncovered a second *H. pylori* induced phenotype consisting of striking formation of stress fibers that does not depend on the *Cag* PAI. Stress fibers are bundles of actin filaments and associated proteins in the cytoplasm that are associated with the lower surface of the cell adjacent to the substratum. This suggests that *H. pylori* has multiple effects on the host-cell cytoskeleton, not all of which are mediated by the *Cag* PAI.

In addition to effects on epithelial cells, *H. pylori* changes the motility of neutrophils. Yoshida *et al.*, described a *H. pylori* neutrophil activating protein (NapA) that increases neutrophil adhesion to endothelial cells.[110] This *H. pylori* activity apparently acts by upregulating the cell surface markers CD18 and CD11b on the neutrophils. Further characterization revealed that NapA is a 15 kD protein that forms a dodecamer and has homology to bacterioferritins and DNA protecting proteins.[111,112] NapA was shown to bind up to 500 atoms of iron per oligomer. A neutrophil receptor for this protein has not been identified. Whether this protein plays a role in epithelial cell migration also remains to be tested. However, these results suggests that *H. pylori* modifies its cellular microenvironment by both chasing out epithelial cells and recruiting neutrophils.

14. CONCLUSION

H. pylori is a remarkable microorganism that inhibits a specialized niche within the stomach of primates, including humans. One can argue whether *H. pylori* is a commensal of humans or if it is a true pathogen. Most infected individuals are asymptomatic, yet one in ten develop ulcer disease and one in 100 develop gastric cancer. Both commensals and pathogens depend on their host for replication and persistence and can be carried asymptomatically. The distinction between these two states is that the pathogen, unlike the commensal, often possesses the ability to either perturb or intoxicate the host's physiology and metabolism and/or to spontaneously cross cellular and anatomic barriers. These barriers normally protect adjacent tissues from bacterial invasion and resulting harm. If host defenses are compromised then the commensal may become an opportunistic pathogen and can often have devastating effects on the host. Hence, the true pathogen consistently mediates overt disease in a significant proportion of infected individuals, unlike the opportunist. We remain largely ignorant of the extent of the interaction between the true commensal microbe and its host as contrasted to those circumstances when the true pathogen is asymptomatically colonizing the host. Unlike most members of the Helicobacter genus, a significant percentage of *H. pylori* form a close association with host cells. In addition, the nature of this interaction differs in two distinct clonal types, type I and type II, one of which more closely resembles the true commensal and the other of which resembles more closely the true pathogen!

It is worthwhile, perhaps, to examine those genetic and molecular attributes of *H. pylori* shared by type I and type II strains that contribute to interactions with the host. Both strains are motile and produce a powerful urease and both of these factors are essential for type I colonization (at least in animal models of infection). Both types produce a neutrophil activating protein, NapA, as well as a form of the VacA cytotoxin. A survey of the adherence properties of *H. pylori* reveal many potential adhesins and receptor molecules but no one seems to be more essential than the other. Indeed, one comes away with the conclusion, that, like many other *Helicobacter* species, adherence is not essential for host colonization. Yet, observations in infected humans, as deduced from biopsy samples, as well as observations in infected primates suggest that at any given moment 20% of the bacteria can be seen in intimate association with the gastric mucosa. Moreover, whether the organism is type I or type II, there is some level of local inflammation. That inflammation is an inevitable consequence of *H. pylori* infection seems to suggest that this is a necessary property of the bacterium's ability to persist within the host for a lifetime. Of course commensals also live in a host for a lifetime, but they do not appear to necessarily modulate the host's defenses to achieve their goal. The distinction between type I and type II *H. pylori* appears to be a matter of degree of host insult and is clearly the result of the inheritance of a defined genetic sequence, the *Cag* PAI. As described above and elsewhere in the book, the *Cag* PAI encodes a secretory apparatus and one or more effector molecules that are delivered into the host cell. There are at least two distinct consequences of the presence of the *Cag* PAI. The first is the induction of a cytokine "storm" in an infected host cell. The second is that type I strains introduce a distinct protein, CagA, into the host cell where it is phosphorylated on a specific tyrosine residue by a host cell enzyme. This interaction results in a rapid and striking change in host cell morphology that seems to be a consequence of the induction of host cell motility. Thus, the direct consequence of the *H. pylori* host cell interaction is a brisk inflammatory response, intoxication by VacA and NapA and a directed cytoskeletal change in some strains that leads to host cell motility. The end result is more instances of serious overt disease in the individual infected with type I strains. One supposes that the inheritance of the *Cag* PAI provides the microbe with a selective advantage. This selective advantage may reflect the ability of the microbe to out-compete its competitors, block the host defenses, or better replicate and persist in its niche.

Both type I and type II *H. pylori* appear able to suppress both the innate and adaptive immune system. Despite a robust immune response, the bacteria persist in the face of phagocytes, inflammatory factors and, antibodies directed against several antigens, including CagA. There is a good deal of information that has been reported about VacA and its effects on the host cell. Yet, despite this wealth of information, the precise role this toxin plays in the biology of the microbe still remains a matter of speculation. There is a need to determine the genetic factors required for colonization, long-term persistence and the actual role of inflammation and induced host-cell motility. It is clear from mouse studies and from the experiments of nature that the *Cag* PAI as well as VacA production increase virulence, but neither are essential for colonization or persistence. The inheritance of *Cag* PAI had important implications for the bacterium as well as for human health. At present the implications for human health are easier to gauge than the importance for the biology of the microbe. One makes the assumption that the type II lineage was the ancestral clone to inhabit the human niche to be followed only later by the inheritance of the *Cag* PAI.

H. pylori infection reflects a particularly intriguing example of a host-pathogen interaction. It has a relatively small genome and the number and nature of the basic set of bacterial tools to adapt and persist in the human host seems almost puny in comparison to the more complex pathogens like *Mycobacterium tuberculosis* or *Salmonella typhi*, which also can persist within infected human hosts for decades or even a life-time. Even the incremental assistance of the *Cag* PAI, gained, we presume, by horizontal gene transfer, surely has profound impact on the human host but is not impressive in terms of the new virulence determinants added to the basic bacterial platform. This highly adapted host-parasite interaction promises to provide one of the most readily accessible models of bacterial disease. Further studies of the effects of this limited set of *H. pylori* virulence factors on host cells should provide new perspectives about the inflammatory response to microbial insult and the steps involved in the evolution of malignancy, the most severe consequence of *H. pylori* infection.

ACKNOWLEDGEMENTS. The authors thank C. Detweiler and E. Strauss for comments on the manuscript.

REFERENCES

1. Hazell S. L., Lee A., Brady L., and Hennessy W., 1986, Campylobacter pyloridis and gastritis: association with intercellular spaces and adaptation to an environment of mucus as important factors in colonization of the gastric epithelium. *J. Infect. Dis.*, **153**:658.

2. Hessey S. J., *et al.*, 1990, Bacterial adhesion and disease activity in Helicobacter associated chronic gastritis [see comments]. *Gut*, **31**:134.
3. Noach L. A., Rolf T. M., and Tytgat G. N. J., 1994, Electron microscopic study of association between Helicobacter pylori and gastric and duodenal mucosa. *Journal of Clinical Pathology (London)*, **47**:699.
4. El-Shoura S. M., 1995, Helicobacter pylori: I. Ultrastructural sequences of adherence, attachment, and penetration into the gastric mucosa. *Ultrastructural Pathology*, **19**:323.
5. Bode G., Malfertheiner P., and Ditschuneit H., 1988, Pathogenetic implications of ultrastructural findings in Campylobacter pylori related gastroduodenal disease. *Scandinavian Journal of Gastroenterology. Supplement*, **142**:25.
6. Chan W. Y., Hui P. K., Leung K. M., and Thomas T. M., 1992, Modes of Helicobacter colonization and gastric epithelial damage. *Histopathology*, **21**:521.
7. Kazi J. L., *et al.*, 1990, Ultrastructural study of Helicobacter pylori-associated gastritis. *Journal of Pathology*, **161**:65.
8. Marshall B. J., and Warren J. R., 1984, Unidentified curved bacilli in the stomach of patients with gastritis and peptic ulceration. *Lancet*, **1**:1311.
9. Goodwin C. S., Armstrong J. A., and Marshall B. J., 1986, Campylobacter pyloridis, gastritis, and peptic ulceration. *Journal of Clinical Pathology*, **39**:353.
10. Falk P., *et al.*, 1993, An in vitro adherence assay reveals that Helicobacter pylori exhibits cell lineage-specific tropism in the human gastric epithelium. *Proceedings of the National Academy of Sciences of the United States of America*, **90**:2035.
11. Caselli M., *et al.*, 1989, Patterns of physical modes of contact between Campylobacter pylori and gastric epithelium: implications about the bacterial pathogenicity. *American Journal of Gastroenterology*, **84**:511.
12. Chan W. Y., *et al.*, 1991, Epithelial damage by Helicobacter pylori in gastric ulcers. *Histopathology*, **19**:47.
13. Bertram T. A., *et al.*, 1991, Gastritis associated with infection by Helicobacter pylori in humans: geographical differences. *Scand. J. Gastroenterol. Suppl.*, **181**:1.
14. Leung K. M., Hui P. K., Chan W. Y., and Thomas T. M., 1992, Helicobacter pylori-related gastritis and gastric ulcer. A continuum of progressive epithelial degeneration [see comments]. *American Journal of Clinical Pathology*, **98**:569.
15. Hui P. K., Chan W. Y., Cheung P. S., Chan J. K., and Ng C. S., 1992, Pathologic changes of gastric mucosa colonized by Helicobacter pylori [see comments]. *Human Pathology*, **23**:548.
16. Doig P., and Trust T. J., 1997, The molecular basis for H. pylori adherence and colonization, in: *The immunobiology of H. pylori: from pathogenesis to prevention*, Ernst P., Michetti P., and Smith P., ed., Lippincott-Raven, Philadelphia.
17. Clyne M., and Drumm B., 1996, Cell envelope characteristics of Helicobacter pylori: Their role in adherence to mucosal surfaces and virulence. *FEMS Immunology and Medical Microbiology*, **16**:141.
18. Watkins W. M., 1980, Biochemistry and Genetics of the ABO, Lewis, and P blood group systems. *Advances in Human Genetics*, **10**:1.
19. Boren T., Normark S., and Falk P., 1994, Helicobacter pylori: Molecular basis for host recognition and bacterial adherence. *Trends in Microbiology*, **2**:221.
20. Boren T., Falk P., Roth K. A., Larson G., and Normark S., 1993, Attachment of Helicobacter pylori to human gastric epithelium mediated by blood group antigens. *Science (Washington DC)*, **262**:1892.
21. Falk P. G., Bry L., Holgersson J., and Gordon J. I., 1995, Expression of a human alpha-1,3/4-fucosyltransferase in the pit cell lineage of FVB/N mouse stomach results in production of Le-b-containing glycoconjugates: A potential transgenic mouse model for studying Helicobacter pylori infection. *Proceedings of the National Academy of Sciences of the United States of America*, **92**:1515.

22. Clyne M., and Drumm B., 1997, Absence of effect of Lewis a and Lewis b expression on adherence of Helicobacter pylori to human gastric cells. *Gastroenterology*, **113**:72.
23. Su B., *et al.*, 1998, Type I Helicobacter pylori shows Lewisb-independent adherence to gastric cells requiring de novo protein synthesis in both host and bacteria. *Journal of Infectious Diseases*, **178**:1379.
24. Ilver D., *et al.*, 1998, Helicobacter pylori adhesin binding fucosylated histo-blood group antigens revealed by retagging. *Science*, **279**:373.
25. Slomiany B., and Slomainay A., 1993, Mucus and gastric mucosal protection, in: *The Stomach*, Domshke W., and Konturek S., ed., Springer-Verlag, Berlin.
26. Tzouvelekis L. S., *et al.*, 1991, In vitro binding of Helicobacter pylori to human gastric mucin. *Infection and Immunity*, **59**:4252.
27. Tomb J.-F., *et al.*, 1997, The complete genome sequence of the gastric pathogen *Helicobacter pylori*. *Nature*, **338**:539.
28. Marais A., Mendz G. L., Hazell S. L., and Megraud F., 1999, Metabolism and genetics of Helicobacter pylori: The genome era. *Microbiology and Molecular Biology Reviews*, **63**:642.
29. Gerhard M., *et al.*, 1999, Clinical relevance of the Helicobacter pylori gene for blood-group antigen-binding adhesin. *Proceedings of the National Academy of Sciences of the United States of America*, **96**:12778.
30. Odenbreit S., Till M., and Haas R., 1996, Optimized BlaM-transposon shuttle mutagenesis of Helicobacter pylori allows the identification of novel genetic loci involved in bacterial virulence. *Mol. Microbiol.*, **20**:361.
31. Odenbreit S., Till M., Hofreuter D., Faller G., and Haas R., 1999, Genetic and functional characterization of the alpAB gene locus essential for the adhesion of Helicobacter pylori to human gastric tissue. *Molecular Microbiology*, **31**:1537.
32. Yamaguchi H., *et al.*, 1997, Heat-shock protein 60 homologue of Helicobacter pylori is associated with adhesion of H. pylori to human gastric epithelial cells. *Journal of Medical Microbiology*, **46**:825.
33. Huesca M., Borgia S., Hoffman P., and Lingwood C. A., 1996, Acidic pH changes receptor binding specificity of Helicobacter pylori: A binary adhesion model in which surface heat shock (stress) proteins mediate sulfatide recognition in gastric colonization. *Infection and Immunity*, **64**:2643.
34. Lingwood C. A., Law H., Pellizzari A., Sherman P., and Drumm B., 1989, Gastric glycerolipid as a receptor for Campylobacter pylori. *Lancet*, **2**:238.
35. Lingwood C. A., Huesca M., and Kuksis A., 1992, The glycerolipid receptor for Helicobacter pylori (and exoenzyme S) is phosphatidylethanolamine. *Infection and Immunity*, **60**:2470.
36. Lingwood C. A., Wasfy G., Han H., and Huesca M., 1993, Receptor affinity purification of a lipid-binding adhesin from Helicobacter pylori. *Infection and Immunity*, **61**:2474.
37. Hazell S. L., Evans D. J. Jr., and Graham D. Y., 1991, Helicobacter pylori catalase. *Journal of General Microbiology*, **137**:57.
38. Odenbreit S., Wieland B., and Haas R., 1996, Cloning and genetic characterization of Helicobacter pylori catalase and construction of a catalase-deficient mutant strain. *Journal of Bacteriology*, **178**:6960.
39. Trust T. J., *et al.*, 1991, High-affinity binding of the basement membrane proteins collagen type IV and laminin to the gastric pathogen Helicobacter pylori. *Infection and Immunity*, **59**:4398.
40. Valkonen K. H., Ringner M., Ljungh A., and Wadstrom T., 1993, High-affinity binding of laminin by Helicobacter pylori: Evidence for a lectin-like interaction. *FEMS Immunology and Medical Microbiology*, **7**:29.
41. Valkonen K. H., Wadstrom T., and Moran A. P., 1994, Interaction of lipopolysaccharides of Helicobacter pylori with basement membrane protein laminin. *Infection and Immunity*, **62**: 2640.

42. Valkonen K. H., Wadstrom T., and Moran A. P., 1997, Identification of the N-acetylneuraminyllactose-specific laminin-binding protein of Helicobacter pylori. *Infection and Immunity*, **65**:916.
43. Evans D. G., Karjalainen T. K., Evans D. J., Graham D. Y., and Lee C.-H., 1993, Cloning, nucleotide sequence, and expression of a gene encoding an adhesin subunit protein of Helicobacter pylori. *Journal of Bacteriology*, **175**:674.
44. Jones A. C., *et al.*, 1997, A flagellar sheath protein of Helicobacter pylori is identical to HpaA, a putative N-acetylneuraminyllactose-binding hemagglutinin, but is not an adhesion for AGS cells. *Journal of Bacteriology*, **179**:5643.
45. O'Toole P. W., *et al.*, 1995, The putative neuraminyllactose-binding hemagglutinin HpaA of Helicobacter pylori CCUG 17874 is a lipoprotein. *Journal of Bacteriology*, **177**:6049.
46. Simon P. M., Goode P. L., Mobasseri A., and Zopf D., 1997, Inhibition of Helicobacter pylori binding to gastrointestinal epithelial cells by sialic acid-containing oligosaccharides. *Infection and Immunity*, **65**:750 .
47. Guruge J. L., *et al.*, 1998, Epithelial attachment alters the outcome of Helicobacter pylori infection. *Proceedings of the National Academy of Sciences of the United States of America*, **95**:3925.
48. Syder A. J., *et al.*, 1999, Helicobacter pylori attaches to NeuAcalpha2,3Galbeta1,4 glycoconjugates produced in the stomach of transgenic mice lacking parietal cells. *Molecular Cell*, **3**:263.
49. Opekun A. R., *et al.*, 1999, Novel therapies for Helicobacter pylori infection. *Alimentary Pharmacology & Therapeutics*, **13**:35.
50. Mysore J. V., *et al.*, 1999, Treatment of Helicobacter pylori infection in rhesus monkeys using a novel antiadhesion compound. *Gastroenterology*, **117**:1316.
51. Münzenmaier A., *et al.*, 1997, A secreted/shed product of Helicobacter pylori activates transcription factor nuclear factor-kappa B. *Journal of Immunology*, **159**:6140.
52. Segal E. D., Cha J., Lo J., Falkow S., and Tompkins L. S., 1999, Altered states: involvement of phosphorylated *Cag*A in the induction of host cellular growth changes by Helicobacter pylori. *Proceedings of the National Academy of Sciences of the United States of America*, **96**:14559.
53. Stein M., Rappuoli R., and Covacci A., 2000, Tyrosine phosphorylation of the Helicobacter pylori *Cag*A antigen after *cag*-driven host cell translocation. *Proc. Natl. Acad. Sci. USA*, **97**:1263.
54. Odenbreit S., *et al.*, 2000, Translocation of Helicobacter pylori *Cag*A into gastric epithelial cells by type IV secretion. *Science*, **287**:1497.
55. Asahi M., *et al.*, 2000, Helicobacter pylori *Cag*A protein can be tyrosine phosphorylated in gastric epithelial cells [see comments]. *J. Exp. Med.*, **191**:593.
56. Ghiara P., *et al.*, 1995, Role of the Helicobacter pylori virulence factors vacuolating cytotoxin, *Cag*A, and urease in a mouse model of disease. *Infect. Immun.*, **63**:4154.
57. Kirschner D. E., and Blaser M. J., 1995, The dynamics of Helicobacter pylori infection of the human stomach. *Journal of Theoretical Biology*, **176**:281.
58. Blaser M. J., and Kirschner D., 1999, Dynamics of Helicobacter pylori colonization in relation to the host response. *Proceedings of the National Academy of Sciences of the United States of America*, **96**:8359.
59. Leunk R. D., Johnson P. T., David B. C., Kraft W. G., and Morgan D. R., 1988, Cytotoxic activity in broth-culture filtrates of *Campylobacter pylori*. *Journal of Medical Microbiology*, **26**:93.
60. Harris P. R., *et al.*, 1996, *Helicobadter pylori* cytotoxin induces vacuolation of primary human mucosal epithelial cells. *Infection and Immunity*, **64**:4867.
61. Cover T. L., Tummuru M. K., Cao P., Thompson S. A., and Blaser M. J., 1994, Divergence of genetic sequences for the vacuolating cytotoxin among Helicobacter pylori strains. *Journal of Biological Chemistry*, **269**:10566.
62. Schmitt W., Odenbreit S., Heuermann D., and Haas R., 1995, Cloning of the Helicobacter pylori recA gene and functional characterization of its product. *Molecular and General Genetics*, **248**:563.

63. Telford J. L., *et al.*, 1994, Gene structure of Helicobacter pylori cytotoxin and evidence of its key role in gastric disease. *Journal of Experimental Medicine*, **179**:1653.
64. Cover T. L., and Blaser M. J., 1992, Purification and characterization of the vacuolating toxin from Helicobacter pylori. *Journal of Biological Chemistry*, **267**:10570.
65. Garner J. A., and Cover T. L., 1995, Analysis of genetic diversity in cytotoxin-producing and non-cytotoxin-productin Helicobacter pylroi strains. *The Journal of Infectious Diseases*, **170**:290.
66. Atherton J. C., *et al.*, 1995, Mosaicism in vacuolating cytotoxin alleles of Helicobacter pylori. Association of specific vacA types with cytotoxin production and peptic ulceration. *J. Biol. Chem.*, **270**:17771.
67. Forsyth M. H., Atherton J. C., Blaser M. J., and Cover T. L., 1998, Heterogeneity in levels of vacuolating cytotoxin gene (vacA) transcription among Helicobacter pylori strains. *Infect. Immun.*, **66**:3088.
68. Pagliaccia C., *et al.*, 1998, The m2 form of the *Helicobacter pylori* cytotoxin has cell type-specific vacuolating activity. *Proceedings of the National Academy of Sciences, USA*, **95**:10212.
69. Lupetti P., *et al.*, 1996, Oligomeric and subunit structure of the *Helicobacter pylori* vacuolatin cytotoxin. *Journal of Cell Biology*, **133**:801.
70. Cover T. L., Hanson P. I., and Heuser J. E., 1997, Acid-induced dissociation of VacA, the Helicobacter pylori vacuolatin cytotoxin, reveals its pattern of assembly. *Journal of Cell Biology*, **138**:759.
71. de Bernard M., *et al.*, 1995, Low pH activates the vacuolating toxin of Helicobacter pylori, which becomes acid and pepsin resistant. *J. Biol. Chem.*, **270**:23937.
72. Reyrat J. M., *et al.*, 1999, 3D imaging of the 58 kDa cell binding subunit of the Helicobacter pylori cytotoxin. *Journal of Molecular Biology*, **290**:459.
73. Ye D., Willhite D. C., and Blanke S. R., 1999, Identification of the minimal intracellular vacuolating domain of the *Helicobacter pylori* vacuolating toxin. *Journal of Biological Chemistry*, **274**:9277.
74. Bernard M. D., *et al.*, 1998, Identification of the *Helicobacer pylori* VacA toxin domain active in the cell cytosol. *Infection and Immunity*, **66**:6014.
75. Vinion-Dubiel A. D., *et al.*, 1999, A dominant negative mutant of Helicobacter pylori vacuolating toxin (VacA) inhibits VacA-induced cell vacuolation. *Journal of Biological Chemistry*, **274**:37736.
76. Cover T. L., Reddy L. Y., and Blaser M. J., 1993, Effects of ATPase Inhibitors on the Response of HeLa Cells to Helicobacter pylori vacuolating toxin. *Infection and Immunity*, **61**:1427.
77. Papini E., *et al.*, 1993, Bafilomycin A1 inhibits *Helicobacter pylori*-induced vacuolization of HeLa cells. *Moleuclar Microbiology*, **7**:323.
78. Papini E., *et al.*, 1994, Cellular vacuoles induced by Helicobacter pylori originate from late endosomal compartments. *Proceedings of the National Academy of Sciences, USA*, **91**:9720.
79. Papini E., *et al.*, 1996, The small GTP binding protein rab7 is essential for cellular vacuolation induced by *Helicobacter pylori* cytotoxin.
80. Molinari M., *et al.*, 1997, Vacuoles induced by *Helicobacter pylori* toxin contain both late endosomal and lysosomal markers. *Journal of Biolgical Chemistry*, **272**:25339.
81. Satin B., *et al.*, 1997, Effect of *Helicobact pylori* vacuolatiing toxin on maturation and extracellular release of porcathepsin D and on epidermal growth factor degredation. *Journal of Biological Chemistry*, **272**:25022.
82. Massari P., *et al.*, 1998, Binding of the *Helicobacter pylori* vacuolatin cytotoxin to target cells. *Infection and Immunity*, **66**:3981.
83. Yahiro K., *et al.*, 1997, *Helicobacter pylori* vacuolating cytotoxin binds to the 140-kDa protein in human gastric cancer cell lines, AZ-521 and AGS. *Biochemical and Biophysical Research Communications*, **238**:629.
84. Yahiro K., *et al.*, 1999, Activation of Helicobacter pylori VacA toxin by alkaline or acid conditions increases its binding to a 250-kDa receptor protein-tyrosine phosphatase beta. *J. Biol. Chem.*, **274**:36693.

85. Padilla P. I., *et al.*, 2000, Morphologic differentiation of HL-60 cells is associated with appearance of RPTPbeta and induction of helicobacter pylori VacA sensitivity [In Process Citation]. *J. Biol. Chem.*, **275**:15200.
86. Luzzi I., *et al.*, 1993, Detection of vacuolating toxin of Helicobacter pylori in human feces. *Lancet (North American Edition)*, **341**:1348.
87. Cover T. L., 1996, The vacuoloting cytotoxin of *Helicbacter pylori. Molecular Microbiology*, **20**:241.
88. Guarino A., *et al.*, 1998, Enterotoxic effects of the vacuolating toxin produced by *Helicobacter pylori* in Caco-2 cells. *Journal of Infectious Diseases*, **178**:1373.
89. Szabo I., *et al.*, 1999, Formation of anion-selective channels in the cell plasma membrane by the toxin VacA of *Helicobacter pylori* is required for its biological activity. *EMBO Journal*, **18**:5517.
90. Tombola F., *et al.*, 1999, *Heliocbacter pylori* vacuolating toxin forms anion-selective channels in planar lipid bilayers: possible implications for the mechanism of cellular vacuolation. *Biophyical Journal*, **76**:1401.
91. Tombola F., *et al.*, 1999, Inhibition of vacuolating and anion channel activities of the VacA toxin of *Helicobacter pylori. FEBS Letters*, **460**:221.
92. de Bernard M., Moschioni M., Napolitani G., Rappuoli R., and Montecucco C., 2000, The VacA toxin of Helicobacter pylori identifies a new intermediate filament-interacting protein. *Embo. J.*, **19**:48.
93. Molinari M., *et al.*, 1998, Selective inhibition of Li-dependent antigen presentatioin by *Helicobacter pylori* toxin VacA. *Journal of Experimental Medicine*, **187**:135.
94. Eaton K. A., Cover T. L., Tummutu M. K. R., Blaser M. J., and Krakowka S., 1997, Role of Vacoulating Cytotoxin in Gastritis Due to *Helicobacter pylori* in Gnotobiotic piglets. *Infection and Immunity*, **65**:3462.
95. Wirth H. P., Beins M. H., Yang M., Tham K. T., and Blaser M. J., 1998, Experimental infection of Mongolian gerbils with wild-type and mutant Helicobacter pylori strains. *Infect. Immun.*, **66**:4856.
96. Brenes F., *et al.*, 1993, Helicobacter pylori causes hyperproliferation of the gastric epithelium: Pre- and post-eradication indices of proliferating cell nuclear antigen. *American Journal of Gastroenterology*, **88**:1870.
97. Hibi K., *et al.*, 1997, Enhanced cellular proliferation and p53 accumulation in gastric mucosa chronically infected with Helicobacter pylori. *American Journal of Clinical Pathology*, **108**:26.
98. Nardone G., *et al.*, 1999, Effect of Helicobacter pylori infection and its eradication on cell proliferation, DNA status, and oncogene expression in patients with chronic gastritis. *Gut*, **44**:789.
99. Fraser A. G., Sim R., Sankey E. A., Dhillon A. P. and Pounder R. E., 1994, Effect of eradication of Helicobacter pylori on gastric epithelial cell proliferation. *Alimentary Pharmacology & Therapeutics*, **8**:167.
100. Cahill R. J., *et al.*, 1995, Effect of eradication of Helicobacter pylori infection on gastric epithelial cell proliferation. *Digestive Diseases and Sciences*, **40**:1627.
101. Lynch D. A. F., *et al.*, 1995, Cell proliferation in Helicobacter pylori associated gastritis and the effect of eradication therapy. *Gut*, **36**:346.
102. Knipp U., Birkholz S., Kaup W., and Opferkuch W., 1996, Partial characterization of a cell proliferation-inhibiting protein produced by Helicobacter pylori. *Infection and Immunity*, **64**:3491.
103. Ricci V., *et al.*, 1996, Effect of *Helicobacter pylori* on gastric epithelial cell migration and proliferation in vitro: role of VacA and *Cag*A. *Infection and Immunity*, **64**:2829.
104. Segal E. D., Falkow S., and Tompkins L. S., 1996, Helicobacter pylori attachment to gastric cells induces cytoskeletal rearrangements and tyrosine phosphorylation of host cell proteins. *Proc. Natl. Acad. Sci. USA*, **93**:1259.
105. Akopyants N. S., *et al.*, 1998, Analyses of the *cag* pahtogenicity island of *Helicobacter pylori. Molecular Microbiology*, **28**:37.

106. Censini S., *et al.*, 1996, *cag*, a pathogenicity island of *Helicobacter pylori*, encodes Type1-specific and disease-associated virulence factors. *Proceedings of the National Academy of Sciences, USA*, in press.
107. Alm R. A., *et al.*, 1999, Genomic-sequence comparison of two unrelated isolates of the human gastric pathogen Helicobacter pylori. *Nature (London)*, **397**:176.
108. Kenny B., *et al.*, 1997, Enteropathogenic E. coli (EPEC) transfers its receptor for intimate adherence into mammalian cells. *Cell*, **91**:511.
109. Segal E. D., Lange C., Covacci A., Tompkins L. S., and Falkow S., 1997, Induction of host signal transduction pathways by Helicobacter pylori. *Proc. Natl. Acad. Sci. USA*, **94**:7595.
110. Yoshida N., *et al.*, 1993, Mechanisms involved in Helicobacter pylori-induced inflammation. *Gastroenterology*, **105**:1431.
111. Evans D. G., *et al.*, 1995, Genetic evidens for host specificity in the adhesin'encoding genes *hxaA* of *Helicobacter acinonyx*, *hnaA* of *H. nemestrinae* and *hpaA* of *H. pylori*. *Gene*, **163**:97.
112. Tonello F., *et al.*, 1999, The Helicobacter pylori neutrophil-activating protein is an iron-binding protein with dodecameric structure. *Molecular Microbiology*, **34**:238.
113. Alkout A. M., *et al.*, 1997, Isolation of a cell surface component of Helicobacter pylori that binds H type 2, Lewis-a, and Lewis-b antigens. *Gastroenterology*, **112**:1179.
114. Angstrom J., *et al.*, 1998, The lactosylceramide binding specificity of Helicobacter pylori. *Glycobiology*, **8**:297.
115. Saitoh T., *et al.*, 1991, Identification of glycolipid receptors for Helicobacter pylori by TLC-immunostaining. *Febs Letters*, **282**:385.
116. Kamisago S., *et al.*, 1996, Role of sulfatides in adhesion of Helicobacter pylori to gastric cancer cells. *Infection and Immunity*, **64**:624.
117. Evans D. G., Evans D. J., Jr., Moulds J. J., and Graham D. Y., 1988, N-acetylneuraminyllactose-binding fibrillar hemagglutinin of Campylobacter pylori: a putative colonization factor antigen. *Infection and Immunity*, **56**:2896.
118. Ringner M., Valkonen K. H., and Wadstrom T., 1994, Binding of vitronectin and plasminogen to Helicobacter pylori. *FEMS Immunology and Medical Microbiology*, **9**:29.
119. Ascencio F., Fransson L. A., and Wadstrom T., 1993, Affinity of the gastric pathogen Helicobacter pylori for the N-sulphated glycosaminoglycan heparan sulfate. *Journal of Medical Microbiology*, **38**:240.
120. Fan X., *et al.*, 1998, The effect of class II major histocompatibility complex expression on adherence of Helicobacter pylori and induction of apoptosis in gastric epithelial cells: A mechanism for T helper cell type 1-mediated damage. *Journal of Experimental Medicine*, **187**:1659.

12

Role of Cytokines in *Helicobacter pylori* Infection

JEAN E. CRABTREE

1. INTRODUCTION

Mucosal damage induced by gastric *Helicobacter pylori* infection will result both from the direct effects of bacterial virulence factors and as a consequence of the inflammatory response elicited by the bacterium. Direct bacterial induced damage will result from the production of urease, phospholipase and the vacuolating cytotoxin. The persistent inflammatory response induced by the bacterium, which includes neutrophil and macrophage activation and induction of Th1 responses, as well as the changes in host physiological responses associated with infection, will also indirectly contribute to mucosal damage.[1] Understanding the mechanisms by which *H. pylori* induces acute and chronic inflammation in the gastric mucosa is important not only in elucidating the pathogenic role of this organism in gastroduodenal disease but also it is an important adjunct to optimizing immunotherapeutic regimes. The clinical importance of *H. pylori* infection has resulted in considerable attention being focused on investigations of host-pathogen interactions and

JEAN E. CRABTREE • Molecular Medicine Unit, St. James University Hospital Leeds LS9 7TF UK.

Correspondence: Dr. J. E. Crabtree Level 7 Clinical Sciences Building St. James's Hospital Leeds LS9 7TF. Tel: 0113-2065267; Fax: 0113-2429722

Helicobacter pylori Infection and Immunity,
Edited by Yamamoto *et al.*, Kluwer Academic/Plenum Publishers, 2002.

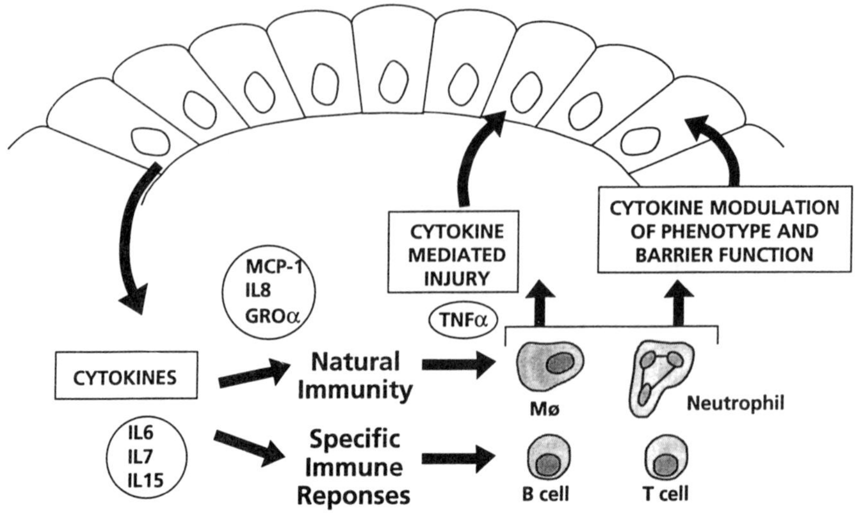

FIGURE 1. The role of the gastrointestinal epithelium in mucosal defense.

the role of cytokines in generation of the chronic inflammatory response.[2] Cytokines have a major role in regulating the extent and characteristics of both innate and specific mucosal inflammatory cellular response and they also contribute to the perturbations in gastric physiological responses associated with infection.[1] Cytokines, directly or indirectly, have a role in promoting gastric epithelial cell proliferation[3,4] and apoptosis[5,8] in *H. pylori* infection and they are also likely to be involved in the regulation of autoimmune responses[9] which can result as a consequence of long term chronic H. *pylori* infection.

2. CYTOKINES AND INNATE HOST RESPONSES

In recent years, the role of the epithelium in mucosal defense has become more fully appreciated.[10,11] The epithelium, the major interface between the host and pathogen, initiates acute mucosal inflammation and interacts with other mucosal cell populations via a cytokine network. The gastrointestinal epithelium will secrete chemokines such as IL-8/GROα.[12–14] Gastrointestinal epithelial cells also expresses transcripts or protein of cytokines with regulatory roles in antigen specific responses such as IL-7,[15] IL-15 [16] and IL-18.[17] The release of cytokines from activated mucosal cell populations will in turn modify epithelial function and phenotype (Figure 1). The capacity of gastrointestinal epithelial cells to secrete chemokines and stimulate innate cellular responses has been the focus of much recent research. The interaction of many bacterial pathogens with epithelial cells results in the secretion of C-X-C chemokines such as IL-8 and GROα, which are major neutrophil chemoattractants.[10,11] In the gastric mucosa, the C-X-C chemokine IL-8 is present in the epithelium and enhanced immunoreactivity is evident in *H. pylori* infection.[18] In addition IL-8 mRNA,[19,20] and transcripts of other C-X-C chemokines such as GROα and ENA-78,[20] are markedly increased in the gastric mucosa in *H. pylori* infection. The increase in epithelial C-X-C chemokines in *H. pylori* infection is thought to play an important role in the recruitment of neutrophils. The basal secretion of chemokines such as IL-8 from gastric epithelial cells induced by *H. pylori* and the binding of chemokines to proteoglycans within the matrix of the lamina propria is likely to be important in generating chemotactic gradients to promote directional migration of neutrophils towards the epithelium (Figure 2). Gastric IL-8 transcript and protein levels and neutrophil infiltration decline rapidly after *H. pylori* eradication demonstrating the direct effect of *H. pylori* infection on IL-8 gene expression.[21,22]

The molecular mechanisms by which *H. pylori* induces epithelial chemokines has been investigated in some detail. Tyrosine kinase inhibitors such as herbimycin[23–25] block *H. pylori*-induced IL-8 secretion and this chemokine response is dependent on activation of NF-kB.[23,26–28] Activated NF-kB has also been identified immuno-histochemically in the gastric epithelial cells of *H. pylori* infected patients.[27,29] Mutational studies in gastric epithelial cell lines have shown that transcriptional regulation of IL-8 by *H. pylori* involves primarily the NFkB site in the promoting region of the IL-8 gene and to a lesser extent the AP-1 site.[23,30] Gastric

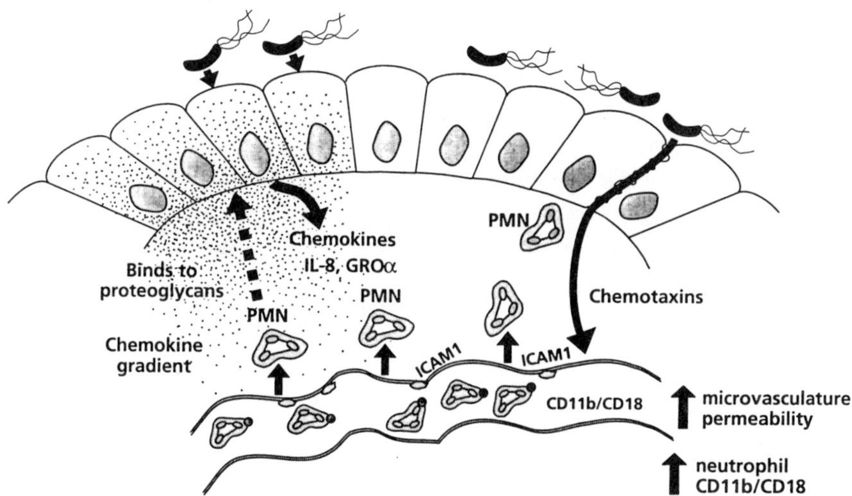

FIGURE 2. Propose model for *H. pylori* stimulation of neutrophils. PMN = polymorphonuclear cells, ICAM-1 = intracellular adhesion molecule 1.

epithelial cell activation by *H. pylori* involves extracellular signal-related kinases (ERK), p38 and c-Jun N-terminal kinase (JNK) MAP kinases.[31] Inhibitors of MAP kinase and p38 block *H. pylori*-induced IL-8 production.[31] There is a marked dichotomy in the ability of *H. pylori* to induce epithelial chemokines. Epithelial IL-8,[12–14] and NF-kB activation[28,32] are only induced by strains carrying the 40 kb *cag* pathogenicity island (PAI).[33,34] Activation of MAP kinases is also induced more strongly by *cag*+ strains than *cag*− strains.[31] The genes encoded by the *cag* PAI are part of a complex secretory system involved in host-pathogen interactions comparable to those previously documented in *Agrobacterium tumefaciens* and *Bordetella pertussis.*[33,34] Mutational studies have shown that multiple genes throughout the whole *cag* PAI are essential for the induction of IL-8 transcription or protein secretion in gastric epithelial cells *in vitro*,[25,33,34] NF-kB activation[32] and activation of MAP kinases.[31]

Examination of gastric chemokine mRNA expression in patients infected with *cag* positive and *cag* negative strains of *H. pylori* has substantiated that *cag* PAI positive *H. pylori* strains induce greater C-X-C chemokine responses.[19,20,35] Enhanced mucosal C-X-C chemokines which correlate with the extent of neutrophil infiltration[20] probably account for the increased neutrophilic infiltration observed in *cag* positive infection.[19,35,36] Such *in vivo* evidence linking enhanced gastric C-X-C chemokines with *cag* positive infection implies that the epithelial chemokine response has a significant role in neutrophil infiltration. Enhanced neutrophil infiltration and activation may contribute to the increased risk of peptic ulceration[36–38] and gastric cancer[39,40] in those infected with *cag* PAI positive strains.

3. CYTOKINES AND ANTIGEN SPECIFIC IMMUNE RESPONSES

The infiltration of neutrophils by disrupting tight junctions will facilitate antigen uptake into the gastric mucosa by the paracellular route and the induction of specific T and B cell responses. *In vitro* H. pylori induces changes in epithelial barrier function[41] and increased gastric permeability is evident in infected patients.[42] Interestingly, changes in gastric permeability are amplified in those with high polymorphonuclear cell infiltration.[42]

T cells have an important role in the generation of *Helicobacter* induced gastric pathology. RAG-$1^{-/-}$ mice fail to develop gastritis with *H. felis* infection[43] and chronic gastritis develops in SCID mice following passive transfer of T cells from infected animals.[44] In contrast, mice with immune deficiency in B cells develop pathology and epithelial hyperplasia with *Helicobacter* infection comparable to wild type mice.[43] Accumulating evidence from both human, primate and murine studies have shown that the T helper response in chronic *Helicobacter* infection has a Th1 profile characterized by gamma interferon secreting effector cells.[45–47] Additionally neither transcripts nor protein of CD30, which is preferentially associated with Th2 responses, is present in the gastric mucosa of *H. pylori* infected patients.[48]

Cytokines are considered to have a critical role in the polarization of T cell responses. In *H. pylori* infection high levels of IL-12, a Th1 stimulating cytokine, in the gastric mucosa may promote Th1 responses. Increased gastric IL-12 (p40) transcripts and IL-12 protein are present in infected subjects.[49,50] Interestingly, IL-12 transcripts are increased in those with *cag* PAI positive infections but not in those infected with *cag*⁻ strains[49] and IL-12 mRNA is also more frequent in patients with duodenal ulcers than in those with only chronic gastritis,[49] suggesting that expression of this important Th1 stimulating cytokine may relate to mucosal damage. Transcripts for IL-18, a cytokine which synergizes with IL-12 in promoting Th1 responses, are also increased in the gastric mucosa in *H. pylori* infection.[51] These two cytokines probably have a crucial role in polarizing gastric Th1 responses. Interestingly IL12, but not IL-18, has recently been shown to significantly increase T-cell mediated tissue injury in human fetal gut explants.[52] IL-12 induced mucosal damage in this experimental system was associated with increases in TNFα, interstitial collagenase and stromelysin-1.[52] Generation of active matrix metalloproteinases by IL-12 activated Th1 cells may thus potentially contribute to gastric mucosal damage in *H. pylori* infection.

The Th1 response and local production of gamma interferon induces important phenotypic and functional changes in gastric epithelial cells. These changes include upregulation of HLA-DR[53,54] and B7-2, a molecule involved in T cell activation[55] and also alterations in epithelial barrier function.[56] TNFα and gamma interferon will also potentiate *H. pylori* induced apoptosis in epithelial cells[6,7] and possibly increase expression of the Fas antigen on gastric epithelial cells in *H. pylori* infection.[5] Such phenotypic and functional changes, which occur in epithelial cells as a consequence of *H. pylori* infection, are likely to be important in the exacerbation of the chronic inflammatory response and the eventual development of atrophic gastritis.

A cytokine which has important immunoregulatory functions inhibiting Th1 responses is IL-10 which acts on accessory cells inhibiting the secretion of IL-12 and thus down regulating cell mediated responses.[57] IL-10 also inhibits the secretion of proinflammatory cytokines and chemokines from macrophages and polymorphs,[58] thereby potentially reducing neutrophil activation and the generation of tissue damaging reactive oxygen metabolites. *H. pylori* infection is associated with increased gastric IL-10 protein production[60] and mRNA expression.[19,49] Gastric IL-10 transcripts are increased in patients infected with *cag*+ *H. pylori* strains[49] who also have elevated IL-12 and C-X-C chemokine mRNA expression.[20,49] These studies suggest the down regulatory cytokine IL-10 is increased in relation to the extent of mucosal damage. Studies with IL-10 deficient mice have confirmed the essential role of IL-10 in down-regulating *Helicobacter* induced gastric inflammatory responses. *H. felis* infection results in rapid development of severe hyperplastic gastritis and loss of corpus physiological function.[3] Thus the balance between proinflammatory cytokines and down-regulatory cytokines, such as IL-10, in the gastric mucosa may influence the extent of mucosal damage and modify epithelial cell proliferation. However, there is no evidence to suggest that impairment in IL-10 relates to ulceration, similar gastric IL-10 transcript levels are observed in ulcer and non-ulcer *H. pylori* infected patients.[49] Further clinical studies have shown that promoter polymorphisms in the IL-10 gene are not associated with risk of atrophy and hypochlorhydria.[59]

4. CYTOKINE MODULATION OF GASTRIC PHYSIOLOGICAL RESPONSES

Gastric mucosal cytokines in addition to being important immunoregulatory molecules controlling the polarity of T cell responses, cellular infiltration and activation may also have a role in disease pathogenesis by modulating gastric physiological responses. Infection with *H. pylori* induces marked changes in gastric physiology, including increased basal and post-prandial plasma gastrin and decreased mucosal somatostatin.[61] Th1 cytokines such as gamma interferon[62] and proinflammatory cytokines IL-1β, TNF-α[63] and IL8[64] induce gastrin secretion from cultured G cells. The effects of IL-8 are markedly potentiated by *H. pylori* extracts.[64] In contrast exposure of isolated D cells to TNF-α results in reduced cellular somatostatin.[65] IL-1β which decreases acid secretion by parietal cells,[66] also decreases histamine release from enterochromaffin cells[67] and inhibits histamine stimulated pepsinogen secretion by human peptic cells.[68] Polymorphisms in IL-1β and the IL-1 receptor antagonist linked to increased IL-1β production have recently been associated with increased risk of developing hypochlorhydria and gastric cancer as a consequence of *H. pylori* infection.[69] Cytokine effects on exocrine and endocrine cell function in the stomach will strongly depend on the distribution of gastritis and *H. pylori* infected subjects with pro-inflammatory IL-1 loci genotypes are more likely to develop corpus atrophy. Analysis of IL-1β and IL-1 receptor polymorphisms may define infected subjects most at risk of developing gastric cancer.

5. CYTOKINES AND PROTECTIVE IMMUNITY

Whether particular gastric cytokine profiles and cellular responses have a protective role in eradicating natural *H. pylori* infection is still under active investigation. Certain genetic polymorphisms may predispose to enhanced innate or specific defenses. Analysis of IL-10 promoter polymorphisms in humans suggests that IL-10 enhancing genotypes may increase the risk of infection,[59] possibly due to immunosuppressive or anti-inflammatory effects.

Cytokine profiles in protective vaccine induced immunity are also under active investigation. Studies in transgenic animals have shown that the protective immune response induced by prophylactic *H. pylori* vaccination is dependent on CD4+ T cells and MHC class II expression.[70] Chronic *Helicobacter* infection however can be eradicated by administration of *Helicobacter* antigen and adjuvant.[71,72] Initial studies suggested that the effector mechanism of therapeutic vaccination in mice involved a switch from Th1 to Th2 responses.[72,73] In the *H. felis* mouse model stimulation of Th2 responses has been associated with a reduction in bacterial load and gastric inflammation.[74] However more recent murine studies have linked enhanced cellular responses to bacterial clearance[75] and emphasized the importance of both IL-12 and gamma interferon in reducing gastric Helicobacter colonization.[76] A balance between Th1 and Th2 responses may thus be important for protection. Direct extrapolation from murine studies to the human situation is however difficult. An understanding of the mechanisms involved and the role of cytokines in the protective mucosal responses to *H. pylori* is important for future clinical use of prophylactic and therapeutic vaccines.

6. CONCLUSIONS

In conclusion, the discovery of *H. pylori* has promoted a great interest in gastric mucosal immune and inflammatory responses. Gastric cytokines induced by *H. pylori* infection are important not only in regulating the inflammatory responses to the bacterium, but also in modulating gastric physiological responses, altering gastric permeability, epithelial differentiation and the induction of autoimmune responses. Cytokines have a major role in the induction of immune mediated mucosal damage. The acquisition of the *cag* pathogenicity island by *H. pylori* has resulted in more severe clinical outcome of infection, which may in part, be explained by the variation in the magnitude and characteristics of the mucosal cytokine responses. Unraveling the effector mechanisms of vaccine induced protective immunity will be an important step for the development of therapeutic alternatives to antibiotic based regimes.

ACKNOWLEDGEMENTS. This work was supported by Yorkshire Cancer Research and the European Commission (contract number ICA4-CT-1999-10010).

REFERENCES

1. Crabtree E., 1998, The role of cytokines in *Helicobacter pylori* induced mucosal damage. *Dig. Dis. Sci.* **43**:46S.
2. Bodger K., and Crabtree J. E., 1998, *Helicobacter pylori* and gastric inflammation. *Brit. Med. Bull.* **54**:139.
3. Berg D. J., Lynch N. A., Lynch R. G. *et al.*, 1998, Rapid development of severe hyperplastic gastritis with gastric epithelial dedifferentiation in *Helicobacter felis* infected IL-10–/–mice. *Am. J. Pathol.* **152**:1377.

4. Yasunaga Y., Shinomura Y., Kanayama S. *et al.*, 1996, Increased production of IL-1β and hepatocyte growth factor may contribute to foveolar hyperplasia in enlarged fold gastritis. *Gut.* **39**:787.
5. Houghton J., Korah R. M., Condon M. R. *et al.*, 1999, Apoptosis in *Helicobacter pylori* associated gastric and duodenal ulcer disease is mediated via the Fas antigen pathway. *Dig. Dis. Sci.* **44**:465.
6. Wagner S., Beil W., Westermann J. *et al.*, 1996, Regulation of gastric epithelial cell growth by *Helicobacter pylori*: evidence for a major role of apoptosis. Gastroenterology **113**:1836.
7. Fan X., Crowe S. E., Behar S. *et al.*, 1998, The effect of class II major histocompatibility complex expression on adherence of *Helicobacter pylori* and induction of apoptosis in gastric epithelial cells: a mechanism of T helper cell mediated damage. *J. Exp. Med.* **187**:1659.
8. Shibata J., Goto H., Arisawa T. *et al.*, 1999, Regulation of tumor necrosis factor (TNF) induced apoptosis by soluble TNF receptors in *Helicobacter pylori* infection. *Gut.* **45**:24.
9. Falcone M., and Sarvetnick N., 1999, Cytokines that regulate autoimmune responses. *Curr. Opin. Immunol.* **11**:670.
10. Kagnoff M. F., and Eckmann L., 1997, Eckmann, Epithelial cells as sensor of microbial infection. *J. Clin. Invest.* **100**:6.
11. McCormick B., Gewirtz A., and Madara J. L., 1998, Epithelial crosstalk with bacteria and immune cells. *Curr. Opin. Gastroenterology* **14**:492.
12. Crabtree J. E., Farmery S. M., Lindley I. J. D. *et al.*, 1994, CagA/cytotoxic strains of *Helicobacter pylori* and interleukin-8 in gastric epithelial cells. *J. Clin. Pathol.* **47**:945.
13. Crabtree J. E., Covacci A., Farmery S. M. *et al.*, 1995, *Helicobacter pylori* induced interleukin-8 expression in gastric epithelial cells is associated with CagA positive phenotype. *J. Clin. Pathol.* **48**:41.
14. Sharma S. A., Tummuru M. K. R., Miller G. G., and Blaser M. J., 1995, Interleukin-8 response of gastric epithelial cell lines to *Helicobacter pylori* stimulation in vitro. *Infect. Immun.* **63**:1681.
15. Watanabe M., Ueno Y., Yijima T. *et al.*, 1995, Interleukin-7 is produced by human intestinal epithelial cells and regulates the proliferation of intestinal mucosal lymphocytes. *J. Clin. Invest.* **95**:2945.
16. Reinecker H. C., MacDermott R. P., Mirau S. *et al.*, 1996, Intestinal epithelial cells both express and respond to interleukin 15. *Gastroenterology* **111**:1706.
17. Pizarro T. T., Michie M. H., Bentz M. *et al.*, 1998, IL-18, a novel immunoregulatory cytokine, is up regulated in Crohn's disease: expression and localization in intestinal cells. *J. Immunol.* **162**:6829.
18. Crabtree J. E., Wyatt J. I., Trejdosiewicz L. K. *et al.*, 1994, Interleukin-8 expression in *Helicobacter pylori*, normal and neoplastic gastroduodenal mucosa. *J. Clin. Pathol.* **47**:945.
19. Peek Jr R. M., Miller G. G., Tham K. T. *et al.*, 1995, Heightened inflammatory response and cytokine expression in vivo to CagA+ *Helicobacter pylori* strains. *Lab. Invest.* **73**:760.
20. Shimoyama T., Everett S., Dixon M., Axon A. T. R., and Crabtree J. E., 1998, Chemokine mRNA expression in gastric mucosa is associated with *Helicobacter pylori cagA* positivity and severity of gastritis. *J. Clin. Pathol.* **51**:765.
21. Ando T., Kusugami K., Ohsuga M. *et al.*, 1998, Differential normalization of mucosal interleukin-8 and interleukin-6 activity after *Helicobacter pylori* eradication. *Infect. Immun.* **66**:4742.
22. Moss S. F., Legon S., Davies J. *et al.*, 1994, Cytokine gene expression in *Helicobacter pylori* associated antral gastritis. *Gut.* **35**:1567.
23. Aihara M., Tsuchimoto D., Takizawa H. *et al.*, 1997, Mechanisms involved in *Helicobacter pylori*-induced interleukin-8 production by a gastric cancer cell line, MKN 45. *Infect. Immun.* **65**:3218.
24. Beales I. L. P., and Calam J., 1997, Stimulation of IL-8 production in human gastric epithelial cells by *Helicobacter pylori*, IL-1β and TNF-a requires tyrosine kinase activity, but not protein kinase C. *Cytokine* **9**:514.
25. Li S. D., Kersulyte D., Lindley I. J. D. *et al.*, 1999, Multiple genes in the left half of the cag pathogenicity island genes of *Helicobacter pylori* are required for tyrosine kinase-dependent transcription of interleukin-8 in gastric epithelial cells. *Infect. Immun.* **67**:3893.
26. Munzenmaier A., Lange C., Glocker E. *et al.*, 1997, A secreted/shed product of *Helicobacter pylori* activates transcription factor nuclear factor-kB. *J. Immunol.* **159**:6140.

27. Keates S., Hitti Y. S., Upton M., and Kelly C. P., 1997, *Helicobacter pylori* infection activates NF-kB in gastric epithelial cells. *Gastroenterol.* **113**:1099.
28. Sharma S. A., Tummuru M. K. R., Blaser M. J. *et al.*, 1998, Activation of IL-8 gene expression by *Helicobacter pylori* is regulated by transcription factor nuclear factor-kB in gastric epithelial cells. *J. Immunol.* **160**:2401.
29. van der Brink G. R., Kate F. J., Ponsioen C. Y. *et al.*, 2000, Expression and activation of NF-kB in the antrum of the human stomach. *J. Immunol.* **164**:3353.
30. Masamune A., Shimosegawa T., Masamune O. *et al.*, 1999, *Helicobacter pylori* dependent ceramide production may mediate interleukin-8 expression in human gastric cancer cell lines. *Gastroenterol.* **116**:1330.
31. Keates S., Keates A., Warny M. *et al.*, 1999, Differential activation of mitogen activated protein kinases in AGS gastric epithelial cells by *cag+* and *cag–* *Helicobacter pylori*. *J. Immunol.* **163**:5552.
32. Glocker E., Lange C., Covacci A. *et al.*, 1998, Proteins encoded by the cag pathogenicity island of *Helicobacter* pylori are required for NF-kB activation. *Infect. Immun.* **66**:2346.
33. Censini S., Lange C., Xiang Z. *et al.*, 1996, *cag*, a pathogenicity island of Helicobacter pylori encodes Type I-specific and disease-associated virulence factors. *Proc. Natl. Acad. Sci. USA* **93**:14648.
34. Akopyants N. S., Clifton S. W., Kersulyte D. *et al.*, 1998, Analyses of the *cag* pathogenicity island of *Helicobacter pylori*. *Mol. Microbiol.* **28**:3754.
35. Yamaoka Y., Kita M., Kodama T. *et al.*, 1996, *Helicobacter pylori cagA* gene and expression of cytokine messenger RNA in gastric mucosa. *Gastroenterology* **110**:1744.
36. Crabtree J. E., Taylor J. E., Wyatt J. I. *et al.*, 1991, Mucosal IgA recognition of *Helicobacter pylori* 120 kDa protein, peptic ulceration and gastric pathology. *Lancet.* **338**:332.
37. van der Hulst R. W. M., Ende van der A., Dekker F. *et al.*, 1997, Effect of *Helicobacter pylori* eradication on gastritis in relation to *cagA*: a prospective 1 year follow up study. *Gastroenterology* **113**:25.
38. Weel J. F. L., van der Hulst R. W. M., Gerrits Y. *et al.*, 1996, The interrelationship between cytotoxin-associated gene A, vacuolating cytotoxin, and *Helicobacter pylori* related disease. *J. Infect. Dis.* **173**:1171.
39. Blaser M. J., Perez-Perez G. I., Kleanthous H. *et al.*, 1995, Infection with *Helicobacter pylori* strains possessing *cagA* associated with an increased risk of developing adenocarcinoma of the stomach. *Cancer Res.* **55**:2111.
40. Parsonnet J., Friedman G. D., Orentreich N. *et al.*, 1997, Risk for gastric cancer in people with *CagA* positive and CagA negative *Helicobacter pylori* infection. *Gut.* **40**:297.
41. Terres A. M., Pajares J. M., Hopkins A. M. *et al.*, 1998, *Helicobacter pylori* disrupts epithelial barrier function in a process inhibited by protein kinase C activators. *Infect. Immun.* **66**:2943.
42. Goodgame R. W., Malaty H. M., El-Zimaity H. M. T. *et al.*, 1997, Decrease in gastric permeability to sucrose following cure of *Helicobacter pylo*ri infection. *Helicobacter* **2**:44.
43. Roth K. A., Kapadia S. B., Martin S. M. *et al.*, 1999, Cellular immune responses are essential for the development of *Helicobacter felis*-associated gastric pathology. *J. Immunol.* **163**:1490.
44. Eaton K. A., Ringler S. R., and Danon S. J., 1999, Murine splenocytes induce severe gastritis and delayed-type hypersensitivity and suppress bacterial colonization in *Helicobacter pylori*-infected SCID mice. *Infect. Immun.* **67**:4594.
45. Bamford K. B., Fan X., Crowe S. E. *et al.*, 1998, Lymphocytes in the human gastric mucosa during *Helicobacter pylori* have a T helper cell 1 phenotype. *Gastroenterol.* **114**:482.
46. Mattapallil J. J., Dandekar S., Canfield D. R. *et al.*, 2000, A predominant Th1 type of immune response is induced early during acute *Helicobacter pylori* infection in rhesus macaques. *Gastroenterol.* **118**:307.
47. Mohammadi M., Czinn S., Redline R. *et al.*, 1998, *Helicobacter*-specific cell-mediated responses display a predominant Th1 phenotype and promote a delayed-type hypersensitivity response in the stomach of mice. *J. Immunol.* 156:472938.

48. D'Elios M. M., Romagnani P., Scaletti C. *et al.*, 1997, In vivo CD30 expression in human diseases with predominant activation of Th2l ike T cells. *J. Leukocyte Biology* **61**:539.
49. Hida N., Shimoyama Jnr T., Neville P. *et al.*, 1999, Increased expression of interleukin 10 and IL-12 (p40) mRNA in *Helicobacter pylori* infection in gastric mucosa: relationship to bacterial *cag* and peptic ulceration. *J. Clin. Pathol.* **52**:658.
50. Bauditz J., Ortner M., Bierbaum M. *et al.*, 1999, Production of IL-12 in gastritis relates to infection with *Helicobacter pylori. Clin. Exp. Immunol.* **117**:316.
51. Tomita T., Jackson A., Hida N. *et al*, Expression of interleukin 18, a Th1 cytokine, is in the human gastric mucosa is increased in *Helicobacter pylori* infection. *J. Infect. Dis.* (in press).
52. Monteleone G., MacDonald T. T., Wathen N. C. *et al.*, 1999, Enhancing lamina propria Th1 cell responses with interleukin 12 produces severe tissue injury. *Gastroenterol.* **117**:1069.
53. Valnes K., Huitfeldt H. S., and Brandtzaeg P., 1990, Relation between T cell number and epithelial HLA class expression quantified by image analysis in normal and inflamed human gastric mucosa. *Gut.* **31**:647.
54. Scheynius A., and Engstrand L., 1991, Gastric epithelial cells in *Helicobacter pylori* associated gastritis express HLA-DR but not ICAM1. *Scand. J. Immunol.* **33**:237.
55. Ye G., Barrera C., Fan X. *et al.*, 1997, Expression of B7-1 and B7-2 costimulatory molecules by human gastric epithelial cells. *J. Clin. Invest.* **99**:1628.
56. Madara J. L., and Stafford J., 1989, Interferon gamma directly affects barrier function of cultured intestinal epithelial cells. *J. Clin. Invest.* **83**:724.
57. De Vries J. E., 1995, Immunosuppressive and anti-inflammatory properties of interleukin 10. *Ann. Med.* **27**:537.
58. Kasama T., Strieter R. M., Lukacs N. W. *et al.*, 1994, Regulation of neutrophil-derived chemokine expression by IL-10. *J. Immunol.* **152**:3559.
59. El-Omar E. M., Wang C. D., McColl K. E. *et al.*, 2000, Interleukin-10 promoter polymorphisms influence risk of chronic *H. pylori* infection. *Gastroenterol.* **118**:A889.
60. Bodger K., Wyatt J. I., and Heatley R. V., 1997, Gastric mucosal secretion of interleukin-10: relations to histopathology, *H. pylori* status and TNF-α secretion. *Gut.* **40**:739.
61. Calam J., 1997, Host mechanisms: are they the key to the various clinical outcomes of *Helicobacter pylori* infection? *Ital. J. Gastroenterol. Hepatol.* **29**:375.
62. Lehmann F. S., Golodner E. H., Wang J. *et al.*, 1996, Mononuclear cells and cytokines stimulate gastrin release from canine antral cells in primary culture. *Am. J. Physiol.* **270**:G783.
63. Weigert N., Schaffer K., Schusdziarra V. *et al.*, 1996, Gastrin secretion from primary cultures of rabbit antral G cells: stimulation by inflammatory cytokines. *Gastroenterol.* **110**:147.
64. Beales I., Blaser M. J., Srinivasin S. *et al.*, 1997, Effect of *Helicobacter pylori* products and recombinant cytokines on gastrin release from cultured canine G cells. *Gastroenterol.* **113**:465.
65. Beales I., Calam J., Post L. *et al.*, 1997, Effect of tumour necrosis factor-α on somatostatin release from canine fundic G cells. *Gastroenterol.* **112**:136.
66. Beales I. L., and Calam J., 1998, Interleukin 1 beta and tumour necrosis factor alpha inhibit acid secretion in cultured rabbit parietal cells by multiple pathways. *Gut.* **42**:227.
67. Prinz C., Neumayer N., Mahr S. *et al.*, 1997, Functional impairment of rat enterochromaffin-like cells by interleukin-1β. *Gastroenterol.* **112**:364.
68. Serrano M. T., Lanas A. I., Lorente S. *et al.*, 1997, Cytokine effects on pepsinogen secretion from human peptic cells. *Gut.* **40**:42.
69. El-Omar E. M., Carrington M., Chow W. H. *et al.*, 2000, Interleukin-1 polymorphisms associated with increased risk of gastric cancer. *Nature* **404**:398.
70. Ermak T. H., Giannasca P. J., Nichols R. *et al.*, 1998, Immunization of mice with urease vaccine affords protection against *Helicobacter pylori* infection in the absence of antibodies and is mediated by MHC class II restricted responses. *J. Exp. Med.* **188**:2277.
71. Corthesy-Theulaz I., Porta N., Glauser M. *et al.*, 1995, Oral immunization of *Helicobacter pylori* urease B subunit as a treatment against *Helicobacter* infection in mice. *Gastroenterol.* **109**:115.

72. Ghiara P., Rossi M., Marchetti M. *et al.*, 1997, Therapeutic intragastric vaccination against *Helicobacter pylori* in mice eradicates an otherwise chronic infection and confers protection against reinfection. *Infect. Immun.* **65**:4997.
73. Saldinger P. F., Porta N., Launois P. *et al.*, 1998, Immunization of BALB/c mice with *Helicobacter pylori* urease B induces a T helper 2 response absent in *Helicobacter* infection. *Gastroenterol.* **115**:891.
74. Mohammadi M., Nedrud J., Redline R. *et al.*, 1997, Murine CD4 T-cell response to *Helicobacter* infection: TH1 cells enhance gastritis and TH2 cells reduce bacterial load. *Gastroenterol.* **113**:1848.
75. Eaton K. A., Ringler S. R., and Danon S. J., 1999, Murine splenocytes induce severe gastritis and delayed-type hypersensitivity and suppress bacterial colonization in *Helicobacter pylori* infected SCID mice. *Infect. Immun.* **67**:4594.
76. Jiang B., Jordan M., Xing Z. *et al.*, 1999, Replication-defective adenovirus infection reduces *Helicobacter felis* colonization in the mouse in a gamma interferon and interleukin-12 dependent manner. *Infect. Immun.* **67**:4539.

13

Animal Models of *Helicobacter pylori* Infection

INGRID L. BERGIN and JAMES G. FOX

1. INTRODUCTION

Early attempts to establish animal models for the study of *Helicobacter pylori* pathogenesis and therapeutics were unsuccessful. In fact, Koch's postulates for *H. pylori* as the causative agent of gastritis were first fulfilled in human volunteers rather than animals.[1,2] Subsequent attempts to develop animal models followed two major strategies. First, gastric *Helicobacter* species other than *H. pylori* were identified in natural or experimental animal hosts and used as models for *H. pylori* infection. In addition, efforts continued to establish colonization with *H. pylori* in an animal host. Animal models that fall into both of these categories will be described below. To adequately assess and utilize an animal model, careful comparison to the pathology and progression of disease in humans must be performed. With this in mind, lesions described below will be compared to those of *H. pylori* infected humans, with distinctions drawn where necessary. The utility of each animal model to the study of human disease will also be discussed.

INGRID L. BERGIN and JAMES G. FOX • Division of Comparative Medicine, Massachusetts Institute of Technology, Cambridge, MA 02139.

Helicobacter pylori Infection and Immunity,
Edited by Yamamoto *et al.*, Kluwer Academic/Plenum Publishers, 2002.

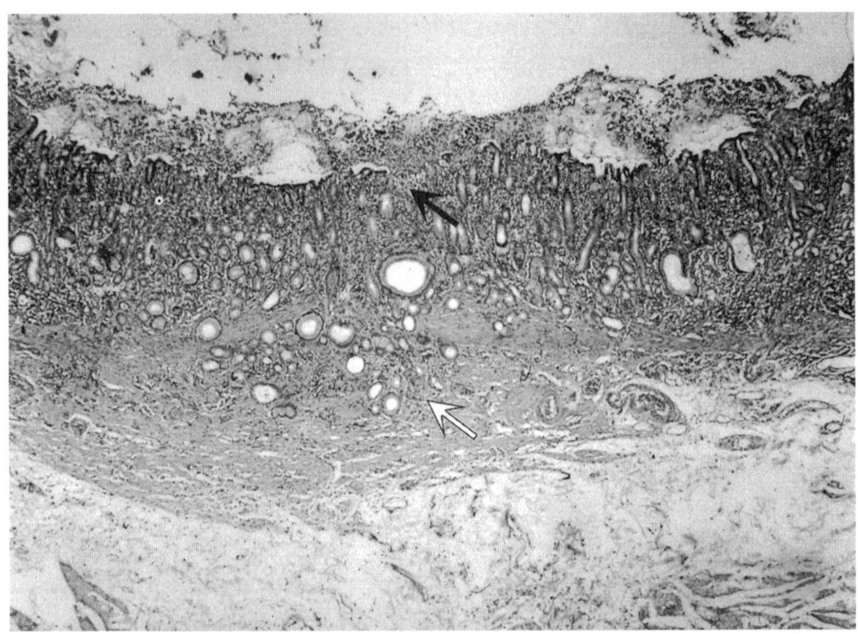

FIGURE 1. Gastritis and a gastric ulcer in the stomach of a *Helicobacter mustelae*-infected ferret. Note that inflammation extends throughout the full thickness of the gastric mucosa (white arrow).

2. FERRETS: *H. mustelae*

H. mustelae was the first naturally occurring gastric helicobacter identified in a species other than the human.[3] It was originally isolated from a ferret with an antral gastric ulcer and has since been established as highly prevalent in U.S., British, Canadian, and Australian ferret populations.[3-8] Attempts have been made to experimentally colonize ferrets with other gastric helicobacters. Limited colonization is seen with *H. felis* but attempts at colonization with *H. pylori* have been unsuccessful.[8]

2.1. Comparison between Human and Ferret Gastric *Helicobacter* Infections

As with human *H. pylori* infection, *H. mustelae* infects ferrets at a young age (5 to 6 weeks in the ferret) and persists throughout life in the absence of treatment. Isolation from infected animals and experimental infection of *H. mustelae*-free ferrets has been performed to fulfill Koch's postulates and establish its causative role in gastritis.[9] Both gastric and, less frequently, duodenal ulceration occur in infected ferrets, making them a suitable model for the study of *Helicobacter*-induced ulcerogenesis (Figure 1). In fact, the ferret is the only non-rodent animal model described to date in which helicobacter infection is highly associated with gastric ulceration. Gastric and duodenal ulcers occur in the ferret infrequently, as in humans where gastric ulcer disease develops only in a small percentage of infected persons. In addition to ulceration, diffuse antral gastritis and parietal cell atrophy, a pre-neoplastic change, are features of gastric helicobacter infection which have been observed in both ferrets and humans.[4,8,9]

Gastric neoplasia is rarely seen in *H. mustelae*-infected ferrets and causality has not been proven. Gastric adenocarcinoma has been reported in *H. mustelae*-infected ferrets both in the presence[10] and absence[11] of chemical carcinogen administration. Additionally, gastric MALT lymphoma has been diagnosed in aged ferrets infected with *H. mustelae* (Figure 2).[12] Despite the rarity of gastric neoplasia, the presence of certain cancer risk factors has been associated with *H. mustelae* infection in ferrets. Infection generates increased cellular proliferation as indicated by immunohistochemical staining of proliferating cell nuclear antigen (PCNA).[13] Increased cell mass and/or increased cellular turnover is theorized to be a necessary precursor to the development of gastric cancer in humans.[14,15] Since gastric cancer in the ferret is an infrequent occurrence, despite the appearance of significant gastritis in virtually all *H. mustelae* infected animals, the organism may be acting as a tumor promotor. A side-by-side comparison of tumor incidence

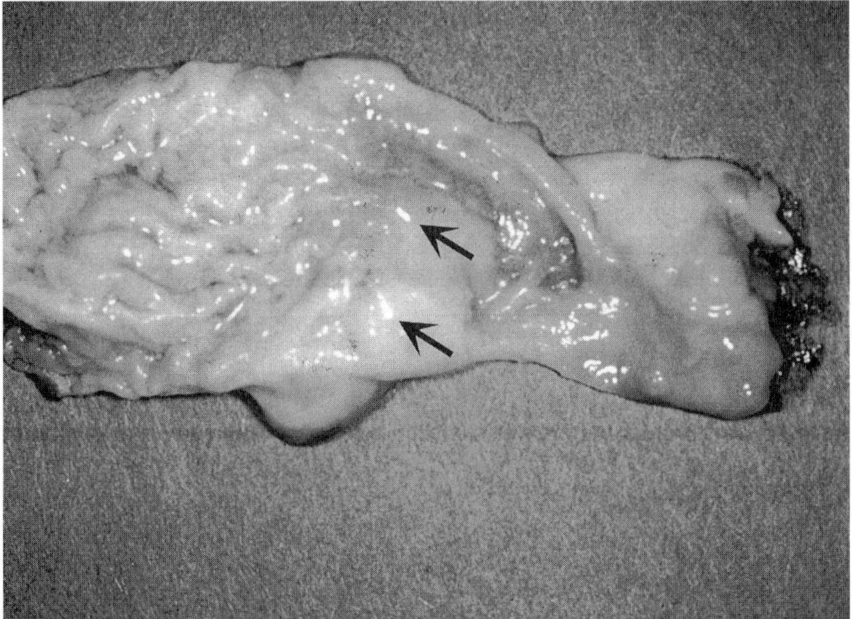

FIGURE 2. Nodular, thickened gastric mucosa in a *Helicobacter mustelae* infected ferret gastric lymphoma.

in carcinogen-treated animals has not been performed using both *H. mustelae* infected and *H. mustelae*-free animals. If the organism is indeed acting as a tumor promoter, infected animals will show more rapid onset of tumors after carcinogen administration.

The type of gastritis seen in ferrets is slightly different from that seen in humans. Both humans and ferrets develop diffuse antral gastritis, but ferrets predominantly show lymphocytic infiltration and lack the strong neutrophilic component seen in humans. Long term *H. mustelae* infection can cause atrophic gastritis, characterized by parietal cell loss, in the ferret. However, *H. mustelae*-infected ferrets do not develop intestinal metaplasia, a pre-neoplastic lesion of *H. pylori* infected humans that is characterized by proliferation of goblet-like cells in the gastric epithelium.

H. pylori and *H. mustelae* show some differences with respect to virulence factors. To date, the pathogenicity island (PAI) encoding the *H. pylori* virulence factors Cag A and Vac A, has not been identified in *H. mustelae*. This is surprising, since *H. mustelae* appears to adhere to the ferret gastric epithelium in a manner similar to the adherence of *H. pylori* in the human stomach.[15] In humans, ulcer development is strongly associated with Type I strains of *H. pylori*, which contain the PAI and express both Cag A and Vac A. However, even if the PAI or its homologue is present in *H. mustelae*, it may be difficult to detect. In *H. pylori*, numerous genomic rearrangements occur, even between strains that show high overall sequence homology.[17] Differences in surrounding sequences or interruptions within the sequence of the PAI itself may make it difficult to identify this region in *H. mustelae* using *H. pylori*-derived PAI probes.

3. UTILITY OF THE FERRET GASTRIC *Helicobacter* MODEL

Ferrets are large enough to allow several manipulations that cannot be performed in rodent models. Gastric changes in histopathology may be monitored over time in individual animals by serial endoscopy. Mucosal biopsies can be taken during this procedure and used for histopathology, culture, or urease assay.[18,19] Reconstructive gastric surgery has also been performed in the ferret.[19,20,21] In *H. pylori*-infected humans, a history of previous gastric surgery such as ulcer resection accompanied by pyloroplasty or gastrojejunostomy has been associated with a higher risk of subsequent adenocarcinoma. Ferrets with surgical gastric reconstruction did not show significant differences from controls in histopathology, gastric emptying, and gastric acidity. They did, however, show a decreased rate of nitrite to nitrate processing although this did not seem to correspond with any change in histopathology.[20,21]

Ferrets are suited for the administration and testing of a variety of treatment regimens. A protocol for the derivation of ferrets that are specific pathogen free

(SPF) of *H. mustelae* has been developed.[18] Eradication of *H. mustelae* in the ferret may be achieved by administration of triple therapy consisting of amoxicillin (10 mg/kg), metronidazole (20 mg/kg), and bismuth subsalicylate (17.5 mg/kg). Drugs are administered in a gelatin capsule or as a mixture with a highly palatable nutritional supplement (Nutri-Cal; Evsco, Buena, N.J.). This regimen can be administered to pregnant female ferrets three times daily beginning two weeks prior to the predicted delivery date and continuing into the post-parturient period for a total of three or four weeks of treatment in order to produce *H. mustelae*-free kits. Other agents used for *H. mustelae* eradication have included enrofloxacin administered with bismuth subsalicylate, ranitidine bismuth citrate, and clarithromycin administered alone or with ranitidine/bismuth citrate. These protocols have been previously reviewed and reportedly achieve between 71–100% efficacy for eradication.[18] In a separate study, several antibiotic protocols used to clear *H. pylori* infection in humans were tested and found to be somewhat less effective at clearing *H. mustelae* infection in ferrets.[22]

In addition to testing antibiotic protocols, *H. mustelae*-infected ferrets have been used in a therapeutic vaccination trial.[23] Therapeutic vaccination is based on the principle that administration of a relevant antigen to an infected animal in combination with a strong adjuvant can generate an immune response that eliminates the existing infection. Ferrets naturally infected with *H. mustelae* were dosed by orogastric gavage with purified recombinant *H. pylori* urease and cholera toxin as adjuvant. Eradication, as determined by urease assay and culture, was achieved in 30% (7 out of 23) of immunized animals at 6 weeks after the last dose. While intriguing, therapeutic vaccination remains a poorly understood concept. The percent of eradication is low when compared to trials using traditional antibiotic eradication.

4. CATS: GASTRIC *Helicobacter*-LIKE ORGANISMS, *H. felis, H. pylori*

Cats are known to carry a number of naturally occurring gastric helicobacter infections. Histological descriptions of spiral-shaped bacteria in the feline stomach were extant long before the discovery of the *Helicobacter* genus.[24] Shortly after the identification of *H. mustelae* in the ferret, a tightly coiled, large, spiral organism was cultured from feline gastric biopsies and was identified as a helicobacter on the basis of its 16S rRNA sequence and other characteristics.[25] It was formally designated *H. felis* after its host species of origin.[26] *H. felis* is longer and more tightly spiraled than *H. pylori*. In contrast to the unipolar flagella of *H. pylori*, *H. felis* has periplasmic fibers in bundles of one to four distributed over the surface of the organism. Since its original isolation, *H. felis* has been found as a naturally occurring gastric infection in both cats and dogs.[24] A serological survey revealed significantly elevated anti-*H. felis* antibody titers in 39% (19 out of 49) of cats surveyed.[27] One significant characteristic of *H. felis* is that it readily colonizes the stomach of susceptible strains of mice (reviewed below) and, in this capacity, serves as an important gastric helicobacter model. Its pathogenicity has also been studied in the cat.[28]

In addition to *H. felis*, other large, spiral bacteria have been observed in histological sections of the feline stomach. Morphologically similar organisms have been described in the stomachs of a variety of host species (Table 1). The nomenclature of these organisms is quite confusing. With rare exceptions,[29] attempts at culture have been unsuccessful. Because of this, it has been difficult to characterize the organisms to the extent necessary to give them an official name. Based on morphology, they were originally referred to as "*Gastrospirillum*". PCR analysis of 16S rRNA sequence from these bacteria showed that they belong to the genus *Helicobacter* and likely represent several distinct but related species.[30] A variety of names have been used to describe similar spiral organisms in many host species. To encompass the existing nomenclature, non-*pylori* gastric spiral organisms of similar morphology can be collectively termed the "large gastric spirals" or gastric Helicobacter-like organisms (GHLOs). GHLOs appear morphologically distinct from *H. pylori* and can readily be distinguished in tissue due to their larger size, tighter spiral pattern, and bipolar multiple flagella. GHLOs resemble *H. felis* but are more tightly spiraled and lack periplasmic fibers.[24] GHLOs are highly preva-

TABLE 1
Gastric helicobacters other than *H. pylori*

Species	Host species	Reference
Named species		
H. mustelae	ferret	3
H. felis	cat	25
H. acinonyx	cheetah	
H. nemestrinae[a]	pig-tailed macaque	96
H. bizzozeroni[b]	human, dog	77
H. salomonis	dog	77
Species with unofficial names[c]		24
"*H. heilmannii*[b]	human, dog, cat non-human primates	30
"*H. suis*"	pig	39

[a]*H. nemestrinae* is genetically similar to *H. pylori* and may be a strain of *H. pylori*.
[b]*H. bizzozeronii* and *H. heilmannii*" may represent strains of the same species.
[c]"Unofficial names have been given to organisms that, by PCR and morphology, are probably helicobacters, but cannot be officially named since they have not been cultured or have not been cultured from more than one individual.

lent in cats, with reports indicating that between 80–100% of clinically normal cats carry these organisms as determined by histopathology, Warthin-Starry staining, Gram staining, or urease testing.[31–33] When culture was used as a detection method, the prevalence of non-*pylori* helicobacters in cats was reported as 13.6%. This probably represents the prevalence *of H. felis* infection since it can be readily cultured unlike the GHLOs.[34]

While infection with GHLOs and, to a lesser degree, *H. felis*, are the most common naturally occurring helicobacter infections of cats, cats supplied to a research institution from a single commercial source were found to be 100% colonized with *H. pylori*.[35,36] Numerous subsequent surveys have failed to turn up *H. pylori* infection in other cat populations.[31,32,37] Since the organism has not been detected in most cat populations surveyed, initial infection of the commercial cat colony may have resulted from exposure to an infected human caretaker.[37] As experimental models, cats can be readily infected with *H. pylori* and develop gastritis with lymphoid follicle formation.[38–40]

The occurrence of helicobacter infections in cats has prompted investigation of zoonotic risks presented by exposure to these animals. A survey of anti-*H. pylori* antibody titers in cat owners did not reveal significant differences from control populations.[41] This finding, coupled with the failure to detect *H. pylori* infection in privately owned cats,[32,37] indicates that the risk to the average cat owner is probably minimal. However, this may not be the case for researchers and animal caretakers working with infected cats. *H. pylori* could be cultured from saliva in 50% (6 out of 12) of experimentally infected cats and from gastric fluid in 91% (11 out of 12).[38] *H. pylori* has also been cultured from saliva, gastric fluid, and feces of naturally infected cats.[39] Exposure to feline bodily secretions may thus represent a risk factor and appropriate protective measures should be taken. In addition to *H. pylori*, the other feline gastric helicobacters may present zoonotic risks. Gastritis caused by GHLO infection is rare in humans, affecting only 0.25–0.60% of the population.[42,43] In contrast to *H. pylori* infection, there is evidence that zoonotic transmission may play a role in these cases. In a survey of patients found to harbor GHLO infections, 70.3% were found to have regular animal contact, compared to 37% of a non-infected control population.[42] There are also several case reports of persons who became clinically ill upon infection with *H. felis* or a GHLO which they had reportedly acquired from contact with pet or research cats.[44,45]

5. COMPARISON BETWEEN HUMAN AND FELINE GASTRIC *Helicobacter* INFECTIONS

H. pylori infection in cats produces diffuse lymphoplasmacytic mucosal infiltration and lymphoid follicle formation. Unlike chronic active gastritis in humans, feline *H. pylori* gastritis lacks a significant neutrophilic component. Gastritis in the cat affects the antrum most severely but also involves the cardia and gastric body.[36,46] Infected animals show distorted glandular architecture owing to extensive lymphocytic infiltration and collapse of the surrounding connective tissue.[46] Gastric or duodenal ulceration and intestinal metaplasia have not been reported. In the duodenum, gastric metaplasia consisting of cells expressing gastric-type mucin has been described.[46] This lesion is associated with duodenal ulcers in humans,[47] although its relation to *H. pylori* infection is unknown. In cats, it is seen in both infected and non-infected animals. Gastric metaplasia may thus be either a non-specific mucosal response[46] or normal duodenal architecture for the cat. *H. pylori*-infected cats have not developed gastric adenocarcinoma or MALT lymphoma. However, they have shown factors such as increased cellular proliferation and apoptosis that are postulated to be necessary precursors for cancer in humans. Since gastric cancer is a rare outcome of infection, the failure to see gastric cancer in *H. pylori* infected cats may simply reflect the low numbers of animals used in most studies. Additionally, other co-factors such as diet may play a role.

6. UTILITY OF THE FELINE GASTRIC *Helicobacter* MODEL

Cats present practical difficulties as models of helicobacter infection since their size and expense limit the number of animals that can be used in a study. Their size can be an advantage in long term studies, however, as they are large enough to permit serial endoscopy for sampling of the gastric mucosa. Although *H. pylori*-infected cats do not show precursor lesions of gastric adenocarcinoma such as intestinal metaplasia, their tendency toward lymphoid follicle formation makes a potential connection with MALT lymphoma particularly interesting. The composition of these lymphoid follicles has been examined in the cat by immunohistochemistry.[40] They contain IgM+ B cells surrounded by CD4+ and CD8+ T cells. Single or aggregate IgA+ and IgM+ B cells are also found in the lamina propria. Anti-*H. pylori* IgA levels are elevated in gastric secretions. Humans infected with *H. pylori* develop similar elevations in local IgA.

Naturally-occurring gastric adenocarcinoma and alimentary lymphoma in cats have both been reported in the veterinary literature.[48–51] Since cats are frequently colonized with GHLOs or *H. felis*, the connection between these infections and subsequent neoplasia is worth considering. However, infection of cats with GHLOs or *H. felis* does not produce as significant gastritis as *H. pylori* infection in these animals.[33,52] The limited extent of gastritis with GHLO or *H. felis* infection may mean that it is less likely that infection with these species will lead to eventual gastric cancer. Co-factors such as concurrent viral infections may also influence disease development.

7. SWINE: GHLOS, *H. pylori*

The first animals successfully experimentally inoculated with *H. pylori* were gnotobiotic piglets.[53] Subsequent studies confirmed that pigs were a susceptible host for *H. pylori* infection.[54–57] Infection of barrier-reared pigs, which are not germ-free but are free of known, specified pathogens demonstrated that *H. pylori* could colonize even in the presence of other organisms.[55] In addition, infected gnotobiotic pigs could be transferred to conventional housing and retain their infected status.[57]

Like cats, pigs can harbor naturally-occurring infections by GHLOs.[58] Pigs are most commonly colonized with an organism that appears morphologically similar to "*H. heilmannii*" but represents a distinct *Helicobacter* species as shown by sequencing of its PCR-amplified 16S rRNA sequence. It is termed "*H. suis*" after its host species of origin.[59] Although this organism cannot be cultured, its presence can be ascertained by PCR,[59,60] histology, or oral inoculation of porcine gastric tissues into mice and subsequent histological examination of the mouse stomach.[61]

8. COMPARISON BETWEEN HUMAN AND PORCINE GASTRIC *Helicobacter* INFECTIONS

While both humans and pigs with persistent *H. pylori* infection have significant gastritis, the character of inflammation differs between the two species. In humans, both the gastric body and antrum are affected and there is a strong neutrophilic component even in chronic infection. Gastritis in pigs experimentally infected with *H. pylori* also affects the gastric body and antrum but is primarily lymphoplasmacytic. Extensive lymphoid follicle formation is also seen. In humans, the development of organized lymphoid follicles is usually not so pronounced, except in a small subset of patients, although lymphoid nodules are regularly seen.[62] In humans, intestinal metaplasia may develop as a pre-neoplastic lesion. In contrast, pigs do not show intestinal metaplasia with *H. pylori* infection. Both species show destruction of the gastric mucosa and epithelial cell vacuolization.[62] The frequency of gastric ulcers with *H. pylori* infection in pigs can be difficult to assess because spontaneously-occurring gastric ulcers commonly occur in this species. However, spontaneous gastric ulcers in the pig usually affect the non-glandular pars esophagea. *H. pylori*, in contrast, is associated with epithelial erosions in the gastric antrum of infected pigs.[63] Gastric cancer has not been reported in the pig model. However, due to their size, *H. pylori* infected pigs are usually only kept for several months, particularly in the case of gnotobiotic piglets, which must be maintained in germ-free isolators. Although infection has been monitored for up to 6 months on occasion, the short course of most studies makes the development of gastric cancer unlikely without the use of additional carcinogens.

9. UTILITY OF THE SWINE GASTRIC *Helicobacter* MODEL

The utility of swine as models for *H. pylori* infection is somewhat limited due to their rapid growth rate, large adult size and, particularly in the gnotobiotic piglet model, special housing requirements. Nevertheless, swine have been used in testing therapeutic and preventative protocols.[55,64,65] Oral vaccination using *H. pylori* sonicate and heat-labile toxin of *E. coli* (LT) suppressed, but failed to prevent infection in gnotobiotic piglets. Interestingly, parenteral vaccination induced a strong, persistent neutrophilic infiltrate in subsequently challenged piglets, in contrast to the usual lymphoplasmacytic gastritis.[64,65] Thus, in the pig, parenteral vaccination may cause a more "pro-inflammatory" response to infection that actually exacerbates gastritis.

Pigs have also been used to study virulence factors for *H. pylori* colonization. Urease is an enzyme that catalyzes the conversion of urea to ammonia and water. Almost all clinical *H. pylori* isolates from humans have high levels of urease activity. An isogenic mutant lacking urease activity failed to colonize gnotobiotic piglets.[66] One explanation for these findings is that urease enables the organism to withstand the acid pH of the gastric environment. However, urease negative mutants of *H. pylori* also failed to colonize pigs with gastric achlorhydria induced by omeprazole and ranitidine.[67] Therefore, protection from acidity cannot be the only role for urease in colonization. It may be that urease plays an important role in *H. pylori* metabolic pathways and its absence puts the organism at a nutritive disadvantage for *in vivo* survival.

In addition to experimental studies of *H. pylori* infection in pigs, recent attention has focused on the potential role of GHLOs, specifically "*H. suis*", in the pathogenesis of naturally-occurring gastric ulcers in swine.[68,69] Since this organism cannot be cultured, work has been limited to epidemiology and diagnostics based on PCR detection[60,70–72] or cultivation of the bacteria in the stomachs of mice.[61,68] Naturally-occurring gastric ulcers occur frequently in pigs. Ulcers most commonly affect the pars oesophagea, or non-glandular area surrounding the gastric cardia, that is not present in the human stomach. Less commonly, ulceration occurs in the glandular mucosa. Non-glandular ulcers can be experimentally produced upon ligation of the bile duct.[73] In several studies, pigs with non-glandular (pars oesophagea) ulcers had a higher prevalence of "*H. suis*" infection than pigs with normal gastric mucosa.[68,69] It should be noted that "*H. suis*" colonizes the glandular stomach as opposed to the non-glandular site of the ulcers. If "*H. suis*" is truly involved in the pathogenesis of these ulcers, it is uncertain as to why the area of colonization is separate from the area of pathology. One possibility is that higher acid production in the glandular area as a result of infection may affect the epithelium of the non-glandular region more markedly due to its lack of a protective mucus layer.[68,74] Humans are infected by the related species "*H. heilmannii*" but this has not shown any correlation with ulcerative disease. Therefore, the relevance of "*H. suis*"—associated ulceration to human pathology is uncertain.

10. DOGS: GHLOS, *H. felis, H. pylori*

10.1. Gastric *Helicobacter* Infections of Dogs

Gnotobiotic dogs were used as experimental hosts for *H. pylori* infection in one early study.[75] All dogs tested were successfully colonized with *H. pylori*. In addition, two sham inoculated dogs co-housed with experimental dogs also became colonized, indicating transmission of infection. The subsequent use of dogs as *H. pylori* models has been limited. One recent study showed that conventionally housed dogs are also susceptible to experimental infection.[76] In addition to experimental studies, efforts have been made to determine the presence of natural gastric helicobacter infections in dogs. Surveys of pet dogs have repeatedly failed to show natural infection with *H. pylori*.[77–79] However, natural infection with other gastric helicobacters commonly occurs. *H. felis*, *H. bilis*, and several GHLOs termed *H. bizzozeronii*, *H. salomonis*, *H. heilmannii*, and "*Flexispira rappini*" have all been identified in surveys of gastric infections in dogs.[77,78,80–82] The pathological significance of these organisms in the dog is currently unknown. A significant association between their presence and the occurrence of gastritis has not been demonstrated.

10.2. Comparison between Human and Canine *Helicobacter* Infections

Experimental infection of gnotobiotic dogs with *H. pylori* results in lower levels of colonization when compared to naturally-occurring human infections. These animals developed antral lymphoid follicles by four weeks post-infection accompanied by scattered neutrophilic infiltration of the lamina propria.[75] Conventionally housed dogs also developed lymphofollicular gastritis of the antrum by four weeks post-infection. Neutrophilic infiltration was most marked at two weeks and was accompanied by increased IL-8 expression, as is the case in human patients.[83] Unlike the gnotobiotic dogs, which remained asymptomatic throughout infection, several of the conventionally housed animals showed vomiting and intermittent diarrhea at one week post-infection. This is similar to dyspeptic symptoms described in human infections. These dogs showed marked hyperemia, edema, and congestion of the gastric mucosa in early infection. Unlike the gnotobiotic dogs, they also developed superficial gastric erosions, although no frank ulcers were seen. This study was hampered by the use of small numbers of animals. In addition, the presence of concurrent infection by GHLOs was not determined.[76]

10.3. Utility of the Canine Model

H. pylori infection in gnotobiotic and conventionally housed dogs produces pathology that correlates fairly well with changes seen in acute infections of humans, although the canine lesions are much less severe. Chronic pathology has not been studied in this model and it is not known whether pre-neoplastic lesions occur. Dogs are large enough so that serial endoscopic sampling may be performed in order to follow the course of infection in the same animal. However, size, expense, housing requirements, and public sensitivity to the use of dogs in research have limited widespread use of this model.

11. NON-HUMAN PRIMATES: GHLOS, *H. felis, H. pylori*

11.1. Natural Infections

Since *H. pylori* naturally colonizes the stomach of humans, non-human primates (NHPs) present a likely animal model for colonization and disease. Indeed, with the exception of the one cat colony discussed previously, NHPs, specifically macaques, are the only animals in which naturally-occurring *H. pylori* infection has been found. Gastric spiral organisms were first described in macaques in 1939.[84] More recently, culture and molecular analyses positively identified *H. pylori* from rhesus macaques (*Macaca mulatta*) with gastritis.[85–90] Infected animals came from multiple colonies so a point source for infection is unlikely. The occurrence of *H. pylori* infection in the wild is unknown. In captive populations, rhesus macaques appear to be most commonly affected although an outbreak of *H. pylori* gastritis was recently reported in a group of cynomolgus macaques (*M. fascicularis*).[91] The prevalence of infection among rhesus, as in humans, appears to increase with age. In rhesus housed in large social groups, seropositivity was lowest (60%) in one-year-old animals and increased to 81% in animals two- to ten-years old.[92] Animals younger than one year were not included in the study so the earliest acquisition of infection could not be determined. Nursery-rearing of animals removed at 24 hours of age has been successfully used to raise rhesus free of *H. pylori* infection.[93]

Natural infections involving helicobacters other than *H. pylori* also occur in NHPs. GHLOs have been observed in gastric tissue of rhesus and cynomolgus macaques.[88,91] Interestingly, 44 of 63 (69.8%) cynomolgus macaques that were infected with GHLOs had concurrent *H. pylori* infection. Gastritis positively correlated with the presence of *H. pylori* but not the GHLOs.[91] This is consistent with GHLO-infected cats, swine, dogs, and humans in which gastritis, if present, is mild to moderate. Despite poor correlation between GHLO infection and gastritis in NHPs, GHLO infection may have other potentially pathogenic consequences. For example, the GHLO "*H. heilmannii*" (previously termed "*Gastrospirillum hominis*") has been reported to invade parietal cells in the gastric epithelium of rhesus monkeys.[94,95] This finding correlates with an increased level of gastric acid secretion. Over-secretion of gastric acid is believed to play a role in the pathogenesis of *H. pylori* infection, and, since many humans are co-infected by "*H. heilmannii*" and *H. pylori*, disease development may involve synergism between the two organisms in some cases.

In addition to the GHLOs, another gastric organism named *H. nemestrinae* was isolated from pig-tailed macaques (*M. nemestrinae*).[96] This species is genetically and morphologically very similar to *H. pylori* and may in fact represent a strain of *H. pylori* rather than a separate species.[97]

11.2. Experimental Infections

Most experimental studies of *H. pylori* infection utilize macaque species including rhesus, cynomolgus, or Japanese macaques.[87,98,99] However, squirrel monkeys (*Saimiri sciureus*), and chimpanzees (*Pan troglodytes*) have also been experimentally infected.[100,101] Although both human-derived and NHP-derived strains have been used, some reports indicate greater success in colonization with NHP-derived strains, which may reflect host adaptation by the bacteria.[87,102] This is similar to the situation in pigs, which show poor colonization upon initial infection with human strains, but improved rates after serial passage of the human isolates through porcine hosts.[103] In a recent study, rhesus monkeys cleared of natural *H. pylori* infection were challenged by simultaneous administration of seven human-derived strains of *H. pylori*.[104] All four animals subjected to challenge became infected, showing that their previous natural *H. pylori* infections had not generated protective immunity. This experiment also revealed strain-dependent differences in colonization. In three of the four challenged animals, multiple strains were present in initial infection, however, one particular strain predominated by four months post-challenge. In the fourth animal, a different strain was predominant from early infection through the seventh month. However, by ten months post-challenge, the predominant strain had changed to the same one as in the other three animals. Therefore, infection is subject to both host and strain variability. Hosts may differ in susceptibility to a particular strain, especially in early infection, but certain strains appear most likely to predominate in long-term infection in a given host species.[104]

11.3. Comparison of Pathology between NHPs and Humans

Both natural and experimental *H. pylori* infections in NHPs result in persistent lymphocytic plasmacytic gastritis. Submucosal and mucosal lymphoid follicle formation can be seen in both cases. This pathology most closely resembles the lesions seen in the subset of human *H. pylori* patients with diffuse antral lymphoid gastritis. As in humans, infection in NHPs generates elevated titers of *H. pylori*-specific serum IgG. Although gastritis is readily detected in histological sections, clinical signs of gastritis such as vomiting have not been reported in experimentally infected animals. The prevalence of symptomatic natural infection is difficult to assess, however, signs suggestive of gastritis such as periodic vomiting and anorexia are common clinical entities in NHPs. In some cases, these may reflect *H. pylori* infections. Gastric ulcers and adenocarcinoma occur spontaneously in macaques but a connection with gastric helicobacter infection has not been determined. In experimental infections with *H. pylori*, ulcers have not been reported although superficial microerosions can be seen.[88] Neoplasia or preneoplastic lesions have not been reported with experimental *H. pylori* infection in NHPs.

11.4. Utility of the NHP Model

Because of their close relation to humans, NHPs provide one of the most physiologically relevant models of *H. pylori* infection. They have been used in studies of pathology, the immune response, and therapeutic trials. Their utility is somewhat hampered, however, by their size and expense. As a result, many studies performed with NHPs utilize very few animals, making results difficult to interpret.

The immune response to infection has been characterized in NHP models. Acute infection (up to 12 weeks) involves increased numbers of CD4+ T cells in the gastric mucosa and the generation of Th1 and pro-inflammatory cytokines such as IFNγ, TNF-α, and MIP-1β.[105] RT-PCR was used to detect mRNA expression for monocyte/macrophage-derived cytokines and showed elevated IL-1β, IL-6, and TNF-α at 7 weeks and in animals persistently infected for 6 years.[106] These results are consistent with mouse models which show that *H. pylori* gastritis is largely T-cell dependent and driven by a Th-1 response.[107,108]

A number of therapeutic trials and vaccination protocols have been tested in NHPs.[109,110] Among these, oral vaccination with recombinant *H. pylori* urease administered with *E. coli* heat-labile toxin (LT) as adjuvant was tested for therapeutic or prophylactic effects in rhesus monkeys.[111] This regimen failed to provide therapeutic benefit, and, although it reduced colonization levels when administered prophylactically, the vaccine failed to cause a statistically significant reduction in gastritis after challenge. Similarly, parenteral administration of recombinant urease with or without a priming oral immunization failed to induce significant protection from gastritis although oral priming followed by parenteral administration did reduce colonization levels.[112] Another trial reported a 31% eradication rate for therapeutic vaccination utilizing recombinant urease and LT.[113] However, this trial utilized culture and histopathology to detect *H. pylori* infection, methods which are not as sensitive as PCR. In addition, animals reported as *H. pylori* negative still showed antral gastritis, although this was less than that reported in *H. pylori* positive animals. Eradication trials based on antibiotic therapy have been more successful. A therapy regimen utilizing omeprazole-clarithromycin-amoxicillin-bismuth subsalicylate administered for ten days cleared *H. pylori* infection in five out of five animals.[114] Three of these animals carried metronidazole-resistant *H. pylori* strains and had previously failed to clear after metronidazole-amoxicillin-bismuth based treatment.

12. RATS, GUINEA PIGS, GERBILS

Because of the difficulty in achieving consistent, reproducible colonization in mice, and because of the size and expense of larger animal models, other small animal species have been tested for their suitability as *H. pylori* infection models.

12.1. Rats: *H. felis*, GHLOs, *H. pylori*

Initial studies using rats were performed with the gastric helicobacter *H. felis*. *H. felis* readily colonized gnotobiotic rats and induced an antral lymphocytic gastritis by 8 weeks post-infection.[115] This lesion is similar to the pattern of gastritis seen in *H. felis*-infected BALB/c mice and the subset of *H. pylori*-infected humans showing diffuse antral gastritis. In contrast, *H. felis*-infected C57BL/6 mice and some *H. pylori*-infected humans develop gastritis that affects both the gastric body and the antrum.

After several unsuccessful attempts,[116,117] researchers achieved colonization of conventionally housed rats with a clinical isolate of *H. pylori* administered in conjunction with omeprazole.[118] These rats developed lymphocytic antral gastritis and showed impaired healing of acetic acid-induced ulcers. A Type II strain of *H. pylori* (Cag A^-, Vac A^-) was utilized. This may have affected the degree of pathology seen, since Type I strains (Cag A$^+$, Vac A$^+$) are associated with increased virulence in humans.

Several GHLOs have also been shown to colonize the rat. In particular, "*Helicobacter suis*", a non-culturable helicobacter of swine, can be studied by oral inoculation of swine gastric secretions into rats.[119] "*Helicobacter heilmannii*", which affects humans, swine, dogs, and cats, can also experimentally infect the rat, causing altered gastric motility.[120] A recent study examined the effects of "*H. heilmannii*" or *H. felis* infection on gastrin secretion and acid production in the rat.[121] Since neither organism causes significant gastritis in the rat, this experiment was intended to determine the direct pathological effects of these organisms, as opposed to the damage that they cause indirectly by inducing inflammation. Neither organism altered gastrin secretion or acid production in infected rats. This was cited as evidence that altered gastrin secretion is caused by inflammation rather than directly by helicobacter infection. However, neither of the two organisms tested contain the Cag pathogenicity island and, therefore, this conclusion cannot be extrapolated to *H. pylori* infection.

12.2. Guinea Pigs: *H. pylori*

Guinea pigs present interesting features as small animal models of *H. pylori* infection. They lack the aglandular forestomach of rats, mice, and gerbils and, in this way, show gastric anatomy more similar to humans. They also possess a homologue to the pro-inflammatory cytokine IL-8, which is not present in rats or mice. IL-8 expression correlates with neutrophilic infiltration in *H. pylori*-infected humans. In addition, guinea pigs, like humans and non-human primates, have a dietary requirement for vitamin C. As an anti-oxidant, vitamin C may provide some protection against *H. pylori*-induced carcinogenesis.[122]

Guinea pigs have been successfully colonized with the Sydney strain of *H. pylori*[123] as well as human clinical isolates.[124] They develop a significant antral lymphohistiocytic gastritis that also extends to the border of the gastric body. There is marked lymphoid follicle formation by 4 weeks post-infection. In addition, polymorphonuclear infiltration[123,124] and crypt abscesses have been reported as well as superficial gastric erosions.[124]

12.3. Gerbils: *H. pylori*

Mongolian gerbils have recently emerged as an exciting new animal model for *H pylori* infection. They are the first rodent shown to develop gastric ulcers upon infection and the first of any animal model to develop adenocarcinoma with chronic infection.[125] The gerbil model is reviewed extensively elsewhere in this volume.

13. MICE: *H. felis* AND *H. pylori*

It is no surprise that efforts to develop animal models of *H. pylori* infection have focused heavily on the use of mice. Their small size and rapid generation time make them an economical choice for an *in vivo* model system. Additionally, the ability to manipulate mouse genetics and immunology allows the examination of various host factors in disease pathogenesis. Both *H. pylori* and *H. felis* have been extensively used in mouse studies focusing on the pathogenesis of helicobacter gastritis as well as vaccination protocols and therapeutic strategies.

13.1. *H. felis* Infections in Mice

H. felis was the first gastric helicobacter successfully used to colonize mice.[126,127] Early studies utilized outbred Swiss-Webster mice kept in a germ-free environment.[127] *H. felis* was found to show specific tissue tropism for the stomach as opposed to other sections of the gastrointestinal tract. Subsequently, non-germ-free Swiss-Webster mice were also shown to become persistently colonized with *H. felis*. These mice developed a predominantly lymphocytic inflammatory cell infiltrate that was most pronounced in the gastric body.[128] More severe gastric pathology was seen in Swiss-Quackenbush mice, which developed parietal cell loss characteristic of atrophic gastritis during a long-term, eighteen month infection.[129]

13.2. Inbred Strains Susceptible to Gastritis

H. felis has since been shown to colonize a variety of inbred strains (Table 2). Interestingly, colonization patterns and gastric pathology vary widely depending on the host strain. C57BL/6, C3H/He, SJL, and DBA/2 mice all become heavily colonized in the antrum.[130] C57BL/6 mice have the highest bacterial densities and become colonized in the gastric body as well as the antrum with time. Low-level colonization of the cardia is also seen. In contrast to the predominantly antral gastritis seen in many animal models, inflammation primarily affects the gastric body in these mice. It is most severe in C57BL/6 and SJL mice. Inflammatory infiltrates are mostly lymphocytic although, in C57BL/6 and DBA/2 mice, there is also a prominent polymorphonuclear component consistent with chronic active gastritis.[108,130] Hyperproliferation of epithelial cells and functional atrophy characterized by loss of parietal cells are seen in all four of these strains. Interestingly, atrophic changes are restricted to the gastric body, despite the fact that colonization is predominantly antral.[130] Mucosal accumulation of goblet-like cells also occurs in the gastric body. This mucus metaplasia may be similar to intestinal metaplasia in humans. Atypically branching glands may also be observed. True neoplasia has not been observed in these strains as a result of *H. felis* infection except in the case of transgenic mice already predisposed to gastric cancer.[131]

TABLE 2
Colonization and pathology with *H. felis* infection in various strains of mice[1]

Strain	Colonization	Gastritis	Atrophy[2]	Mucus Metaplasia[3]	Erosions[4]	Ref.
Outbred strains						
Swiss-Webster (germ-free)	Stomach	B; Lymphocytes, PMNs	no	No	no	127
Swiss-Quackenbush	Stomach	B, A Lymphocytes, PMNs	yes	NR	no	129
Inbred strains						
C57BL/6	High: A, C, B	B; Lymphocytes, PMNs	yes	Yes	no	108, 130
C3H/He	High: A, C Low: B	B; Lymphocytes, PMNs	yes	Yes	yes	130
SJL	Low: A, C, B	B; Lymphocytes, PMNs	yes	Yes	no	130
DBA/2	High: A, C, B	B; Lymphocytes, PMNs	yes	No	no	130
BALB/c	High: A Low: C	Minimal; A, B; Lymphocytes; MALToma-like lesions	no	No	no	108, 130, 132, 133
CBA	High: A Low: C	Minimal	no	No	no	130

[1]Abbreviations: A = antrum, C = cardia, B = body, A/B = antrum/body transitional zone, B/C = body/cardia transitional zone, PMNs = polymorphonuclear cells, NR = not reported.
[2]Atrophy refers here to parietal cell loss and resultant loss of glandular architecture.
[3]Mucus metaplasia refers to the proliferation of mucus-producing cells in the gastric mucosa that is sometimes seen with or following parietal cell loss.
[4]Erosions are defined as loss of epithelial integrity with preservation of the muscularis mucosa. This is distinct from ulceration which is a deeper lesion involving disruption of the muscularis mucosa.

Gastric ulcers are not seen with *H. felis* infection in any mouse strain, although superficial gastric erosions have been reported in C3H mice.[108]

13.3. Inbred Strains Resistant to Gastritis

In contrast to the extensive pathology and heavy colonization seen in the strains above, BALB/c and CBA mice exhibit less severe effects.[108,130,132,133] Both strains colonize predominantly in the antrum although there is also limited colonization of the cardia in the BALB/c.[132,133] Colonization levels for the BALB/c have been variably reported as heavy[130] to low,[108] however, gastritis is consistently described as minimal in this strain.[108,130,132,133] CBA mice also show minimal gastritis.[130] Where present, inflammation is predominantly lymphocytic and has been variably reported as restricted to the antrum[130] or affecting the antrum and body.[108] Atrophic changes and mucus metaplasia have not been reported in the BALB/c. However, in infections of 22 months or greater, *H. felis*-infected BALB/c mice developed accumulations of large mucosal and submucosal lymphoid follicles accompanied by hyperplastic to dysplastic changes in the adjacent epithelium.[133] These lesions bore similarities to mucus-associated lymphoid tissue (MALT) lymphomas in humans.

13.4. *H. pylori* Infections in Mice

Despite the ease of colonization and significant pathology induced in mouse models with *H. felis* infection, there are several factors that make it desirable to have a mouse model of infection with *H. pylori*. Most strains of *H. pylori* that have been associated with ulcer development are Type I strains, meaning that they have the virulence factors Cag A and Vac A. These factors may play a role in epithelial cell destruction and, potentially, carcinogenesis. *H. felis*, on the other hand, does not have these factors. This may explain why epithelial erosions are rarely seen with *H. felis* infection. In contrast, administration of sonicate or purified antigens from Type I strains of *H. pylori* was found to produce superficial erosions and epithelial vacuolization in mice while administration of sonicate or antigen from a Type II (cag A^-, vac A^-) strain failed to produce these lesions.[134,135] Other differences between *H. pylori* and *H. felis* include their preferred colonization niches. *H. felis* resides in the gastric mucus layer, while *H. pylori* can be found in the mucus layer or adhering to gastric epithelium. *H. felis* also colonizes deeper in the gastric pits than *H. pylori*, which resides primarily on the mucosal surface. The significance of these differences for disease pathogenesis is unknown. They may indicate that *H. felis*, while useful in studying helicobacter gastritis, colonization, and host immune response, is less suited for studies involving ulcer development or carcinogenesis.

13.5. Early Studies with Clinical Isolates

The first successful *H. pylori* mouse model utilized fresh isolates from human patients to infect germ-free athymic and euthymic ICR mice.[136,137] These isolates were found to colonize only transiently in euthymic mice that were not germ-free, an effect attributed to competing natural gastric infection by *Lactobacillus* species.[137] Subsequently, conventionally housed BALB/c and CD1 mice were successfully colonized using human clinical isolates administered in high concentration (10^9 CFU/ml).[138] For the most part, these studies showed low levels of colonization and minimal pathology, consisting mainly of scattered lymphocytic infiltration of the lamina propria and distortion of the glandular architecture. Gastric epithelial erosions were also reported by eight weeks post-infection.[138]

13.6. Standardized Strain for Mouse Models: The Sidnay Strain

The use of fresh clinical isolates makes interpretation and comparisonof infection studies difficult. Variation between studies may be due to differing genetic properties of the isolates or aspects of their cultivation. To avoid these difficulties, a standardized *H. pylori* strain that readily colonizes mice was developed. This strain, termed the Sydney strain (SS1), was derived from fresh clinical isolates that were serially passaged through mice.[139]

Interestingly, *H. pylori* SS1 also shows host strain-dependent differences in colonization although the pattern is different from that seen in *H. felis* mouse models. *H. pylori* SS1 will colonize the inbred strains C57BL/6, BALB/c, DBA/2, and C3H/He[130,139] (Table 3) as well as outbred Swiss mice.[140] Bacterial counts are high in C57BL/6 mice and lower in BALB/c, C3H, and DBA/2 mice. In all mouse strains tested, *H. pylori* SS1 colonizes the transitional zone between the antrum and body and, to a lesser extent, the body/cardia. However, C57BL/6 mice show more extensive colonization encompassing the entire glandular stomach.[139] Gastritis develops most rapidly in the C57BL/6 mouse and affects both the antrum and body. BALB/c mice, although colonized primarily in the antro-oxynctic transitional zone, also develop inflammation affecting both the antrum and the body. Gastritis occurs more slowly in this strain, becoming significant at eight months post-infection as opposed to six months post-infection in the C57BL/6. The extent of gastritis in the BALB/c is greater with *H. pylori* SS1 infection than with *H. felis*, which elicits minimal gastritis confined to the antrum. Inflammation in response to *H. pylori* infection is predominantly lymphocytic in most strains, although a significant polymorphonuclear component is present in the C57BL/6. Functional atrophy characterized by parietal cell loss develops in the body of both BALB/c and C57BL/6 mice, unlike the *H. felis* model which does not induce these changes in the BALB/c.[139] Superficial epithelial erosions have been reported[141] but are uncommon in mice infected with *H. pylori* SS1 alone. However, infection delays ulcer healing in an acetic-acid induced mouse ulcer model.[142] Unlike *H. felis*, *H. pylori* SS1 forms attachments to the gastric epithelium with associated "adhesion pedestals" similar to those seen in infected humans.[139] Despite this close association with the epithelium, and despite the presence of gastritis and parietal cell atrophy, further lesions such as mucosal metaplasia and gastric neoplasia have not been reported in *H. pylori* SS1 mouse models.

TABLE 3
Colonization and pathology with *H. pylori* SS1 infection in various strains of mice[1]

Strain	Colonization	Gastritis	Atrophy[2]	Mucus Metaplasia	Erosions[4]	Ref.
Outbred strains						
Swiss	High: A Low: B	B; Lymphocytes, PMNs	no	No	no	140
Inbred strains						
C57BL/6	High: A, A/B, B/C Low: B, C	Rapid: A/B, A, B Lymphocytes, PMNs	yes	No	no	130, 139, 140
DBA/2	High: A/B Low: A	NR	NR	NR	NR	139
C3H/He	Low: A Minimal: A/B, B/C	NR	NR	NR	NR	130, 139
BALB/c	Low: A/B, B/C Minimal: B, A	Slow: A/B, A, B Lymphocytes, PMNs	yes	No	no	139, 140

[1]Abbreviations: A = antrum, C = cardia, B = body, A/B = antrum/body transitional zone, B/C = body/cardia transitional zone, PMNs = polymorphonuclear cells, NR = not reported.
[2]Atrophy refers here to parietal cell loss and resultant loss of glandular architecture.
[3]Mucus metaplasia refers here to the proliferation of mucus-producing cells in the gastric mucosa that is sometimes seen with or following parietal cell loss.
[4]Erosions are defined as loss of epithelial integrity with preservation of the muscularis mucosa. This is distinct from ulceration which is a deeper lesion involving disruption of the muscularis mucosa.

14. UTILITY OF *H. pylori* AND *H. felis* MOUSE MODELS

14.1. Role of Th1 and Th2 Responses

As described above, both *H. pylori* and *H. felis* show distinct differences in colonization and severity of disease depending on the mouse strain infected. These differences have been used to determine host immune factors that affect pathogenesis. Although helicobacter gastritis involves a significant neutrophilic component in humans, it also generates lymphoid nodule formation with the accumulation of centrally located B cells surrounded by $CD4^+$ T cells.

Similar lesions are seen in mice[128] leading to the speculation that adaptive immunity plays an important role in pathogenesis. In fact, *H. felis*-infected transgenic mice lacking T cells fail to develop gastritis, despite significant colonization.[107] This underlies the importance of T cells in directing inflammation and thus generating pathology. Since humans with gastritis show a predominant

Th-1 cytokine polarization in the gastric mucosa, and since an extensive inflammatory cell infiltrate is seen throughout infection, it has been postulated that pathology is due to an exuberant, non-protective Th-1 response. This is supported by findings in mouse models. The C57BL/6, a "pro-inflammatory" strain, is most susceptible to helicobacter gastritis. Its susceptibility may stem from its propensity to mount a Th-1 or inflammatory response to infection. BALB/c mice, although they may be colonized, are more resistant to gastritis. This strain generally mounts strong humoral responses and has been shown to generate higher serum IgG levels upon *H. pylori* SS1 infection than C57BL/6 mice.[140] Its resistance to gastritis may be due to polarization of the immune response toward a Th-2 phenotype.

While strong evidence exists in mouse models for the role of a Th-1 response in pathogenesis[107,108,143,144] the role of the Th-2 response is more complicated. Adoptive transfer of either Th-1 or Th-2 cell lines into naïve C57BL/6 recipients resulted in exacerbation of gastritis upon subsequent *H. felis* challenge. Based on this finding, a Th-2 response was not protective against gastritis.[143] However, in this experiment, mice receiving the Th-2 cell line did show a decreased bacterial load. These investigators postulated that Th-1 responses are involved in the pathogenesis of gastritis while Th-2 controls bacterial load. However, subsequent studies report conflicting results. In particular, a Th-2 response was recently reported to protect against gastric pathology but allow increased colonization.[144] This study used the novel approach of infecting C57BL/6 mice with the intestinal nematode *Heligmosomoides polygyrus*, inducing a Th-2 response. Upon subsequent infection with *H. felis*, mice with concurrent helminth infection showed less gastric pathology but were more heavily colonized than mice infected with *H. felis* alone. This strategy was designed to investigate one possible explanation for the so-called "African enigma". This term refers to countries which show high levels of *H. pylori* infection in the population but low levels of gastric ulcers and gastric cancer.[145] Since these countries also tend to show high levels of endemic parasitism, one explanation for this paradox is that *H. pylori* infection occurs concurrently with strongly Th-2 polarizing parasitic infections, preventing the development of Th-1-mediated pathology.[144] The potentially protective role of Th-2 polarization requires further investigation. Interestingly, relatively few studies have been performed in altering the immune response to helicobacter infection in BALB/c mice. If a Th-2 response truly conveys resistance, monoclonal antibodies against the inhibitory cytokine IL-10 or treatment with IL-12, which drives a Th-1 response, may exacerbate gastritis or alter colonization in this strain.

14.2. Role of Cytokines

Knockout mice have been used to investigate the role of particular cytokines in disease pathogenesis (Table 4). IFNγ is a major Th-1 associated, CD4+ T-cell-generated cytokine that induces MHC II expression and activation of

TABLE 4
Gastric helicobacter infections in mice with altered cytokine expression

Helicobacter Species	Cytokine alteration	Strain background	Pathology as compared to wild-type or untreated mice: *Colonization*	Gastritis	Other	Reference
H. felis	Anti-IFNγ mAb	C57BL/6	no change	↓		108
H. felis	IL-4$^{-/-}$	C57Bl/6	↑	↓		143
H. felis	IL-10$^{-/-}$	129/SvEv	NR[1]	↑		147
H. pylori	IFNγ$^{-/-}$	C57Bl/6	↑	↓↓		141
H. pylori	IL-4$^{-/-}$	C57Bl/6J	no change	no change		146
H. pylori	IL-4 transgenic (overexpression)	C3H	no change	no change	↑ IgA, ↑ IgG	146
H. pylori	IL-10$^{-/-}$		↓	earlier onset		148

[1]NR: Not reported.

macrophages and natural killer cells. It is believed to play a key role in the pathogenesis of *H. pylori* gastritis since high levels of expression are associated with severe gastritis in both human patients and mouse models of disease. In support of this, treatment of C57BL/6 mice with anti-IFNγ monoclonal antibodies ameliorated gastritis in response to *H. felis* infection.[143] Furthermore, IFNγ knockout mice on a C57BL/6 background were colonized with *H pylori* but failed to develop gastritis even by 15 months post-infection.[141] Despite the absence of inflammation, IFNγ knockout animals exhibited higher levels of colonization with *H. pylori* than wild-type mice. From this study, it would appear that IFNγ has both harmful and protective roles as it induces significant gastritis but is also necessary to limit bacterial colonization. This is also consistent with the observation that *H. felis*-infected mice with a pre-existing Th2 immune polarization show decreased levels of IFNγ and higher levels of colonization.[144]

The role of the Th2 cytokines IL-10 and IL-4 has also been investigated using transgenic mice. IL-4 knockouts, wild-type mice, and mice over-expressing IL-4 were inoculated with *H. pylori* SS1.[146] No statistically significant difference in levels of gastric inflammation or colonization were seen, although mice over-expressing IL-4 had significantly elevated titers of *H. pylori*-specific IgA and IgG. Thus it would seem that, although IL-4 is required for efficient antibody production, it has little effect on disease manifestation or colonization levels in *H. pylori* SS1 infection. Interestingly, in a mouse model of *H. felis* infection, IL-4 knockout mice were found to have increased gastritis and increased levels of colonization.[143] This may represent a true difference in the role of IL-4 between the two types of bacterial infection or may result from methodological differences in the analysis of colonization levels.[146] Differentiating the two possibilities awaits a side-by-side comparison of *H. felis* and *H. pylori* SS1 infection in IL-4 knockout mice of the same background strain. IL-10 is a Th-2 cytokine that primarily functions to down-regulate Th-1 responses. IL-10 knockout mice show spontaneously occurring inflammatory bowel disease. It would seem likely that IL-10 knockout mice would show exacerbation of a Th-1-associated disease such as *Helicobacter* gastritis. Indeed, *H. felis* infected IL-10 knockout mice on a 129/SvEv background showed more severe gastritis with altered glandular architecture in comparison to wild-type by four weeks post-infection.[147] IL-10 knockout mice also show earlier onset of gastritis with *H. pylori* SS1 infection yet, interestingly, decreased colonization compared to wild-type mice.[148]

Several other cytokines may play a role in *H. pylori* infection and have not yet been investigated in mouse models. These include IL-8 which is known to be elevated in human *H. pylori* infection. Mice do not have an IL-8 homologue but have a cytokine known as MIP-2 which performs some of the biological activities of IL-8.[140] The role of this cytokine in mouse models of *Helicobacter* infection remains to be determined. Protective cytokines that warrant investigation include TGFβ. Although produced by a variety of cell types including, to some degree, both Th1 and Th2 $CD4^+$ T cells, TGFβ is strongly expressed by Th3 cells. Th-3 polarized $CD4^+$ T cells are regulatory T cells and diminish the immune response to an antigen. They are known to be important in tolerance. Abnormalities of these cells or a lack of Th-3 cytokines may play a role in syndromes such as inflammatory bowel disease. The role of Th-3 cells in *Helicobacter* gastritis is currently unknown. Interestingly, a significant increase in TGFβ in the gastric mucosa was seen in mice protected from *H. felis* gastritis in the *H. polygyrus* co-infection model.[144]

15. IMMUNIZATION TRIALS

Both *H. felis* and *H. pylori* mouse infection models have been extensively used in immunization trials. Successful immunization against challenge has been achieved using oral administration of *H. pylori* or *H. felis*[149,150] sonicate or lysate accompanied by the adjuvant cholera toxin (CT). Purified or recombinant helicobacter antigens such as urease[151–154] have also been used in vaccination strategies with some success. Additionally, antigenic cross-reactivity has been demonstrated since *H. pylori* antigens administered with CT convey protection against *H. felis* challenge when administered orally.[150,151] Successful parenteral immunization strategies are less common but have also been reported.[155,156] Despite these reported successes, the percent of protected mice in immunization trials is highly variable. Some studies achieved protection in only 30% of immunized animals[150] while others have reported protection as high as 80%.[151]

To compare and interpret immunization trials, it is important to understand the difficulties in defining and assessing protection from challenge. Some studies define protection by stringent criteria such as failure to detect bacteria in challenged animals.[150] Other immunization trials consider decreased colonization and diminished gastritis as sufficient criteria for protection. The wide variation in percent protection among different trials may be partially explained by the methods used to assess colonization. Colonization has been assessed by histology,[150–153] urease testing,[150–154] and culture.[151,153] Depending on the technique and on the amount of gastric tissue tested, sensitivity of detection can vary widely, with false negatives being common. An assessment of urease testing, histology, and quantitative culture revealed that culture was the most sensitive of these three methods.[157] Some animals showing bacterial counts of 10^5 CFU/g upon quantitative culture were reported as negative when colonization was assessed solely by histology and urease assay. PCR is an even more sensitive technique and can detect levels as low as 100 bacterial cells per stomach.[158] PCR detection, however, has the disadvantage of increased likelihood of contamination (for example, at necropsy) and also does not reflect bacterial viability. Another factor to consider in assessing vaccination trials is that gastric lymphoid infiltration may occur as a result of immunization itself.[152,153] Whether this is necessary for protection or whether this phenomenon itself could be harmful is currently unknown.

In addition to prophylactic immunization trials, therapeutic immunization strategies have been tested in mouse models.[159–162] Administration of *H. felis* sonicate and CT to *H. felis* infected BALB/c mice eradicated infection in 94% of treated animals by 3 months post-immunization.[159] Subsequently, recombinant *H. pylori* antigens Vac A or Cag A were administered with attenuated heat-labile toxin of *E. coli* (LT) to *H. pylori* infected CD1 mice. Eradication was reportedly achieved in 82.1% of therapeutically vaccinated mice. However, success of immunization was only assayed at one week after the last immunization and whether these animals remained free of detectable infection at later time-points is unknown. In addition, eradication was determined by culture, which is not a highly sensitive detection method.

One possible mechanism behind successful prophylactic and therapeutic vaccination is induction of a Th-2 response and generation of protective IgA antibodies.[162] IgA may coat luminal bacteria and facilitate their removal or prevent their interaction with epithelial cells. This hypothesis is supported by the observation that passive administration of anti-*H. felis* IgA protects against disease.[163] The adjuvants CT and LT[154,164] are known to induce Th-2 responses and are the most commonly used adjuvants in immunization trials. CT has also been used alone, without helicobacter antigen, to provide some degree of protection against challenge, possibly through non-specific Th-2 induction. Gastric production of IgG has also been demonstrated in response to *H. felis* vaccination and this has been postulated to play a role in protection.[165] However, this mechanism would not account for the fact that both prophylactic and therapeutic immunization have reduced colonization by *H. felis* in μMT mice which lack antibodies and mature B cells.[166,167]

Although several immunization trials have shown decreased colonization, protection from gastritis has been more difficult to establish. Mechanisms leading to decreased gastritis may require down-regulation of the normally robust helicobacter-specific Th-1 response. This immune regulation could proceed through IL-10 (a Th-2 cytokine) or by the action of Th-3 cells that secrete TGF-β and are regulatory in nature. This corresponds with elevation of IL-10 and TGF-β in mice protected against *H. felis* infection by concurrent helminth infection.[144] Protection from gastritis may involve several of the above mechanisms or others, as yet undescribed. It is likely that knockout mice with specific immune system abnormalities will continue to be used in investigation of these mechanisms.

16. THERAPEUTIC AGENTS

Mouse models of *H. felis* and *H. pylori* have been used extensively to test the efficacy of anti-helicobacter therapeutic regimens. Triple therapy protocols, consisting of bismuth subsalicylate, metronidazole or another imidazole, and an antibiotic such as amoxicillin, clarithromycin, or tetracycline, have been tested using *H. felis*[168,169] or *H. pylori* infection in the nude mouse.[170] A variety of therapeutic regimens used in humans were tested in Swiss Webster mice infected by *H. felis*. Good correspondence was shown between eradication results in humans and those in the mouse model, demonstrating its efficacy as a screening tool for therapeutic agents.[171] A triple therapy regimen utilizing tetracycline, bismuth, and metronidazole was also successful in clearing *H. pylori* SS1 from both C57BL/6 and BALB/c mice.[139] In addition to antibiotics, other alternative strategies for eradication have been tested in mouse models. For example, *Lactobacillus salivarius* has been used as a probiotic. This bacteria was shown to have inhibitory effects on *H. pylori* growth and to suppress the development of gastritis.[172,173]

17. DISEASE PATHOGENESIS

The availability of knockout mice deficient in various cytokines has allowed examination of immunological factors involved in *H. pylori* infection. Similarly, transgenic mice, which show overexpression or inducible expression of certain molecules, can be used to explore the pathogenesis of *H. pylori*-induced gastric changes. One such example is the INS-GAS mouse which has been used to study the connection between hypergastrinemia and gastric epithelial alterations.[131,174,175] This mouse carries a transgene coding for human gastrin under the control of a rat insulin promoter that restricts expression to pancreatic beta cells. Gastrin is secreted from these cells into the general circulation. By five months of age, INS-GAS mice show serum gastrin levels twice as high as those seen in wild-type control mice. Correspondingly, gastric acid secretion is two to three times as high in INS-GAS mice compared to controls. This correlates with increased parietal cell numbers in early life, however, by 10–12 months of age, parietal cell numbers in INS-GAS mice are significantly lower than in controls. At 20 months or older, parietal cells are almost completely depleted and, most significantly, all mice show significant epithelial dysplasia. The majority of mice followed to 20 months or older develop invasive gastric carcinomas affecting the mucosa, submucosa, muscularis, and vasculature. The development of gastric cancer in the INS-GAS mouse is a long process, taking almost the entire lifetime of the mouse. However, when INS-GAS mice were infected with *H. felis* at seven weeks of age, carcinogenesis was accelerated with carcinomas developing by four to six months after inoculation. Indeed, the study could not be followed past seven months post-inoculation due to the extremely rapid and debilitating progression of the gastric carcinomas.[131] These findings provide strong evidence for a gastric helicobacter acting as a tumor promoter. The initiating event is due to another genetic or environmental factor but the presence of the organism accelerates subsequent tumor development.

18. CONCLUSIONS AND FUTURE PROSPECTS

Despite early difficulties, many animal models have been developed for the study of *H. pylori* gastritis. Some of these models utilize gastric helicobacters other than *H. pylori*. In addition, comparison of the pathology seen in these animal models to that occurring in humans reveals some differences in the distribution of lesions and their cellular composition. However, in almost all cases, lesions reflect inflammatory or immune cell infiltration into the stomach, which is normally relatively free of these components. The host immune response to infection plays a large role in the severity of disease. Accordingly, examination of those factors influencing host immune response has been and will continue to be an important focus for research. The mouse will probably continue to play a major role in these studies due to the availability of a wide variety of genetically modified animals. However, certain types of research may more effectively utilize a larger animal model. For example, in NHPs or cats, comparison of lesions in the same animal before and after a therapeutic intervention can be achieved by serial endoscopy. Also, some studies may require the presence of a particular lesion. For instance, although pre-neoplastic lesions are seen in multiple species, the *H. pylori*-infected Mongolian gerbil may be particularly well-suited for studies of factors influencing gastric adenocarcinoma development.

In the future, characterization of pathology on a molecular scale may play a larger role. One common problem with animal models is that histologically similar lesions may develop through dissimilar pathways in different hosts. Examination of gene expression patterns would allow greater insight into disease pathogenesis on a molecular level. Techniques such as RT-PCR and immunostaining are already being used to look at expression of individual genes in human gastric cancer, most notably p53.[176,177] However, more recent technologies such as microchip gene arrays would allow many more genes to be examined at a time. In addition, expression patterns could be compared between human patients and animals with experimental lesions to determine similarities and differences. This technique has been used to classify human tumor types based on gene expression patterns.[178] This would bring new sophistication to the use of animal models as it would allow more accurate assessment of whether microscopically similar lesions reflect the same genetic changes across species. This technology holds great promise for increasing our accuracy at determining whether an animal model of disease can be confidently compared to its human counterpart.

REFERENCES

1. Marshall B. J., Armstrong J. A., McGechie D. B., and Glancy R. J., 1985, Attempt to fill Koch's postulates for pyloric *Campylobacter*, *Med. J. Aust.* **142**:436.
2. Morris A., and Nicholson G., 1987, Ingestion of *Campylobacter pyloridis* causes gastritis and raised fasting gastric pH, *Am. J. Gastroenterol.* **82**:192.
3. Fox J. G., Edrise B. M., Cabot E., Beaucage C., Murphy J. C., and Prostak K. S., 1986, *Campylobacter*-like organisms isolated from gastric mucosa of ferrets, *Am. J. Vet. Res.* **47**:236.
4. Fox J. G., Cabot E. B., Taylor N. S., and Laraway R., 1988, Gastric colonization of *Campylobacter pylori* subsp. *mustelae* in ferrets, *Infect. Immun.* **56**:2994.
5. Fox J. G., Chilvers T., Goodwin C. S., *et al.*, 1989, *Campylobacter mustelae*, a new species resulting from the elevation of *Campylobacter pylori* subsp. *mustelae* to species status, *Int. J. Syst. Bact.* **39**:301.
6. Goodwin C. S., Armstrong J. A., Chilvers T., Peters M., Collins M. D., Sly L., McConnell W., and Harper W. E. S., 1989, Transfer of *Campylobacter pylori* and *Campylobacter mustelae* to *Helicobacter* gen. nov. as *Helicobacter pylori* comb. nov. and *Helicobacter mustelae* comb. nov., respectively. *Int. J. Syst. Bacteriol.* **39**:397–405.
7. Tompkins D. S., Wyatt J. I., Rathbone B. J., and West A. P., 1988, The characterization and pathological significance of gastric *Campylobacter*-like organisms in the ferret: a model for chronic gastritis? *Epidemiol. Infect.* **101**:269.
8. Fox J. G., Otto G., Murphy J. C., Taylor N. S., and Lee A., 1991, Gastric colonization of the ferret with *Helicobacter* species: natural and experimental infections. *Rev. Inf. Dis.* **13**(Suppl 8):S671.
9. Fox J. G., Otto G., Taylor N. S., Rosenblad W., and Murphy J. C., 1991, *Helicobacter mustelae*-induced gastritis and elevated gastric pH in the ferret (*Mustela putorius furo*). *Infect. Immun.* **59**:1875.
10. Fox J. G., Wishnok J. S., Murphy J. C., Tannenbaum S., and Correa P., 1993, MNNG-induced gastric carcinoma in ferrets infected with *Helicobacter mustelae. Carcinogenesis.* **14**:1957.
11. Fox J. G., Dangler C. A., Sager W., Borkowski R., and Gliatto J. M., 1997, *Helicobacter mustelae*-associated gastric adenocarcinoma in ferrets (*Mustela putorius furo*). *Vet. Pathol.* **34**:225.

12. Erdman S. E., Correa P., Coleman L. A., Schrenzel M. D., Li X., and Fox J. G., 1997, *Helicobacter mustelae*-associated gastric MALT lymphoma in ferrets. *Am. J. Vet. Path.* **151**:273.
13. Yu J., Russell R. M., Saloman R. N., Murphy J. C., Palley L. S., and Fox J. G., 1995, Effect of *Helicobacter mustelae* infection on ferret gastric epithelial cell proliferation. *Carcinogenesis.* **16**: 1927.
14. Lipkin M., 1988, Biomarkers of increased susceptibility to gastrointestinal cancer; new application to studies of cancer prevention in human subjects. *Adv. Cancer. Res.* **50**:1.
15. Lipkin M., Correa P., Mikol Y. B., Higgins P. J., Cuello C., Zarama G., Fontham E., and Savala D., 1985, Proliferative and antigenic modifications in epithelial cells in chronic atrophic gastritis. *J. Natl. Cancer Inst.* **75**:613.
16. O'Croinin T., Clyne M., and Drumm B., 2000, *Helicobacter mustelae* infection of the ferret as a natural animal model for helicobacter adherence studies. *Gut.* **47**(Suppl. 1):A4.
17. Aim R. A., Ling L.-S. L., Moir D. J., King B. L., *et al.*, 1999, Genomic sequence comparison of two unrelated isolates of the human gastric pathogen *Helicobacter pylori*, *Nature*, **397**:176.
18. Marini R. P., Fox J. G., 1999, Animal models of *Helicobacter* (ferrets), in: *Handbook of Animal Models of Infection*, Eds. O. Zak, M. Sande, Academic Press, London.
19. Cabot E. B., and Fox J. G., 1990, Bile reflux and the gastric mucosa: an experimental ferret model, *J. Investig. Surg.* **3**:177.
20. Fox J. G., 1994, Gastric disease in ferrets: effects of *Helicobacter mustelae*, nitrosamines, and reconstructive gastric surgery, *Eur. J. Gastroenterol. Hepatol.* **6**(Suppl. 1):S57.
21. Ryden E. B., Licht W. R., Cabot E. B., and Fox J. G., 1990, Gastric nitrite processing in the surgically altered maximal and minimal bile duct reflux ferret model, *carcinogenesis.* **11**:405.
22. Alder J. D., Ewing P. J., Mitten M. J., Oleksjiew A., and Tanaka S. K., 1996, Relevance of the ferret model of *Helicobacter*-induced gastritis to evaluation of antibacterial therapies, *Am. J. Gastroenterol.* **91**:2347.
23. Cuenca R., Blanchard T. G., Czinn S. J., Nedrud J. G., Monath T. P., Lee C. K., and Redline R. W., 1996, Therapeutic immunization against *Helicobacter mustelae* in naturally infected ferrets, *Gastroenterology.* **110**:1770.
24. Fox J. G., 1997, The expanding genus of *Helicobacter*, *Semin. Gastrointest. Dis.* **8**:124.
25. Lee A., Hazell S. L., O'Rourke J., and Kouprach S., 1988, Isolation of a spiral-shaped bacterium from the cat stomach. *Infect. Immun.* **56**:2843.
26. Paster B. J., Lee A., Fox J. G., Dewhirst F. E., Tordoff L. A., Fraser G. J., O'Rourke J. L., Taylor N. S., and Ferrero R., 1991, Phylogeny of *Helicobacter felis* sp. nov., *Helicobacter mustelae*, and related bacteria. *Int. J. Syst. Bacteriol.* **41**:31.
27. Seidel K. E., Stolte M., Lehn N., and Bauer J., 1999, Antibodies against *Helicobacter felis* in sera of cats and dogs, *Zentralbl. Veterinarmed.* **46**:181.
28. Simpson K. W., Strauss-Ayali D., Scanziani E., Straubinger B. K., McDonough P. I., Straubinger A. F., Chang Y. F., Domeneghini C., Arebi N., and Cahan J., 2000, *Helicobacter felis* infection is associated with lymphoid follicular hyperplasia and mild gastritis but normal gastric secretory function in cats, *Infect. Immun.* **68**:779.
29. Hanninen M. C., Happonen I., Saari S., and Jalava K., 1996, Culture and characterization of *Helicobacter bizzozeronii*, a new canine *Helicobacter* sp., *Int. J. Syst. Bacteriol.* **46**:160.
30. Solnick J. V., O'Rourke J. L., Lee A., Paster B. J., Dewhirst F. E., and Tomkins L. S., 1993, An uncultured gastric spiral organism is a newly identified *Helicobacter* in humans, *J. Infect. Dis.* **168**:379.
31. Yamasaki K., Suematsu H., and Takahashi T., 1998, Comparison of gastric lesions in dogs and cats with and without gastric spiral organisms, *J. Am. Vet. Med. Assoc.* **212**:529.
32. Neiger R., Dieterich C., Burnens A., Waldvogel A., Corthesy-Theulaz I., Halter F., Lauterburg B., and Schmassmann A., 1998, Detection and prevalence of *Helicobacter* infection in pet cats, *J. Clin. Microbiol.* **36**:634.

33. Norris C. R., Marks S. L., Eaton K. A., Torabian S. Z., Munn R. I., and Solnick J. V., 1999, Healthy cats are commonly colonized with "*Helicobacter heilmannii*" that is associated with minimal gastritis, *J. Clin. Microbiol.* **37**:189.
34. Jalava K., On S. L. W., Vandamme P. A., Happonen I., Sukura A., and Hanninen M. L., 1998, Isolation and identification of *Helicobacter* spp. from canine and feline gastric mucosa, *Appl. Environ. Microbiol.* **64**:3998.
35. Handt L. K., Fox J. G., Dewhirst F. E., Fraser G. J., Paster B. J., Yan L. L., Rozmiarek H., Rufo R., and Stalis I. H., 1994, *Helicobacter pylori* isolated from the domestic cat: public health implications, *Infect. Immun.* **62**:2367.
36. Handt L. K., Fox J. G., Stalis I. H., Rufo R., Lee G., Linn J., Li X., and Kleanthous H., 1995, Characterization of feline *Helicobacter pylori* strains and associated gastritis in a colony of domestic cats, *J. Clin. Microbiol.* **33**:2280.
37. El-Zaatari F. A., Woo J. S., Badr A., Osato M. S., Serna H., Lichtenberger L. M., Genta R. M., and Graham D. Y., 1997, Failure to isolate *Helicobacter pylori* from stray cats indicates that *H. pylori* in cats may be an anthroponosis—an animal infection with a human pathogen, *J. Med. Microbiol.* **46**:372.
38. Fox J. G., Batchelder M., Marini R. P., Yan L., Handt L., Li X., Shames B., Hayward A., Campbell J., and Murphy J. C., 1995, *Helicobacter pylori*-indcued gastritis in the domestic cat, *Infect. Immun.* **63**:2674.
39. Fox J. G., Perkins S., Yan L., Shen Z., Attardo L., and Pappo J., 1995, Local immune response in *Helicobacter pylori*-infected cats and identification of *H. pylori* in saliva, gastric fluid, and feces, *Immunology*. **88**:400.
40. Yan L. L., Shen Z., Hayward A., Murphy J. C., and Fox J. G., 1996, Use of PCR and culture to detect *Helicobacter pylori* in naturally infected cats following triple antimicrobial therapy, *Antimicrob. Agents. Chemother.* **40**:1486.
41. Ansorg R., Von Heinegg E. H., and Von Recklinghausen G., 1995, Cat owners' risk of acquiring a *Helicobacter pylori* infection, *Zentralbl. Bakteriol.* **283**:122.
42. Stolte M., Wellens E., Bethke B., Ritter M., and Eidt M., 1994, *H. heilmannii* (formerly *Gastrospirillum hominis*) gastritis: an infection transmitted by animals? *Scand. J. Gastroenterol.* **29**:1061.
43. Heilmann K. L., and Borchard F., 1991, Gastritis due to spiral shaped bacteria other than *H. pylori*: clinical, histological, and ultrastructural findings, *Gut.* **32**:137.
44. Lavelle J. P., Landas S., Mitros F. A., and Conklin J. L., 1994, Acute gastritis associated with spiral organisms from cats, *Dig. Dis. Sci.* **39**:744.
45. Dieterich C., Wiesel P., Neiger R., Blum A., and Corthesy-Theulaz I., 1998, Presence of multiple "*Helicobacter heilmannii*" strains in an individual suffering from ulcers and in his two cats, *J. Clin. Microbiol.* **36**:366.
46. Esteves M. I., Schrenzel M. D., Marini R. P., Taylor N. S., Xu S., Hagen S., Feng Y., Shen Z., and Fox J. G., 2000, *Helicobacter pylori* gastritis in cats with long-term natural infection as a model of human disease, *Am. J. Pathol.* **156**:709.
47. Lee A., 1995, *Helicobacter* infections in laboratory animals: a model for gastric neoplasia, *Ann. Med.* **27**:575.
48. Turk M. A., 1981, Nonhematopoietic gastrointestinal neoplasia in cats: a retrospective study of 44 cases, *Vet. Pathol.* **18**:614.
49. Brodey R. S., 1966, Alimentary tract neoplasms in the cat: a clinicopathologic survey of 46 cases, *Zahnarztl. Prax.* **17**:74.
50. Mahony O. M., Moore A. S., Cotter S. M., Engler S. J., Brown D., and Penninck D. G., 1995, Alimentary lymphoma in cats: 28 cases (1988–1993), *J. Am. Vet. Med. Assoc.* **207**:1593.
51. Holmberg C. A., Manning J. S., Osburn B. I., 1976, Feline malignant lymphomas: comparison of morphologic and immunologic character, *Am. J. Vet. Res.* **37**:1455.

52. Otto G., Hazell S. H., Fox J. G., Howlett C. R., Murphy J. C., O'Rourke J. L., and Lee A., 1994, Animal and public health implications of gastric colonization of cats by *Helicobacter*-like organisms. *J. Clin. Micro.* **32**:1043.
53. Krakowka S., Morgan D. R., Kraft W. G., and Leunk R. D., 1987, Establishment of gastric *Campylobacter pylori* infection in the neonatal gnotobiotic piglet, *Infect. Immun.* **55**:2789.
54. Lambert J. R., Borromes M., Pinkard K. J., Turner H., Chapman C. B., and Smith M. L., 1987, Colonization of gnotobiotic piglets with *Campylobacter pyloridis*—an animal model? *J. Infect. Dis.* **155**:1344.
55. Engstrand L., Gustavsson S., Jorgensen A., Schwan A., and Scheynius A., 1990, Inoculation of barrier-born pigs with *Helicobacter pylori*: a useful animal model for gastritis Type B, *Infect. Immun.* **58**:1763.
56. Eaton K. A., Morgan D. R., and Krakowka S., 1989, Virulence factors for *Campylobacter pylori* infection in gnotobiotic piglets, *Infect. Immun.* **57**:1119.
57. Eaton K. A., Morgan D. R., and Krakowka S., 1990, Persistence of *Helicobacter pylori* in conventionalized piglets, *J. Infect. Dis.* **161**:1299.
58. Queiroz D. M., Rocha G. A., Mendes E. N., Cage A. P., Carualho A. C., and Barbosa A. J., 1990, A spiral microorganism in the stomach of pigs, *Vet. Microbiol.* **24**:199.
59. DeGroote D., van Doorn L. J., Ducatelle R., Verschuuren A., Haesebrouck F., Quint W. G., Jalava K., and Vandamme P., 1999, "*Candidatus Helicobacter suis*", a gastric helicobacter from pigs, and its phylogenetic relatedness to other gastrospirilla, *Int. J. Syst. Bacteriol.* **49**:1769.
60. DeGroote D., Ducatelle R., van Doorn L. J., Tilmant K., Vershuuren A., and Haesebrouck F., 2000, Detection of "*Candidatus Helicobacter suis*" in gastric samples of pigs by PCR: comparison with other invasive diagnostic techniques, *J. Clin. Microbiol.* **38**:1131.
61. Mendes E. N., Queiroz D. M., Moura S. B., and Rocha G. A., 1998, Mouse inoculation for the detection of non-cultivable gastric tightly spiraled bacteria, *Braz. J. Med. Biol. Res.* **31**:373.
62. Bertram T. A., Krakowka S., and Morgan D. R., 1991, Gastritis associated with infection by *Helicobacter pylori*: comparative pathology in humans and swine, *Rev. Inf. Dis.* **13**(Suppl. 8):S714.
63. Krakowka S., Eaton K. A., and Rings D. M., 1995, Occurrence of gastric ulcers in gnotobiotic piglets colonized by *H. pylori*, *Infect. Immun.* **63**:2352.
64. Eaton K. A., and Krakowka S., 1992, Chronic active gastritis due to *H. pylori* in immunized gnotobiotic piglets, *Gastroenterol.* **103**:1580.
65. Eaton K. A., Ringler S. S., Krakowka S., 1998, Vaccination of gnotobiotic piglets against *Helicobacter* species, *J. Infect. Dis.* **178**:1399.
66. Eaton K. A., Brooks C. L., Morgan D. R., and Krakowka S., 1991, Essential role of urease in pathogenesis of gastritis induced by *Helicobacter pylori* in gnotobiotic piglets, *Infect. Immun.* **59**:2470.
67. Eaton K. A., and Krakowka S., 1994, Effect of gastric pH on urease-dependent colonization of gnotobiotic piglets, *Infect. Immun.* **62**:3604.
68. DeMagalhaes Queiroz D. M., Rocha G. A., Mendes E. N., de Moura S. B., de Oiveira A. M. R., and Miranda D., 1996, Association between *Helicobacter* and gastric ulcer disease of the pars esophagea in swine, *Gastroenterology.* **111**:19.
69. Barbosa A. J. A., Silva J. C. P., and Nogueira A. M. M. F., 1995, Higher incidence of *Gastrospirillum sp.* in swine with gastric ulcer of the pars esophagea, *Vet. Pathol.* **32**:134.
70. Cantet F., Magras C., Marais A., Federighi M., and Megraud F., 1999, *Helicobacter* species colonizing pig stomach: molecular characterization and determination of prevalence, *Appl. Environ. Microbiol.* **65**:4672.
71. Utriainen M., and Hanninen M. L., 1998, Detection of *Helicobacter*-like bacteria in porcine gastric biopsy samples by amplification of 16S rRNA, ureB, vacA, and cagA genes by PCR, *Vet. Res. Commun.* **22**:373.
72. Roosendaal J. H., Vos T., Roumen R., van Vugt G., Cottoli A., Bart H. L., Klaasen E. J., Kuipers, Vandenbroucke, and Kusters J. G., 2000, Slaughter pigs are commonly infected

by closely related but distinct gastric ulcerative lesion-inducing gastrospirilla. *J. Clin. Microbiol.* **38**:2661.

73. Mall A. S., Hickman R., Terblanche J., and Kahn D., 1997, The pig as ulcer model, *Gastroenterol.* **113**:366.
74. Lee A., 2000, Animal models of gastroduodenal ulcer disease, *Bailliere's Best. Pract. Res. Clin. Gastroenterol.* **14**:75.
75. Radin M. J., Eaton K. A., Krakowka S., Morgan D. R., Lee A., Otto G., and Fox J. G., 1990, *Helicobacter pylori* gastric infection in gnotobiotic beagle dogs, *Infect. Immun.* **58**:2606.
76. Rossi G., Rossi M., Vitali C. G., Fortuna D., Burroni D., Pancotto L., Capecchi S., Sozzi S., Renzoni G., Braca G., Del Giudice G., Rappuoli R., Ghiara P., and Taccini E., 1999, A conventional beagle dog model for acute and chronic infection with *Helicobacter pylori*, *Infect. Immun.* **67**:3112.
77. Happonen I., Linden J., Saari S., Karjalainen M., Hanninen M. L., Jalava K., and Westermarck E., 1998, Detection and effects of helicobacters in healthy dogs and dogs with signs of gastritis, *J. Am. Vet. Med. Assoc.* **213**:1767.
78. Eaton K. A., Dewhirst F. E., Paster B. J., Tzellas N., Coleman B. F., Paola J., and Sherding R., 1996, Prevalence and varieties of *Helicobacter* species in dogs from random sources and pet dogs: animal and public health implications, *J. Clin. Microbiol.* **34**:3165.
79. Marini R. P., Labato M. A., Taylor N. S., Schrenzel M. D., Xu S., Speilman B., Shen Z., Yan L., Feng L., and Fox J. G., 2000, Failure to detect *Helicobacter pylori* in gastric endoscopic biopsies from dogs and cats, Contemp. *Topics Lab. Anim. Sci.* **39**:52.
80. Cattoli G., van Vugt R., Zanoni R. G., Sanguinetti V., Chiocchetti R., Gualtieri M., Vandenbroucke-Graals W., and Kusters J. G., 1999, Occurrence and characterization of gastric *Helicobacter spp.* in naturally-infected dogs, *Vet. Microbiol.* **70**:239.
81. Peyrol S., Lecoindre P., Berger I., Deleforge J., and Chevallier M., 1998, Differential pathogenic effect of two *Helicobacter*-like organisms in dog gastric mucosa, *J. Submicrosc. Cytol. Pathol.* **30**:425.
82. Happonen I., Saari S., Castren L., Tyni O., Hanninen M. L., and Westermarck E., 1996, Occurrence and topographical mapping of gastric *Helicobacter*-like organisms and their association with histological changes in apparently healthy dogs and cats, *Zentralbl. Veterinarmed.* **43**:305.
83. Crabtree J. E., Peichl P., Wyatt J. L., Stachl U., and Lindley I. J., 1993, Gastric interleukin-8 and IgA IL-8 antibodies in *Helicobacter pylori* infection, *Scand. J. Immunol.* **37**:65.
84. Doenges J. L., 1939, Spirochetes in the gastric glands of macacas rhesus and of man without related disease, *Arch. Pathol.*, **27**:469.
85. Baskerville A., and Newell D. G., 1988, Naturally ocurring chronic gastritis and *C. pylori* infection in the rhesus monkey: a potential model for gastritis in man, *Gut.* **29**:465.
86. Newell D. G., Hudson M. J., and Baskerville A., 1988, Isolation of a gastric campylobacter-like organism from the stomach of four rhesus monkeys and identification as *Campylobacter pylori*, *J. Med. Microbiol.* **27**:41.
87. Euler A. R., Zurenko G. E., Moe J. B., Ulrich R. G., and Yagi Y., 1990, Evaluation of two monkey species (*Macaca mulatta* and *Macaca fascicularis*) as possible models for human *Helicobacter pylori* disease, *J. Clin. Microbiol.* **28**:2285.
88. Dubois A., Fiala N., Heman-Ackah L. M., Drazek E. S., Tarnawski A., Fishbein W. N., Perez-Perez G. I., and Blaser M. J., 1994, Natural gastric infection with *Helicobacter pylori* in monkeys: a model for spiral bacteria infection in humans, *Gastroenterology.* **106**:1405.
89. Drazek E. S., Dubois A., and Holmes R. K., 1994, Characterization and presumptive identification of *Helicobacter pylori* isolates from rhesus monkeys, *J. Clin. Microbiol.* **32**:1799.
90. Handt L. K., Fox J. G., Yan L. Y., Shen Z., Pouch W. J., Ngai D., Motzel S. L., Nolan T. E., and Klein H. J., 1997, Diagnosis of *Helicobacter pylori* infection in a colony of rhesus monkeys (*Macaca mulatta*), *J. Clin. Microbiol.* **35**:165.

91. Reindel J. F., Fitzgerald A. L., Breider M. A., Gough A. W., Yan C., Mysore J. V., and Dubois A., 1999, An epizootic of lymphoplasmacytic gastritis attributed to *Helicobacter pylori* infection in cynomolgus monkeys (*Macaca fascicularis*), *Vet. Pathol.* **36**:1.
92. Dubois A., Fiala N., Weichbrod R. H., Ward G. S., Nix M., Mehlman P. T., Taub D. M., Perez-Perez G. I., and Blaser M. J., 1995, Seroepizootiology of *Helicobacter pylori* gastric infection in nonhuman primates housed in social environments, *J. Clin. Microbiol.* **33**:1492.
93. Solnick J. V., Canfield D. R., Yang S., and Parsonnet J., 1999, Rhesus monkey (*Macaca mulatta*) model of *Helicobacter pylori*: noninvasive detection and derivation of specific-pathogen-free monkeys, *Lab. Anim. Sci.* **49**:197.
94. Sato T., and Takeuchi T. A., 1982, Infection by spirilla in the stomach of the rhesus monkey, *Vet. Pathol.* **19**(Suppl 7):17.
95. Dubois A., Tarnawski A., Newell D. G., Fiala N., Dabros W., Stachura J., Krivan H., and Heman-Ackah L. M., 1991, Gastric injury and invasion of parietal cells by spiral bacteria in rhesus monkeys, *Gastroenterology.* **100**:884.
96. Bronsdon M. A., Goodwin C. S., Sly L. I., Chilvers T., and Schoenkrecht F. D., 1991, *Helicobacter nemestrinae* sp. nov., a spiral bacterium found in the stomach of a pigtailed macaque, *Int. J. Syst. Bacteriol.* **41**:148.
97. Fox J. G., and Suerbaum S., unpublished observations.
98. Fujioka T., Kubota T., Shuto R., Kodama R., Murakami K., Perparim K., and Nasu M., 1994, Establishment of an animal model for chronic gastritis with *Helicobacter pylori*: potential model for long-term observations, *Eur. J. Gastroenterol. Hepatol.* **6**(Suppl 1):S7.
99. Fujiyama K., Fujioka T., Murakami K., and Nasu M., 1995, Effects of *Helicobacter pylori* infection on mucosal defense factors in Japanese monkeys, *J. Gastroenterol.* **30**:441.
100. Stadtlander C. T., Gangemi J. D., Stutzenberger F. J., Lawson J. W., Lawson B. R., Khanolkar S. S., Elliott-Raynor K. E., Farris H. E., Fulton L. K., Hill J. E., Huntington F. K., Lee C. K., and Monath T. P., 1998, Experimentally induced infection with *Helicobacter pylori* in squirrel monkeys (*Saimiri spp*): clinical, microbiological, and histopathological findings, *Lab. Anim. Sci.* **48**:303.
101. Hazell S. L., Eichberg J. W., Lee D. R., Alpert L., Evans D. G., Evans D. J., and Graham D. Y., 1992, Selection of the chimpanzee over the baboon as a model for *Helicobacter pylori* infection, *Gastroenterol.* **103**:848.
102. Dubois A., Berg D. E., Incecik E. T., Fiala N., Heman-Ackah L. M., PerezPerez G. I., and Blaser M. J., 1996, Transient and persistent experimental infection of nonhuman primates with *Helicobacter pylori*: implications for human disease, *Infect. Immun.* **64**:2885.
103. Akopyants N. S., Eaton K. A., and Berg D. E., 1995, Adaptive mutation and co-colonization during *Helicobacter pylori* infection of gnotobiotic piglets, *Infect. Immun.* **63**:116.
104. Dubois A., Berg D. E., Incecik E. T., Fiala N., Heman-Ackah L. M., Del Valle J., Yang M., Wirth H. P., Perez-Perez G. I., and Blaser M. J., 1999, Host specificity of *Helicobacter pylori* strains and host responses in experimentally challenged nonhuman primates, *Gastroenterology.* **116**:90.
105. Mattapallil J. J., Dandekar S., Canfield D. R., and Solnick J. V., 2000, A predominant Th1 type of immune response is induced early during acute *Helicobacter pylori* infection in rhesus macaques, *Gastroenterology.* **118**:307.
106. Harris P. R., Smythies L. E., Smith P. D., and Dubois A., 2000, Inflammatory cytokine mRNA expression during early and persistent *Helicobacter pylori* infection in nonhuman primates, *J. Infect. Dis.* **181**:783.
107. Roth K. A., Kapadia S. B., Martin S. M., and Lorenz R. G., 1999, Cellular immune responses are essential for the development of *Helicobacter felis*-associated gastric pathology, *J. Immunol.* **163**:1490.
108. Mohammadi M., Czinn S., Redline R., and Nedrud J., 1996, Helicobacter-specific cell-mediated immune responses display a predominant Th1 phenotype and promote a delayed-type hypersensitivity response in the stomachs of mice, *J. Immunol.* **156**:4729.

109. Mysore J. V., Wigginton T., Simon P. M., Zopf D., Heman-Ackah L. M., and Dubois A., 1999, Treatment of *Helicobacter pylori* infection in rhesus monkeys using a novel antiadhesion compound. *Gastroenterology.* **117**:1316.
110. Solnick J. V., Canfield D. R., Hansen L. M., and Torabian S. Z., 2000, Immunization with recombinant *Helicobacter pylori* urease in specific-pathogen-free rhesus monkeys (*Macaca mulatta*), *Infect. Immun.* **68**:2560.
111. Lee C. K., Soike K., Hill J., Georgakopoulos K., Tibbitts T., Ingrassia J., Gray H., Boden J., Kleanthous H., Giannasca P., Ermak T., Weltzin R., Blanchard J., and Monath T. P., 1999, Immunization with recombinant *Helicobacter pylori* urease decreases colonization levels following experimental infection of rhesus monkeys, *Vaccine.* **17**:1493.
112. Lee C. K., Soike K., Giannasca P., Hill J., Weltzin R., Kleanthous H., Blanchard J., and Monath T. P., 1999, Immunization of rhesus monkeys with a mucosal prime, parenteral boost strategy protects against infection with *Helicobacter pylori*, *Vaccine.* **17**:3072.
113. Dubois A., Lee C. K., Fiala N., Kleanthous H., Mehlman P. T., and Monath T., 1998, Immunization against natural *Helicobacter pylori* infection in nonhuman primates, *Infect. Immun.* **66**:4340.
114. Dubois A., Berg D. E., Fiala N., Heman-Ackah L. M., Perez-Perez G. I., and Blaser M., 1998, Cure of *Helicobacter pylori* infection by omeprazole-clarithromycin-based therapy in non-human primates, *J. Gastroenterol.* **33**:18.
115. Fox J. G., Lee A., Otto G., Taylor N. S., and Murphy J. C., 1991, *Helicobacter felis* gastritis in gnotobiotic rats: an animal model of *Helicobacter pylori* gastritis. *Infect. Immun.* **59**:785.
116. Ehlers S., Warrelman M., and Hahn H., 1988, In search of an animal model for experimental *Campylobacter pylori* infection: administration of *Campylobacter pylori* to rodents, *Zentralbl. Bakteriol. Mikrobiol. Hyg.* **268**:341.
117. Cantorna M. T., and Balish E., 1990, Inability of human clinical strains of *Helicobacter pylori* to colonize the alimentary tract of germfree rodents. *Can. J. Microbiol.* **36**:237.
118. Li H., Kalies I., Meligard B., and Helander M. F., 1998, A rat model of chronic *Helicobacter pylori* infection: studies of epithelial cell turnover and gastric ulcer healing, *Scand. J. Gastroenterol.* **33**:370.
119. Mendes E. N., Queiroz D. M., Coimbra R. S., Moira S. B., Barbosa A. J., and Rocha G. A., 1996, Experimental infection of Wistar rats with *Gastrospirillum suis*, *J. Med. Microbiol.* **44**:105.
120. Duval-Araujo I., De-Magalhaes Queiroz D. M., Magnago A. G., Simal G. J., Marino V. S., Carvalho S. D., DaSilva Machado L. A., and Miranda D., 2000, Increased gastric emptying induced by *Helicobacter heilmannii* type 1 infection in rats, *J. Med. Microbiol.* **49**:627.
121. Danon S. J., Moss N. D., Larsson H., Arvidsson S., Ottosson S., Dixon M. F., and Lee A., 1998, Gastrin release and gastric acid secretion in the rat infected with either *Helicobacter felis* or *Helicobacter heilmannii*, *J. Gastroenterol. Hepatol.* **13**:95.
122. Goodman K. J., Correa P., Tengana Aux H. J., Delany J. P., and Collazos T., 1997, Nutritional factors and *Helicobacter pylori* infection in Colombian children, *J. Pediatr. Gastroenterol. Nutr.* **25**:507.
123. Shomer N. H., Dangler C. A., Whary M. T., and Fox J. G., 1998, Experimental *Helicobacter pylori* infection induces antral gastritis and gastric mucosa-associated lymphoid tissue in guinea pigs, *Infect. Immun.* **66**:2614.
124. Sturegard E., Sjunnessson H., Ho B., Willen R., Alleljung P., Ng H. C., and Wadstrom T., 1998, Severe gastritis in guinea pigs infected with *Helicobacter pylori*, *J. Med. Microbiol.* **47**:1123.
125. Watanabe T., Tada M., Nagai H., Sasaki S., and Nakao M., 1998, *Helicobacter pylori* infection induces gastric cancer in Mongolian gerbils, *Gastroenterol.* **115**:641.
126. Dick E., Lee A., Watson G., and O'Rourke J., 1989, Use of the mouse for the isolation and investigation of stomach-associated, spiral-helical shaped bacteria from man and other animals, *J. Med. Microbiol.* **29**:55.
127. Lee A., Fox J. G., Otto G., and Murphy J. C., 1990, A small animal model of *Helicobacter pylori* active chronic gastritis, *Gastroenterology.* **99**:1315.

128. Fox J. G., Blanco M., Murphy J. C., Taylor N. S., Lee A., Kabok Z., and Pappo J., 1993, Local and systemic immune responses in murine *Helicobacter felis* active chronic gastritis, *Infect. Immun.* **61**:2309.
129. Lee A., Chen M. H., Coltro N., O'Rourke J., Hazell S., Hu P., and Li Y., 1993, Long term infection of the gastric mucosa with *Helicobacter* species does induce atrophic gastritis in an animal model of *Helicobacter pylori* infection, *Zentralbl. Bakteriol.* **280**:38.
130. Sakagami T., Dixon M., O'Rourke J., Howlett R., Alderuccio F., Vella J., Shimoyama T., and Lee A., 1996, Atrophic gastric changes in both *Helicobacter felis* and *Helicobacter pylori* infected mice are host dependent and separate from antral gastritis, *Gut.* **39**:639.
131. Wang T. C., Dangler C. A., Chen D., Goldenring J. R., Koh T., Raychowdury R., Coffey R. J., Ito S., Varro A., Dockray G. J., and Fox J. G., 2000, Synergistic interaction between hypergastrinemia and *Helicobacter* infection in a mouse model of gastric cancer, *Gastroenterology*. **118**:36.
132. Danon S. J., O'Rourke J. L., Moss N. D., and Lee A., 1995, The importance of local acid production in the distribution of *Helicobacter felis* in the mouse stomach, *Gastroenterology.* **108**:1386.
133. Enno A., O'Rourke J. L., Howlett C. R., Jack A., Dixon M. F., and Lee A., 1995, MALToma-like lesions in the murine gastric mucosa after long-term infection with *Helicobacter felis*, *Am. J. Path.* **147**:217.
134. Telford J. L., Ghiara P., Dell'Orco M., Comanducci M., Burroni D., Bugnoli M., Tecce M. F., Censini S., Covacci A., Xiang Z., Papini E., Montecucco C., Parente L., and Rappuoli R., 1994, Gene structure of the *Helicobacter pylori* cytotoxin and evidence of its key role in gastric disease, *J. Exp. Med.* **179**:1653.
135. Ghiara P., Marchetti M., Blaser M. J., Tummuru M. K. R., Cover T. L., Segal E. D., Tompkins L. S., and Rappuoli R., 1995, Role of the *Helicobacter pylori* virulence factors vacuolating cytotoxin, CagA, and urease in a mouse model of disease, *Infect. Immun.* **63**:4154.
136. Karita M., Kouchiyama T., Okita K., and Nakazawa T., 1991, New small animal model for human gastric *Helicobacter pylori* infection in both nude and euthymic mice, *Am. J. Gastroenterol.* **86**:1596.
137. Karita M., Li Q., Cantero D., and Okita K., 1994, Establishment of a small animal model for human *Helicobacter pylori* infection using germ-free mouse, *Am. J. Gastroenterol.* **89**:208.
138. Marchetti M., Arico B., Burroni D., Figura N., Rappuoli R., and Ghiara P., 1995, Development of a mouse model of *Helicobacter pylori* infection that mimics human disease, *Science.* **267**:1655.
139. Lee A., O'Rourke J., de Ungria M. C., Robertson B., Daskalopoulos G., and Dixon M. F., 1997, A standardized mouse model of *Helicobacter pylori* infection: introducing the Sydney strain, *Gastroenterology.* **112**:1386.
140. Ferrero R. L., Thiberge J.-M., Huerre M., and Labigne A., 1998, Immune responses of specific-pathogen-free mice to chronic *Helicobacter pylori* (strain SS1) infection, *Infect. Immun.* **66**:1349.
141. Sawai N., Kita M., Kodama T., Tanahashi T., Yamaoka Y., Tagawa Y.-I., Iwakura Y., and Imanishi J., 1999, Role of gamma interferon in *Helicobacter pylori*-induced gastric inflammatory response in a mouse model, *Infect. Immun.* **67**:279.
142. Konturek P. C., Brzozowski T., Konturek S. J., Stachura J., Karczewska E., Pajdo R., Ghiara P., and Hahn E. G., 1999, Mouse model of *Helicobacter pylori* infection: studies of gastric function and ulcer healing, *Aliment. Pharmacol. Ther.* **13**:333.
143. Mohammadi M., Nedrud J., Redline R., Lycke N., and Czinn S. J., 1997, Murine CD4 T-cell response to *Helicobacter* infection: Th1 cells enhance gastritis and Th2 cells reduce bacterial load, *Gastroenterology*. **113**:1848.
144. Fox J. G., Beck P., Dangler C. A., Whary M. T., Wang T. C., Shi H. N., and Nagler-Anderson C., 2000, Concurrent enteric helminth infection modulates inflammation, gastric immune responses, and reduces *Helicobacter*-induced gastric atrophy, *Nature Med.* **6**:536.
145. Holcombe C., 1992, *Helicobacter pylori*: the African enigma, *Gut.* **33**:429.

146. Chen W., Shu D., and Chadwick V. S., 1999, *Helicobacter pylori* infection in interleukin-4 deficient and transgenic mice, *Scand. J. Gastroenterol.* **34**:987.
147. Berg D. J., Lynch N. A., Lynch R. G., and Lauricella D. M., 1998, Rapid development of severe hyperplastic gastritis with epithelial cell de-differentiation in *Helicobacter felis*-infected IL-10 (−/−) mice, *Am. J. Pathol.* **152**:1377.
148. Whary M. T., and Fox J. G., 2000, IL-10 deficiency reduces *Helicobacter pylori* colonization in C57Bl/6 mice, *Gut.* **47**(Suppl. 1):A36.
149. Chen M., Lee A., and Hazell S., 1992, Immunisation against gastric helicobacter infection in a mouse/*Helicobacter felis* model, *Lancet.* **339**:1120.
150. Lee A., and Chen M., 1994, Successful immunization against gastric infection with *Helicobacter* species: use of a cholera toxin B-subunit whole cell vaccine, *Infect. Immun.* **62**:3594.
151. Michetti P., Corthesy-Theulaz I., Davin C., Haas R., Vaney A.-C., Heitz M., Bille J., Kraehenbuhl J.-P., Saraga A., and Blum A. L., 1994, Immunization of BALB/c mice against *Helicobacter felis* infection with *Helicobacter pylori* urease, *Gastroenterology.* **107**:1002.
152. Ferrero R. L., Thiberge J.-M., Huerre M., and Labigne A., 1994, Recombinant antigens prepared from the urease subunits of *Helicobacter* spp.: evidence of protection in a mouse model of gastric infection, *Infect. Immun.* **62**:4981.
153. Pappo J., Thomas W. D., Kabok Jr. Z., Taylor N. S., Murphy J. C., and Fox J. G., 1995, Effect of oral immunization with recombinant urease on murine Helicobacter felis gastritis, *Infect. Immun.* **63**:1246.
154. Lee C. K., Weltzin R., Thomas W. D., Kleanthous Jr. H., Ermak T. H., Soman G., Hill J. E., Ackerman S. K., and Monath T. P., 1994, Oral immunization with recombinant *Helicobacter pylori* urease induces secretory IgA antibodies and protects mice from challenge with *Helicobacter felis*, *J. Inf. Dis.* **172**:161.
155. Guy B., Hessler C., Fourage S., Haensler J., Vialon-Lafay E., Rokbi B., and Millet M. J., 1998, Systemic immunization with urease protects mice against *Helicobacter pylori* infection, *Vaccine.* **16**:850.
156. Guy B., Hessler C., Fourage S., Rokbi B., and Millet M. J., 1999, Comparison between targeted and untargeted systemic immunizations with adjuvanted urease to cure *Helicobacter pylori* infection in mice, *Vaccine.* **17**:1130.
157. Sutton P., Wilson J., and Lee A., 2000, Further development of the *Helicobacter pylori* mouse vaccination model, *Vaccine.* **18**:2677.
158. Kong L., Smith J. G., Bramhill D., Abruzzo G. K., Bonfiglio C., Cioffe C., *et al.*, 1996, A sensitive and specific PCR method to detect *Helicobacter felis* in a conventional mouse model, *Clin. Diag. Lab. Immunol.* **3**:78.
159. Doidge C., Gust I., Lee A., Buck F., Hazell S., and Manne U., 1994, Therapeutic immunization against *Helicobacter* infection, *Lancet.* **343**:914.
160. Ghiara P., Rossi M., Marchetti M., DiTommaso A., Vindigni C., Ciampolini F., Covacci A., Telford J. L., DeMagistris M. T., Pizza M., Rappuoli R., and Del Giudice G., 1997, Therapeutic intragastric vaccination against *Helicobacter pylori* in mice eradicates an otherwise chronic infection and confers protection against reinfection, *Infect. Immun.* **65**:4996.
161. Crabtree J. E., 1998, Eradication of chronic *Helicobacter pylori* infection by therapeutic vaccination, *Gut.* **43**:7.
162. Ikewaki J., Nishizono A., Goto T., Fujioka T., and Mifune K., 2000, Therapeutic oral vaccination induces mucosal immune response sufficient to eliminate long-term *Helicobacter pylori* infection, *Microbiol. Immunol.* **44**:29.
163. Czinn S. J., Cai A., and Nedrud J. G., 1993, Protection of germ-free mice from infection by *Helicobacter felis* after oral or passive IgA immunization, *Vaccine.* **11**:637.
164. Marchetti M., Rossi M., Giarrelli V., Giuliani M. M., Pizza M., Censini S., Covacci A., Massiri P., *et al.*, 1998, Protection against *Helicobacter pylori* infection in mice by intragastric vaccination

with *Helicobacter pylori* antigens is achieved using a non-toxic mutant of *E. coli* heat-labile toxin LT as adjuvant, *Vaccine.* **16**:33.

165. Ferrero R. L., Thiberge J. M., and Labigne A., 1997, Local immunoglobulin G antibodies in the stomach may contribute to immunity against *Helicobacter* infection in mice, *Gastroenterology.* **113**:185.
166. Blanchard T. G., Czinn S. J., Redline R. W., Sigmund N., Harriman G., and Nedrud J. G., 1999, Antibody-independent protective mucosal immunity to gastric helicobacter infection in mice, *Cell. Immunol.* **191**:74.
167. Sutton P., Wilson J., Kosaka T., Wolowczuk I., and Lee A., 1998, Therapeutic immunization against *Helicobacter pylori* infection in the absence of antibodies, *Immunol. Cell. Biol.* **78**:28.
168. Dick-Hegedus E., and Lee A., 1991, Use of a mouse model to examine anti-*Helicobacter pylori* agents, *Scand. J. Gastroenterol.* **26**:909.
169. Hook-Nikanne J., Aho P., Karkkainen P., Kosunen T. U., and Salaspuro M., 1996, The *Helicobacter felis* mouse model in assessing anti-*Helicobacter* therapies and gastric mucosal prostaglandin E_2 levels, *Scand. J. Gastroenterol.* **31**:334.
170. Karita M., Li Q., and Okita K., 1993, Evaluation of new therapy for eradication of *H. pylori* infection in nude mouse model, *Am. J. Gastroenterol.* **88**:1366.
171. Smith J. G., Kong L., Abruzzo G. K., Gill C. J., Flattery A. M., Scott P. M., Silver L., Kropp H., and Bartizal K., 1997, Evaluation of experimental therapeutics in a new mouse model of *Helicobacter felis* utilizing 16S rRNA polymerase chain reaction for detection, *Scand. J. Gastroenterol.* **32**:297.
172. Aiba Y., Suzuki N., Kabir A. M., Takagi A., and Koga Y., 1998, Lactic acid-mediated suppression of *Helicobacter pylori* by the oral administration of *Lactobacillus salivarius* as a probiotic in a gnotobiotic murine model, *Am. J. Gastroenterol.* **93**:2097.
173. Kabir A. M. A., Aiba Y., Takagi A., Kamiya S., Miwa T., and Koga Y., 1997, Prevention of *Helicobacter pylori* infection by lactobacilli in a gnotobiotic murine model, *Gut.* **41**:49.
174. Wang T. C., Bonneir-Weir S., Oates P. S., Chulak M. B., Simon B., Merlino G. T., Schmidt E. V., and Brand S. J., 1993, Pancreatic gastrin stimulates isolet differentiation of TGF-alpha-induced ductular precursor cells, *J. Clin. Invest.* **92**:1349.
175. Wang T. C., Koh T. J., Varro A., Cahill R. J., Dangler C. A., Fox J. G., and Dockray G. J., 1996, Processing and proliferative effects of human progastrin in transgenic mice, *J. Clin. Invest.* **98**:1918.
176. Moss S. F., 1998, Cell markers in the gastric precancerous process, *Aliment. Pharmacol. Ther.* **12**(Suppl 1):91.
177. Wu M. S., Shun C. T., Lee W. C., Chen C. J., Wang H. P., Lee W. J., Sheu J. C., and Lin J. T., 1998, Overexpression of p53 in different subtypes of intestinal metaplasia and gastric cancer, *Br. J. Cancer.* **78**:971.
178. Golub T. R., Slonim D. K., Tamayo P., Huard C., Gaasenbeek M., Mesirov J. P., Coller H., Loh M. L., Downing J. R., Caligiuri M. A., Bloomfield C. D., and Lander E. S., 1999, Molecular classification of cancer: class discovery and class prediction by gene expression monitoring, *Science.* **286**:531.

14

Mongolian Gerbils Model

TAKASHI SHIMOYAMA,[1] TAKASHI SAKAGAMI,[1] NORIYASU YAMAMOTO,[1] YUKIO SAWADA,[1] YOSHIHIRO FUKUDA,[1] NORITOSHI TANIDA,[1] HIROKO SASHIO,[2] and KAZUO TAMURA[2]

1. INTRODUCTION

Since the isolation of *Helicobacter pylori* (*H. pylori*), much clinical and experimental effort has been spent on this bacterium to clarify the relationship with gastroduodenal disorder. The results, especially in the clinical field, have led to the recognition of *H. pylori* as a causal pathogen of gastroduodenal diseases, such as gastritis and peptic ulcer. Statements of management for peptic ulcer related to *H. pylori* infection were issued worldwide.[1,2] The International Agency for Research on Cancer (IARC), a working group of WHO, acknowledged *H. pylori* as a definite carcinogen of gastric cancer (Group 1 carcinogen) in 1994.[3] What needs to be emphasized at this juncture is that this decision was based on epidemiological data alone. Little was known about animal experimental data for gastric carcinogenesis related to *H. pylori*. The scarceness in animal data was explained by the lack of appropriate animal models of *H. pylori* infection. However, we have seen drastic

TAKASHI SHIMOYAMA, TAKASHI SAKAGAMI, NORIYASU YAMAMOTO, YUKIO SAWADA, YOSHIHIRO FUKUDA, and NORITOSHI TANIDA • Internal Medicine 4. HIROKO SASHIO and KAZUO TAMURA • Institute Advanced Medical sciences, Laboratory Hereditary Tumor, Hyogo College of Medicine, 1-1 Mukogawacho, Nishinomiya, Hyogo 663-8501, Japan.

Helicobacter pylori Infection and Immunity,
Edited by Yamamoto *et al.*, Kluwer Academic/Plenum Publishers, 2002.

changes. An appropriate animal model to investigate *H. pylori* infection was established in 1996 in Japan. Hirayama *et al.* established an animal model infected with *H. pylori* using Mongolian gerbils.[4] In this model, *H. pylori* infection persisted over a long term and caused gastric lesions. In addition, the processes of gastric mucosal changes resembled those of humans. In this chapter, we examine the serial changes in gastric lesions including gastric carcinogenesis in this model.

2. MONGOLIAN GERBILS

Mongolian gerbils (*Meriones unguiculatus*) were captured in Mongolia by Japanese in 1935. This gerbil was established as an experimental animal particularly for investigating the cerebral metabolism. We can use 2 strains of Mongolian gerbils in Japan, namely MGS/Sea, purchased by Seac Yoshitomi, and MON/J ms/G bs, purchased by SLC Japan.

There are significant differences in the gastric pathology, including the incidence of gastric cancer, between Mongolian gerbil and mouse models infected with *H. pylori.* Genetic factors are likely to be important in understanding this phenomenon. Unfortunately Mongolian gerbils have been poorly characterized as an experimental animal model compared with mice. Few reagents (for example, antibodies, immune marker, etc.) are available for detailed investigation. Further investigation in this area will contribute to clarifying the mechanism of gastric pathology, including carcinogenesis related to *H. pylori* infection.

3. GASTRITIS AND GASTRIC ULCER

To be appropriate for investigating *H. pylori* infection, an animal model should have a persistent *H. pylori* infection over a long term and a resemblance to human in the course of gastric mucosal changes. A lot of effort was spent trying to establish such a model using gnotobiotic piglet, barrier bone pig, gnotobiotic dog and mouse.[5–8] However these animal models were by no means satisfactory. In 1991 Yokota *et al.*, first reported an animal model infected with *H. pylori* (ATCC43504) using Mongolian gerbils.[9] They demonstrated a persistent *H. pylori* infection for 2 months and infiltration of inflammatory cells in the stomach due to *H. pylori* infection in this model. This was the first reported persistent infection by a standard *H. pylori* strain. In 1996, Hirayama *et al.* reported results from a longer observation period in Mongolian gerbils.[4] In addition, the progression of gastric mucosal changes resembled those of humans. Therefore, this model seems to be the best for investigating *H. pylori* infection at present.

We also investigated the pathology of gastro-duodenal mucosa infected with *H. pylori* in detail using this model.[10] Thus, 8-week-old male Mongolian gerbils (MGS/Sea, purchased by Seac Yoshitomi, Fukuoka, Japan) were orally inoculated with ATCC43504 (1.5×10^8 CFU), the standard *H. pylori* strain with *cagA* gene and vacuolating cytotoxin. Subsequently, animals were sacrificed every 2 weeks for 48 weeks to examine gastric mucosal pathological changes, status of infection of *H. pylori* and systemic serum antibody against *H. pylori*. Mild infiltration of neutrophils and lymphocytes were observed in the lamina propria in week 2 after inoculation. Acute gastritis and gastric erosion developed in week 4, and progressed to chronic active gastritis in week 8. Neutrophil infiltration decreased in week 10; the dominant infiltration cells were lymphocytes. Lymphocyte aggregations and follicles were observed with time. These findings were especially conspicuous in the deep portion of the mucosa and the submucosal layer. The border of pyloric gland area and fundic gland area were moved from the anal to oral side by aging, fundic specialized cells were decreased and replaced with pseudopyloric gland. These findings resemble the process of atrophy of gastric mucosa in humans. Incomplete intestinal metaplasia in week 20 and peptic ulcer in week 32 developed (Figure 1). The incidence of gastric ulcer was about 30%. The mucine of surface mucosal cells decreased by *H. pylori* infection, whereas the thickness of the surface mucosal gel layer increased in the inflamed pyloric mucosa. Ikeno *et al.* examined the consistency of the surface mucosal gel layer in detail in this model.[11] The surface mucosal gel layer consisted of two types of gastric mucine originating from the surface mucosal cells and from the gland mucosal cells. This finding resembles those of humans.[12] At 48 weeks, gastric mucosal nodular changes were observed. Microscopically this lesion showed hypertrophic mucosal changes. Slight-to-moderate neutrophil infiltration was persistently observed in the mucosa and submucosal layer throughout the experiment. Gastric cancer was not observed during the whole experimental period (48 weeks). However, gastric mucosal cell proliferation was accelerated. On the other hand, no significant change in the duodenal mucosa was observed throughout. Culture of *H. pylori* in resected glandular stomach specimens revealed a mean count of about 10^6 CFUs during the entire observation period. The serum *H. pylori* antibody titer was higher in the

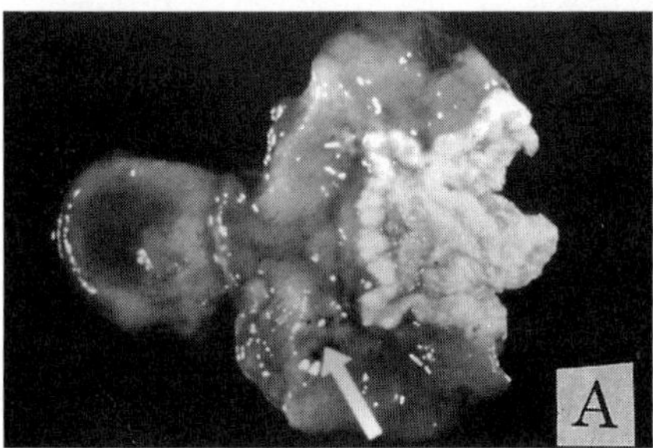

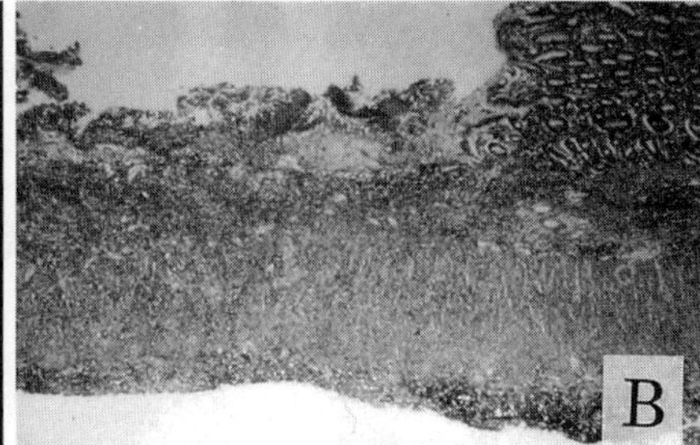

FIGURE 1. Gastric ulcer induced by infection with *H. pylori* (ATCC43504) in Mongolian gerbils (MGS/sea) at week 34 after inoculation A: Macroscopic findings: Gastric ulcer (arrow), B: Microscopic findings.

H. pylori-inoculated animals than in the normal control animals. The antibody titer gradually increased with the period after inoculation.

Peptic ulcer infection has not been developed in *H. pylori* infection models using other animals. Therefore, the Mongolian gerbil model is the first to show the development of peptic ulcer and intestinal metaplasia induced by infection with *H. pylori* in animals. In 1997, Lee *et al.*, isolated a new *H. pylori* strain named Sydney strain 1 (SS1) which can infect various strains of mice and induce gastric mucosal changes.[13]

This strain also colonizes Mongolian gerbils, producing persistent infection over a long term and gastric mucosal changes. The severity of gastric mucosal inflammation in C57BL/6 mice infected with *H. pylori* SS1 is less prominent than that in the Mongolian gerbils model. Such a difference in susceptibility of the mouse and Mongolian gerbils may serve to clarify the role of *H. pylori* in gastric diseases.

4. GASTRIC CANCER

In 1998, gastric carcinogenesis in an animal model due to *H. pylori* infection alone was first reported by Watanabe *et al.*, using 5-week-old male Mongolian gerbils (MGS/Sea).[14] *H. pylori* TN2GF4 ($10^{7.54}$ CFU), which was isolated from a patient with gastric ulcer, was used to orally inoculate gerbils. TN2GF4 had *cagA* gene and vacuolating cytotoxin. Subsequently, animals were sacrificed at 6, 26, 39, 52 and 62 weeks after inoculation to examine gastric mucosal pathological changes and status of *H. pylori* colonization. The result is shown in Table 1. Thirty seven percent of infected animals had adenocarcinoma at 62 weeks after inoculation. All cancers were located in the pyloric region with intestinal metaplasia. In addition, all cancers had well-differentiated intestinal type epithelium. Thus, the authors suggested that the development of these tumors, closely related to intestinal metaplasia, formed in the chronically inflamed mucosa.

In 1998, Honda *et al.*, also reported the development of gastric cancer in *H. pylori* infected Mongolian gerbils.[15] They used 5-week-old male Mongolian gerbils (MGS/Sea) and oral inoculation with ATCC43504 (10^9 CFU). They found that of the animals infected, 2 of 5 had well differentiated adenocarcinoma at the end of an 18-month experiment period. On the other hand, Hirayama *et al.*, reported the development of poorly differentiated adenocarcinoma due to *H. pylori* infection in this model.[16] They used same strain of Mongolian gerbils and *H. pylori* ATCC43504 and examined the pathological changes over a 24 month period. Only one animal (2%) had adenocarcinoma for the whole experimental period. In addition, this carcinoma was poorly differentiated adenocarcinoma arising from non intestinal metapastic gastric mucosa. Sugiyama *et al.* reported that no carcinoma was detected for 40 weeks in the same manner of experiment.[17]

TABLE 1
Sequential microbiological and histopathologic changes in the glandular stomach of Mongolian gerbils infected with *H. pylori* (TN2GF4)[14]

Duration after HP inoculation (wk)	6	26	39	52	62
No. of animals examined	5	5	5	5	27
Microbiology					
Bacterial count (log CFU/gastric wall)	5.17	5.33	5.89	4.59	5.40
Histopathology					
Active chronic gastritis	5[a] (100)	5 (100)	5 (100)	5 (100)	27 (100)
Ulcer	0 (0)	5 (100)	5 (100)	2 (40)	16 (59)
Regenerative hyperplasia	5 (100)	5 (100)	5 (100)	5 (100)	27 (100)
Invagination of glands	0 (0)	5 (100)	5 (100)	5 (100)	27 (100)
Hyperplastic polyp	0 (0)	0 (0)	0 (0)	3 (60)	4 (15)
Intestinal metaplasia	0 (0)	3 (60)	4 (80)	5 (100)	23 (85)
Adenocarcinoma	0 (0)	0 (0)	0 (0)	0 (0)	10 (37)
Carcinoid	0 (0)	0 (0)	0 (0)	0 (0)	3 (11)

[a]Incidence with percentage in parentheses Watanabe *et al.* Gastroenterology. 1998 Sep;115(3):642–8.

In Watanabe's experiment all animals had gastric ulcer at week 26 and intestinal metaplasia at week 52. Similarly, all animals had gastric ulcer and intestinal metaplasia at 18 months after infection in Honda's experiment. In contrast, only about 30%, 10% and 20% of the animals had gastric ulcer in ours, Hirayama's and Sugiyama's experiments, respectively. The differences in the rates of gastric ulcer and severity of gastric mucosal lesions between the former group and the latter group suggested that the severity and the period of gastric inflammation had an important role in gastric carcinogenesis. In addition, the difference of *H. pylori* strains might have contributed to this phenomenon.

Tatematsu *et al.*, had demonstrated N-methyl-N-nitrosourea (MNU) and N-methyl-N′-nitrosoguanidine (MNNG) could induce glandular stomach carcinoma in Mongolian gerbils.[18] In 1998, Sugiyama *et al.* reported *H. pylori* infection enhanced susceptibility of chemical gastric carcinogenesis in Mongolian gerbils applying Tatematsu's result.[17]

They used 7-week-old male Mongolian gerbils (MGS/Sea) and *H. pylori* ATCC43504. The first group of animals were inoculated with *H. pylori* and one week later they were administered N-methyl-N-nitrosourea (MNU) in drinking water at 10 ppm concentration for 20 weeks continuously to test the co-initiative effect of *H. pylori* infection for chemically gastric carcinogenesis. The second group of animals were first administrated 30 ppm MNU in drinking water for 6 weeks continuously, and then were inoculated with *H. pylori* at 1 week after finishing MNU treatment to test the promotive effect of *H. pylori* infection for chemically gastric carcinogenesis. Controls were administrated MNU in the same fashion without *H. pylori* infection. These animals were sacrificed at 40 weeks and gastric

TABLE 2
Incidence of adenocarcinoma in Mongolian gerbils given MNU and infected with *H. pylori* (ATCC43504)[17]

Group	Animal number	Cancer number	Histopathology		
			Well	Poor	Signet
promotive effect					
HP + MNU (10 ppm 20 w)	19	7 (36.8%)	1	1	5
MNU (10 ppm 20 w)	18	1	0	0	0

Modified from Sugiyama A *et al.* Cancer Res. 1998 May 15;58(10):2067–69.

pathological changes evaluated. The result is shown in Table 2. *H. pylori* infected animals had significantly higher incidence of gastric carcinogenesis, showing that *H. pylori* infection influenced the susceptibility of the chemical gastric carcinogenesis in Mongolian gerbils. A further important point was that not only well differentiated adenocarcinoma but also poorly differentiated adenocarcinoma and signet ring cell carcinoma were induced in this model. This finding supported the epidemiological data that both intestinal type cancer and diffuse type cancer had an almost equal association with *H. pylori* infection.

So far we have related gastric carcinogenesis to *H. pylori* infection in Mongolian gerbils. It is concluded that *H. pylori* infection induced gastric cancer, and the gastric chronic inflammation due to *H. pylori* infection (i.e., atrophic gastritis and intestinal metaplasia) had an important role in gastric carcinogenesis. The result also suggested that host factors and *H. pylori* strain difference may have some roles in development of gastric disease by *H. pylori*. As an example, the presence of other *Helicobacter* species may be studied in the Mongolian gerbils, because it has been reported that dysplasia and gastric carcinoma were caused by natural *Helicobacter* infection using a conventional Quankenbush Swiss strain (QS strain) mouse model by Lee *et al.* in 1998.[19]

They concluded that natural *Helicobacter* infection had a major role in gastric carcinogenesis in this model. Therefore we investigated the co-existence of other *Helicobacter* species status in two strains of Mongolian gerbils (MGS/Sea, purchased by Seac Yoshitomi, Fukuoka, Japan and MON/J ms/G bs purchased by SLC Japan) using the PCR technique.[20] Naturally occurring *H. hepaticus* was detected only in the gastro-intestinal tract of MGS/Sea (Figure 2), but not in MON/J ms/G bs. All previous reports relating gastric pathology and gastric carcinogenesis to *H. pylori* used MGS/Sea as an experimental animal. Thus, it seems important to study the influence of this bacterium on gastric carcinogenesis in this model.

Peek *et al.*, investigated the state of gastric mucosal apoptosis and cell proliferation in *H. pylori* infected Mongolian gerbils.[21] They describe that apoptosis

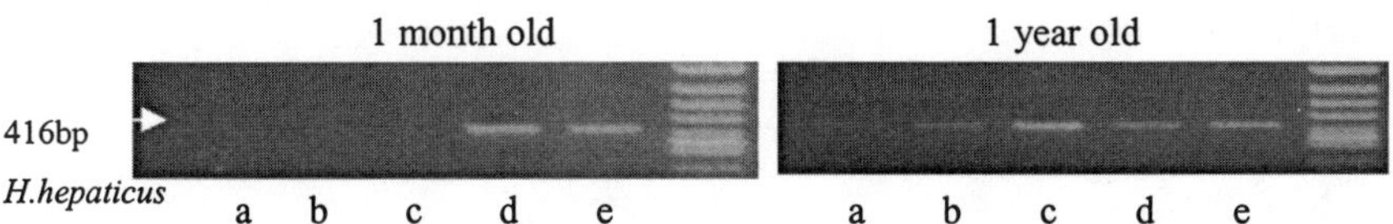

FIGURE 2. The status of *H. hepaticus* in Mongolian gerbils (MGS/sea) detected by PCR. a. stomach, b. jejunum, c. ileum, d. cecum, e. colon.

increases in an early phase after infection. In contrast to apoptosis, gastric epithelial cell proliferation peaks later and is related to gastrin levels, suggesting that epithelial cell growth with *H. pylori* may be mediated by a gastrin-dependent mechanism. Further studies are warranted using Mongolian gerbils to evaluate gastric mucosal changes, especially gastric carcinogenesis due to *H. pylori* infection.

5. SUMMARY

Animal models have an important role in clarifying the pathogenicity of *H. pylori*. A desirable animal model must have a resemblance to humans in the course of gastric mucosal changes due to *H. pylori* infection. Only the Mongolian gerbils model suffices for this condition, because acute gastritis and chronic active gastritis were induced followed by the development of gastric ulcer and then intestinal metaplasia and gastric carcinoma due to *H. pylori* infection alone. So this model has a considerable impact on the investigation of the exact mechanism in development of gastritis, gastric ulcer and gastric carcinoma. In addition, this model may be useful to establish new treatments of gastroduodenal disorder related to *H. pylori*. Indeed, the efficacy of some treatments for gastric disorder due to *H. pylori* infection have been documented using this model.[21,22] Therefore, this model seems to be the best for investigating *H. pylori* infection at present. However, there are several key questions that remain unanswered in this model. For example, the incidences of gastric cancer were different between TN2GF4 infected animals and ATCC43504 infected animals, which suggested that some bacterial factors have a role in gastric carcinogenesis. The role of naturally colonized *H. hepaticus* in their gastro-intestinal tract should be studied in relation to gastric carcinogenesis. The most important question to be addressed may be why this animal is especially susceptible to *H. pylori* infection. Also, detailed studies of both host and bacterial factors may disclose the exact role of *H. pylori* in gastritis, gastric ulcer and gastric carcinogenesis.

Mongolian gerbils have opened a way to investigate *H. pylori* in the field of pathogenicity and treatment in the future.

REFERENCES

1. European Helicobacter Pylori Study Group, 1997, Current European concepts in the management of *Helicobacter pylori* infection. The Maastricht Consensus Report. *Gut.*; **41**(1):8–13. Review.
2. NIH Consensus Conference. Helicobacter pylori in peptic ulcer disease. NIH Consensus Development Panel on *Helicobacter pylori* in Peptic Ulcer Disease. *JAMA.*; 6;**272**(1):65–69. Review (1994).
3. International Agency for Research on Cancer, World Health Organization, 1994, Schisosomes, liver flukus and *Helicobacter pylori*: IARC Monogr Eval Carcinog Risks Hum **61**:177–241.
4. Hirayama F., Takagi S., Yokoyama Y., Iwao E., and Ikeda Y., 1996, Establishment of gastric *Helicobacter pylori* infection in Mongolian gerbils. *J. Gastroenterol.*; 31 Suppl **9**:24–28.
5. Krakowka S., Morgan D. R., Kraft W. G., Leunk R. D., 1987, Establishment of gastric Campylobacter pylori infection in the neonatal gnotobiotic piglet. *Infect. Immun.*; **55**(11): 2789–2796.
6. Engstrand L., Gustavsson S., Jorgensen A., Schwan A., and Scheynius A., 1990, Inoculation of barrier-born pigs with Helicobacter pylori: a useful animal model for gastritis type B. *Infect. Immun.*; **58**(6):1763–1768.
7. Radin M. J., Eaton K. A., Krakowka S., Morgan D. R., Lee A., Otto G., and Fox J., 1990, *Helicobacter pylori* gastric infection in gnotobiotic beagle dogs. *Infect. Immun.*; **58**(8):2606–2612
8. Karita M., Li Q., Cantero D., and Okita K., 1994, Establishment of a small animal model for human *Helicobacter pylori* infection using germ-free mouse. *Am. J. Gastroenterol.*; **89**(2):208–213.
9. Yokota K., Kurebayashi Y., Takayama Y., Hayashi S., Isogai H., Isogai E., Imai K., Yabana T., Yachi A., and Oguma K., 1991, Colonization of *Helicobacter pylori* in the gastric mucosa of Mongolian gerbils. *Microbiol. Immunol.*; **35**(6):475–480.
10. Sawada Y., Kuroda Y., Sashio H., Yamamoto N., Tonokatsu Y., Sakagami T., Fukuda Y., Shimoyama T., Nishigami T., and Uematsu K., 1998, Pathological changes in glandular stomach of *Helicobacter pylori*-infected Mongolian gerbil model. *J. Gastroenterol.*; 33 Suppl **10**:22–25.
11. Ikeno T., Ota H., Sugiyama A., Ishida K., Katsuyama T., Genta R. M., and Kawasaki S., 1999, *Helicobacter pylori*-induced chronic active gastritis, intestinal metaplasia, and gastric ulcer in Mongolian gerbils. *Am. J. Pathol.*; **154**(3):951–960.
12. Ota H., and Katsuyama T., 1992, Alternating laminated array of two types of mucin in the human gastric surface mucous layer. *Histochem. J.*; **24**(2):86–92.
13. Lee A., O'Rourke J., De Ungria M. C., Robertson B., Daskalopoulos G., and Dixon M. F., 1997, A standardized mouse model of *Helicobacter pylori* infection: introducing the Sydney strain. *Gastroenterology.*; **112**(4):1386–1397.
14. Watanabe T., Tada M., Nagai H., Sasaki S., and Nakao M., 1998, *Helicobacter pylori* infection induces gastric cancer in mongolian gerbils. *Gastroenterology.*; **115**(3):642–648.
15. Honda S., Fujioka T., Tokieda M., Satoh R., Nishizono A., and Nasu M., 1998, Development of *Helicobacter pylori*-induced gastric carcinoma in Mongolian gerbils. *Cancer Res.*; **58**(19):4255–4259.
16. Hirayama F., Takagi S., Iwao E., Yokoyama Y., Haga K., and Hanada S., 1999, Development of poorly differentiated adenocarcinoma and carcinoid due to long-term *Helicobacter pylori* colonization in Mongolian gerbils. *J. Gastroenterol.*; **34**(4):450–454.
17. Sugiyama A., Maruta F., Ikeno T., Ishida K., Kawasaki S., Katsuyama T., Shimizu N., and Tatematsu M., 1998, *Helicobacter pylori* infection enhances N-methyl-N-nitrosourea-induced stomach carcinogenesis in the Mongolian gerbil. *Cancer Res.*; 15;**58**(10):2067–2069.
18. Tatematsu M., Yamamoto M., Shimizu N., Yoshikawa A., Fukami H., Kaminishi M., Oohara T., Sugiyama A., and Ikeno T., 1998, Induction of glandular stomach cancers in *Helicobacter pylori*-sensitive Mongolian gerbils treated with N-methyl-N-nitrosourea and N-methyl-N′-nitro-N-nitrosoguanidine in drinking water. *Jpn. J. Cancer Res.*; **89**(2):97–104.

19. Lee A., Correa P., Roa J., Leung V., O'Rourke J., and Dixon M. F., 1998, The first evidence of dysplasia and possibly gastric cancer caused by natural Helicobacter infection in an animal model. *Gut.* Suppl **2**:A66–A67 (abstract).
20. Sakagami T., 2000, Helicobacter hepaticus naturally colonizes in a strain of Mongolian gerbils (MGS/Sea). In preparation.
21. Peek R. M., Wirth H. P., Moss S. F., Yang M., Abdalla A. M., Tham K. T., Zhang T., Tang L. H., Modlin I. M., and Blaser M. J., 2000, Helicobacter pylori Alters Gastric Epithelial Cell Cycle Events and Gastrin Secretion in Mongolian Gerbils. *Gastroenterology.*; **118**(1):48–59.
22. Keto Y., Takahashi S., and Okabe S., 1999, Healing of *Helicobacter pylori*-induced gastric ulcers in Mongolian gerbils: combined treatment with omeprazole and clarithromycin. *Dig. Dis. Sci.*; **44**(2):257–265.
23. Suzuki H., Mori M., Kai A., Suzuki M., Suematsu M., Miura S., and Ishii H., 1998, Effect of rebamipide on *H. pylori*-associated gastric mucosal injury in Mongolian gerbils. *Dig. Dis. Sci.*; **43**(9 Suppl):181S–187S.

15

Vaccine Development

THOMAS G. BLANCHARD and STEVEN J. CZINN

1. NEED FOR A *H. pylori* VACCINE

It has been nearly two decades since Marshall and Warren discovered the relationship between *Helicobacter pylori* (*H. pylori*) and chronic active gastritis and peptic ulcer disease.[1,2] Following their initial reports, many studies ultimately confirmed the presence of *H. pylori* in association with antral gastric inflammation and peptic ulcer disease. It is now clear that a significant percentage of gastritis and peptic ulcer disease is in part due to this infectious disease. However, individuals with a documented peptic ulcer are the only agreed upon clinical entity for which eradication therapy for *H. pylori* infection is currently recommended.[3] During the past decade it has been estimated that peptic ulcer disease affects 4 million people annually. Fortunately, in a compliant patient, antimicrobial therapies in combination with proton pump inhibitors are now available that can provide a cure rate greater than 80%. But despite the significant progress that has been made during the last five years to develop simple inexpensive antimicrobial therapies, there continues to be a number of significant drawbacks to this approach.

To date, these pharmacologic therapies require a minimum of three agents to provide reproducible cure rates greater than 80%. Although the length of treatment has dramatically decreased from 4 weeks to 7 to 14 days, three agents

THOMAS G. BLANCHARD and STEVEN J. CZINN • Case Western Reserve University School of Medicine, Department of Pediatrics, Division of Pediatric Gastroenterology, Rainbow Babies & Children's Hospital, 11100 Euclid Avenue, Cleveland, OH 44106.

Helicobacter pylori Infection and Immunity,
Edited by Yamamoto *et al.*, Kluwer Academic/Plenum Publishers, 2002.

continue to be required. A typical, recommended eradication therapy for *H. pylori* incorporates 14 days of amoxicillin (1 gram bid), clarithromycin (500 mg bid), and a proton pump inhibitor such as omeprazole (20 mg bid). Alternatively equally good eradication rates can be achieved by replacing the clarithromycin with metronidazole (500 mg bid). Lengthy, complicated treatments such as these often lead to poor patient compliance and increase the risk of adverse side effects due to the pharmaceutical agents.

Barring problems with patient cooperation however, there are more far-reaching issues that warrant the development of a *H. pylori* vaccine. Antimicrobial resistance, particularly to clarithromycin and metronidazole, have recently become significant clinical problems diminishing our ability to eradicate this infection.[4] The emergence of such antibiotic resistant strains increases with poor patient compliance. Additionally, since *H. pylori* is so prevalent worldwide, aggressive programs using antibiotics to eradicate *H. pylori* infection in large numbers of individuals could also foster the development of antibiotic resistance in other bacterial pathogens, leading to further public health complications.

A further shortcoming of pharmacologic therapy to treat *H. pylori* infection is lack of immunity to subsequent infection with *H. pylori*. As described, natural and acquired immune responses to *H. pylori* infection fail to eradicate the organism from the gastric mucosa. Both humans and animal models of *H. pylori* infection confirm that patients are vulnerable to re-infection following successful eradication therapy.[5–7] This could be a problem for children and adults living in areas that are endemic for *H. pylori*.

If in fact chronic *H. pylori* infection resulted only in the development of peptic ulcer disease and could easily be eradicated using a one or two-week treatment regimen it may still be possible to argue effectively against the need for a vaccine. But in addition to peptic ulcer disease and gastritis, chronic long-lasting *H. pylori* infection, particularly when acquired in childhood can significantly increase the risk of developing gastric cancer.[8] Although the prevalence of *H. pylori* infection appears to be dropping in developed countries, in part related to improved socioeconomic status, the worldwide prevalence of *H. pylori* infection appears to be approximately 50%. At the time of initial infection the patient may develop abdominal pain and/or vomiting. However, symptoms such as dyspepsia or abdominal pain resolve rapidly and are not sufficiently sensitive to reliably predict the presence of *H. pylori*. Once infected, most individuals do not experience symptoms or manifest signs of disease, and in fact are unaware of the infection their entire life. Depending upon variations in the host response and bacterial virulence factors of the organism, this chronic inflammatory response leads to peptic ulcer disease or gastric cancer in a small subset of individuals. Studies supporting a role for *H. pylori* as a risk factor in the development of gastric cancer have been so compelling that in 1994 the World Health Organization classified *H. pylori* as a Class I human carcinogen.[9]

While the incidence of gastric cancer varies greatly from one geographic region to another, there are many regions of the world where gastric cancer continues to cause significant morbidity and mortality. The majority of these cancer patients have been infected for most of their lives with *H. pylori* without overt symptoms. Treatment for *H. pylori* by antibiotic therapy fails to identify these asymptomatic individuals who are at risk for developing gastric cancer later in life. Therefore, attention has once again focused on the development of a preventative or therapeutic vaccine. Vaccines have historically been used for disease prevention. Therefore, the ultimate scientific goal of a *H. pylori* vaccine would be to prevent this extremely common infection of mankind and ultimately not only prevent peptic ulcer disease but dramatically decrease the development of non-cardia gastric adenocarcinoma. As discussed below, it may also be possible to apply a vaccine to asymptomatic individuals chronically infected with *H. pylori* and prevent development of peptic ulcer disease gastric adenocarcinoma later in life.

Scientific studies have been reviewed which confirm the feasibility of developing a prophylactic and/or therapeutic vaccine to prevent or cure *H. pylori* infection. However, in this day and age a new vaccine must not only be efficacious, it must also be cost effective. One major factor hindering the development of a *H. pylori* vaccine is that epidemiologic studies continue to confirm that *H. pylori* infection is dramatically decreasing in the developed world. In addition, as the socio-economic conditions improve in developing countries the prevalence of *H. pylori* will also begin to decline. Although it does appear that *H. pylori* infection is slowly but surely disappearing, recent mathematical models presented by Rupnow *et al.*[10] calculate that the disappearance of *H. pylori* in the United States will take in excess of a century. In the United States, less than 1% of infected individuals are at risk for the development of gastric cancer. However, economic studies have been published by Fendrick *et al.*,[11] and Rupnow *et al.*,[10] suggesting that therapeutic interventions such as a vaccination or antimicrobial therapy which results in a 20–30% reduction of gastric cancer would in fact be cost effective in the United States. Therefore, if a safe, effective and inexpensive *H. pylori* vaccine were developed, it would not only be scientifically viable, but economically viable as well.

2. EARLY *H. pylori* VACCINE SUCCESS STORIES

Helicobacter vaccine research was bolstered in 1990 by the development of a murine model for Helicobacter infection. Previously, *H. pylori* infection of germ-free canine pups, barrier-born piglets, and nonhuman primates had been described (reviewed in).[12] In addition *H. mustelae* and *H. felis* had been isolated from ferrets and cats respectively.[12] However, no cost-effective, practical model had been described that would enable large-scale vaccine studies. In 1990 Lee *et al.* demonstrated that *H. felis* readily infects mice and induces gastric inflammation, thus opening the door for a wave of seminal studies on Helicobacter vaccines.[13] Most of those early reports employed an oral vaccination protocol developed by Czinn and Nedrud in which antigen was delivered in combination with the mucosal adjuvant cholera toxin (CT) to induce mucosal immune responses.[14] Two groups initially reported that protective immunity against *H. felis* could be induced in mice using whole cell extracts of *H. felis* as an antigen.[15,16] Protection was also demonstrated to be long-lived as mice immunized 15 months prior to challenge with *H. felis* were protected from challenge.[17]

Soon after these reports were published, other groups took vaccination a step further by using the same oral immunization strategy but with purified or recombinant Helicobacter proteins. The urease enzyme was found to be an effective vaccine candidate antigen conferring protection on 80% of immunized mice.[18,19] This was accomplished with both *H. felis* urease and *H. pylori* urease. *H. pylori* heat shock protein A (hspA) was also shown to be a protective antigen for *H. felis* by the oral route.[20] However, by combining urease with hspA, 100% of immunized mice were protected from challenge with *H. felis* suggesting that a vaccine for use in humans might require multiple subunits to optimize efficacy.

Perhaps one of the most surprising events in these early studies was the discovery that mice chronically infected with *H. felis* could be cured by administering the vaccine therapeutically.[21,22] The observation was made using both *H. felis* whole cell sonicate and the urease enzyme as antigens. A similar study was performed in the ferret against chronic *H. mustelae* infection demonstrating that therapeutic immunity also works against endogenous Helicobacter infections.[23] Collectively, these studies provoked much enthusiasm for the Helicobacter community since over half the world's population is already infected with *H. pylori.*

The murine model of Helicobacter infection also raised some serious concerns about the potential for immunization as a means of controlling Helicobacter infections. Challenge of immunized mice with *H. felis* resulted in histologic gastritis equivalent to, and sometimes in excess of that observed from chronic infection.[18,24] This inflammation has been termed "post-immunization gastritis". Therefore, while bacteria were often absent, the tissue still resembled the disease state that vaccination was intended to ameliorate. This has been a universal finding for prophylactic immunization studies and raises several issues. First, it is not clear that in this context all inflammation is harmful. Second, while there have been some reports that suggest the intensity of post-immune gastritis declines over time, it is not known how long it takes the post immunization gastritis to completely resolve or indeed if it ever does. It is possible that like the intestine, the gastric mucosa lacks lymphoid tissue until stimulated by bacterial flora, in this case Helicobacter organisms. Post-immune gastritis may represent a permanent form of diffuse mucosal-associated lymphoid tissue designed to provide for future immune surveillance, regulation, and protection. Finally, the presence of the post-immune gastritis, even in the absence of any detectable organisms may indicate that protection is not complete. Two independent studies have shown that treatment of mice with post-immunization gastritis with antibiotic therapy results in a significant decrease in inflammation.[25,26] These findings indicate that there may be Helicobacter organisms that escape immunity and continue to drive the inflammatory response.

3. TRANSLATION TO *H. pylori* MODELS AND HUMANS

Early successes with oral immunization observed in the *H. felis* mouse model translated very well to newly developed mouse models of *H. pylori* infection. Within a short time of the initial description of the murine *H. pylori* model effective immunization routes were expanded from oral to include intranasal, rectal, and parental (see below). Additionally, other virulence factors were found to be effective vaccine antigens such as catalase, cytotoxin, and the cytotoxin associated gene protein CagA.[27,28] Similar to the *H. felis* model, protection from *H. pylori* infection could be achieved by either prophylactic or therapeutic immunization,[29] and was also accompanied by post-immunization gastritis. However, whereas many of the *H. felis* immunizations often resulted in the lack of any detectable organisms by urease detection, culture, or histology, few if any *H. pylori* mouse immunizations have achieved complete protection. In the *H. pylori* model protection is frequently reported as a significant reduction in bacterial load. This lends credence to the theory that post-immunization gastritis in the *H. felis* model is due to residual bacteria.

Success in mice has not translated well to larger animal models. Initial reports of natural *H. pylori* infection in a domestic cat colony garnered much enthusiasm among the Helicobacter community.[30,31] Subsequent reports of the successful adaptation of specific *H. pylori* isolates to the cat suggested the possibility of performing significant vaccine studies.[32] However, early attempts at prophylactic immunization of cats were disappointing and there has been no further reports indicating any real success in this model. As mentioned above, the canine model of *H. pylori* infection was one of the earliest models. Recently there has been a renewed effort to develop this model further but actual immunizations have not been reported.[33]

H. pylori infection of barrier born piglets has proven to be a valuable albeit somewhat cumbersome model for the investigation of *H. pylori* associated pathogenesis and virulence factors. It was also one of the first animal models in which prophylactic immunization was attempted. Unfortunately, no protective immunity was obtained by either the oral or parental route of immunization.[34] Despite these early results, Eaton *et al.* have recently reported renewed efforts at *H. pylori* immunization and were able to demonstrate complete protection in a subset of animals following parental immunization.[35] These results are encouraging but will require continued and expanded experimentation. The results of nonhuman primate immunization against *H. pylori* have been mixed but encouraging. Thus while some efforts have failed to obtain any degree of protection in Rhesus monkeys, others have reported protection in as many as 31% of immunized animals and in another study an overall significant reduction in bacterial load. Caution must be used in interpreting immunization studies performed in non-human primates because the overwhelming majority of non-human primates in captivity are infected with gastric Helicobacters at a very young age. In order to perform an *H. pylori* prophylactic immunization study, these animals are first treated with "triple antimicrobial therapy" to eradicate the gastric Helicobacter infection. Therefore, strictly speaking these studies generally do not employ naive animals, rather they utilize non-human primates recently cured of Helicobacter infection. Until a Helicobacter-free colony of non-human primates is available this model has limited utility for predicting the success or failure of a human *H. pylori* vaccine.

The successful use of therapeutic immunization in mice and ferrets described above were significant in that greater than half of the world's population is chronically infected with *H. pylori* and therapeutic vaccination would provide a more cost effective means than antimicrobial therapy for *H. pylori* eradication. Therapeutic immunization has already been attempted in human volunteers infected with *H. pylori*.[36] The vaccine consisted of recombinant *H. pylori* urease in combination with the mucosal adjuvant *E. coli* heat labile toxin (LT). The results were encouraging but resembled those of the *H. pylori* animal models but not the *H. felis* model in that subjects receiving the test vaccine had significant reductions in gastric *H. pylori* density relative to those receiving placebo controls but did not clear the infection. Additionally, urease specific IgA-producing cells from the circulation were significantly elevated in patients receiving the vaccine compared to controls. Although a significant number of patients experienced diarrhea due to the LT, and complete bacterial eradication was not observed in any subjects, this study was an encouraging first step suggesting that improved vaccine formulations and safer adjuvants may achieve satisfactory outcomes. Other human studies are currently in progress. Recombinant, attenuated strains of *Salmonella typhi* (*S. typhi*),[37] and *S. enterica*[38] expressing the *H. pylori* urease subunits are well tolerated by human volunteers and a single oral dose of the live bacteria induced seroconversion to *H. pylori* in half of the subjects. A whole cell *H. pylori* vaccine has also been clinically tested in humans. It is well tolerated and induces both serum and mucosal immune responses. The efficacy of both the Salmonella and whole cell vaccines formulations have yet to be tested.

4. MECHANISMS OF PROTECTION

Many laboratories have now demonstrated that, at least in rodents, prophylactic and therapeutic immunity against *H. pylori* is readily achieved by vaccination. The immune mechanisms that contribute to protective immunity however have remained elusive. In fact, antibody profiles and inflammatory infiltrates of the gastric mucosa are remarkably similar between chronically infected mice and mice that have been protectively immunized against subsequent challenge. Since *H. pylori* reside primarily in the mucus lining the gastric epithelium and do not invade the tissue, few described immune mechanisms would actually have access to the bacteria. Thus, a reasonable assumption was that secreted antibody must be an important aspect of protective immunity. Recent studies by our laboratory and others employing mice genetically deficient in their ability to generate antibodies have now demonstrated that protective immunity can be achieved in the complete absence of any antibodies.[39,40] Thus, while antibodies may contribute to protective immunity, in mice these antibodies are not necessary for protection.

While the mechanism(s) by which protection is accomplished remains unknown, and in part as a result of the studies demonstrating protection in the absence of antibody, several laboratories have demonstrated the important role of T cells both for Helicobacter-associated disease and for protection. Immunodeficient mice such as SCID and *rag*$^{-/-}$ mice, and mice deficient in T cells, infected with *H. felis* fail to develop appreciable amounts of inflammation[41,42] while fully immunocompetent mice or mice lacking B cells develop gastritis within several weeks of infection.[39,42] However, reconstitution of these mice with T cells from immunocompetent donor mice prior to challenge results in the rapid onset of Helicobacter-associated gastritis (author's unpublished observations). Similar studies have been performed in *H. pylori* infected mice. Therefore, recruitment of T cells to the stomach seems to be required even for the induction of the acute phase inflammation. Examination of peripheral blood mononuclear cells and gastric lymphocytes from *H. pylori* infected patients have consistently shown that IFN- is the predominant cytokine produced by these cells in the virtual absence of non-inflammatory cytokines such as IL-4 and IL-5.[43–49] Interleukin-12 in gastric biopsies has also been detected. Although IL-12 is produced primarily by macrophages, it can regulate the generation of specific cellular immune responses. These results suggest that *H. pylori* infection induces a Th1 mediated proinflammatory response.

It has been much more difficult to define the role of specific cells and cytokines in the protective immune response. Two independent groups have demonstrated mice deficient in $CD4^+$ helper T cells (MHC class II deficient) are not protected from Helicobacter challenge following immunization, while mice deficient in $CD8^+$ T cells (MHC class I deficient) could be protected to the same degree as fully immunocompetent animals.[40,50] Consistent with these observations, we have shown that adoptive transfer of $CD4^+$ T cells from *H. felis*-immunized mice to immunodeficient *rag*$^{-/-}$ mice is sufficient to transfer protective immunity.[51] $CD4^+$ T cells from mice immunized with an irrelevant antigen such as ovalbumin failed to transfer protective immunity.

The effector mechanism of these protective T cells remains unknown. Previous studies suggested that protection might be the result of Th2 immune responses induced by immunization. This theory was initiated by Mohamaddi *et al.* who transferred spleen cells from immunized/protected mice (containing IL-4 producing lymphocytes) or a Helicobacter-specific Th2 cell line into naive C57BL/6 recipients prior to challenge with *H. felis*. The mice benefited by a striking drop in bacterial load relative to control mice.[52] No such reduction in bacterial load was observed in mice that received cells from chronically infected mice or a *H. felis* specific Th1 cell line. Additionally gene targeted IL-4 knockout mice (with compromised Th2 immunity) exhibit higher bacterial loads than wild type control mice following challenge with *H. felis* and are not well protected from *H. felis* infection following immunization.[52,53] However, there is now evidence to suggest that the dichotomy between Th1 and Th2 immunity is not sufficient to explain how immunization confers protection in mice. The recent report described above in which immune responses have been polarized towards Th1 and Th2 immunity following immunization reveal that Th1 responding mice are protected with the same efficacy as Th2 responding mice in both the *H. felis* and *H. pylori* mouse models.[51,54]

As described above, $CD4^+$ T cells from mice immunized with *H. felis* whole cell lysate were sufficient to transfer protective immunity to otherwise immunodeficient $rag^{-/-}$ mice.[51] Since $CD4^+$ T cells do not possess direct bactericidal activity, and since $rag^{-/-}$ mice lack lymphocytes, The transferred T cells must mediate help by regulating some form of innate immune effector mechanism(s). Such mechanisms may be provided by macrophages, polymorphonuclear leukocytes, or even epithelial cells and could be the accomplished by either secreted products or cell to cell contact. While these mechanisms have yet to be described, it appears likely that they are not induced, or at least not induced sufficiently in the inflammatory response to chronic Helicobacter infection. T cells activated by antigen at the gastric mucosa during chronic infection may be activated in such a way as to result in a nonprotective phenotype. Antigen presentation may occur by leakage of antigen across the epithelial border and uptake by macrophages, by direct uptake by epithelial cells or by dendritic cells that might span the tight junctions. Regardless, primary activation of the T cell under these circumstances does not induce the T cell help signals required for protective immunity. Alternatively, T cells receiving proper primary activation distal from the stomach must be fundamentally different from those activated in the stomach. These cells subsequently respond to infection based on inflammatory signals and upon arrival in the stomach, further exposure to antigen results in help that is sufficient to activate the mechanisms required for protection. As more research on innate defense mechanisms such as Defensins, nitric oxide synthase, and other mechanisms is performed, this picture should become clearer.

5. OPTIMIZING SUBUNIT VACCINES

Early animal vaccine studies in mice and piglets used killed Helicobacter organisms or whole cell sonicates as immunogens. However, a human use vaccine will most likely require the use of purified proteins in order to insure safety, consistency, and proper characterization. As described above, many early studies have been performed using the *H. pylori* urease enzyme complex, a highly conserved, surface exposed antigen that represents up to 6% of the total cell mass.[55] Its functions to convert urea to ammonia and carbon dioxide to help survive in the gastric mucosa. Michetti *et al.* made the first demonstration that purified *H. pylori* urease could be used to provide prophylactic immunity to *H. felis* infection in mice.[18] Lee *et al.* have performed a series of immunizations in which it was demonstrated that as little as 5 μg doses of recombinant *H. pylori* urease can be used to induce protective immunity in mice.[56] Urease now represents the most commonly used antigen for Helicobacter vaccine research in both animals and clinical trials.[36–38]

Several other *H. pylori* proteins have now been demonstrated to provide protective immunity to mice against *H. pylori* challenge. Early studies in the mouse model indicate that several different proteins may be required in order to induce complete protection. Ferrero *et al* performed oral immunizations with a combination of recombinant *H. pylori* hspA and urease in mice to demonstrate that the combination of antigens was more efficacious than either antigen alone.[20] By combining the two antigens, 100% protection from challenge with *H. felis* could be achieved where as either component individually induced only 80% protection. The initial clinical trial in humans using recombinant urease and LT for therapeutic immunization which reduced the bacterial load but did not completely eradicate the *H. pylori* may be improved by adding a second or third antigen component. Other antigens that have been tested in the mouse model include catalase, cytotoxin, and CagA.[27,29]

6. DEVELOPING AN EFFECTIVE MUCOSAL ADJUVANT OR DELIVERY SYSTEM

It has long been appreciated that immunity at mucosal surfaces such as the intestines is best achieved by local stimulation. Therefore, oral immunization is traditionally used to induce protective immunity against enteric pathogens. Initial studies in the piglet model of *H. pylori* infection seemed to establish that similarly, immunity at the gastric mucosa could not be achieved through systemic immunization.[34] Thus early attempts at inducing protective immunity against *H. pylori* in the mouse focused primarily on oral immunization. However, proteins are weak immunogens by the oral route and generally must be administered in large doses.

Exceptions to this rule included proteins or organisms with specificity for the intestinal mucosa such as Streptococcal M protein, Reovirus, and some lectins. Therefore, *H. pylori* vaccine research, similar to other enteric pathogen vaccine research, is very much concerned with the development of "mucosal adjuvants." To date, CT has proven to be the most effective mucosal adjuvant for use in animal studies using rodents, ferrets and non-human primates and it has greatly facilitated vaccine research for *H. pylori*. Unfortunately, even the low doses of CT and LT used for immunization of mice are toxic when administered to humans.

Several laboratories have developed technologies designed to avoid the toxic effects of CT and LT. The most straightforward method is to directly conjugate a candidate protein antigen to the nontoxic B subunit of CT or LT that retains its GM1 ganglioside binding property and therefore continue to target the intestinal epithelium. The use of CTB and LTB as "carriers" has been exploited in numerous animal model systems.[57] Alternatively, some investigators have simply combined the candidate protein with biochemically purified B subunit in place of CT holotoxin for immunization. Interpretation of these studies is complicated since commercially purified CTB is typically contaminated with small amounts of holotoxin that may synergize with CTB. Two studies using the *H. felis* rodent model have indicated that whereas commercially prepared CTB could enhance protection versus Helicobacter infection, holotoxin free recombinant CTB does not possess adjuvant activity.[58,59] This is consistent with a recent study in which recombinant LTB was ineffective as an adjuvant by the oral route.[60]

Investigators have also developed genetic constructs encoding for CT or LT with decreased or absent toxicity in the A subunit, but normal cell binding activity in the B subunit. Many such mutant CT and LT molecules have been described by a number of laboratories around the world. Testing for the adjuvanticity of all these mutant molecules has not been completed and most often the test antigens are model proteins with no infectious challenge model. However, while some of these mutants might lose adjuvant activity completely when given via the oral route, some retain adjuvanticity for intranasal immunization. Such adjuvants may hold significant promise since intranasal immunization has been employed successfully as an effective means of Helicobacter immunization in mice.[61–63] At least one successful LT mutant construct devoid of toxicity has been described recently where the A subunit is resistant to the cleavage that is required for toxicity. Yet it has been used to protect mice against *H. pylori* by both prophylactic and therapeutic immunization.[28,29]

In addition to the bacterial toxins described above several other alternative mucosal adjuvants and delivery systems are now being investigated. Muramyl dipeptide, a potent adjuvant for systemic immunization has been tested as an adjuvant for oral immunization of ferrets against *H. mustelae*. No protection was achieved and the ferrets actually suffered from increased gastritis upon challenge.[64] However, it is important to remember that adjuvants that fail to elicit immunity by oral immunization could possibly be successful when administered by alternative routes (see below). More recently, poly (D,L-lactide-co-glycolide) microparticles containing *H. pylori* whole cell lysate have been used to orally immunize mice.[65] While these mice were not challenged, immunization did induce a significant mucosal and serum antibody response suggesting potent adjuvanticity.

7. ALTERNATIVE STRATEGIES TO MUCOSAL ADJUVANTS

Unlike bacterial toxin adjuvants, attenuated recombinant bacterial strains such as *S. typhi*, BCG, and *V. cholerae* have already been demonstrated to be effective, safe delivery vehicles for the induction of local and systemic immunity by the oral route in humans. In fact these strains have actually been in use as successful vaccines against infectious diseases for decades. Their use has several distinct advantages. Infection with these attenuated strains of bacteria leads to prolonged presence in the body compared to toxin adjuvants and this would lead to enhanced immunogenicity and increased vaccine efficacy. Additionally, several recombinant proteins from the same or several different heterologous pathogens can be expressed in a single bacterial vector to create multivalent vaccines with stronger efficacy, or to immunize against multiple pathogens with one recombinant organism. Also, these vectors can be administered by the oral route, circumventing the number of intramuscular injections required to immunize children, and providing a means of inducing mucosal immunity against enteric and urogenital pathogens.

Several studies have already been published examining the potential use of attenuated, recombinant *S. typhimurium* strains for vaccination of mice against *H. Pylori*.[63,66] and *S typhi* and *S. enterica* for use in humans.[37,38] In the *S. typhimurium* 3261 strain (*aroA* mutation), plasmid encoded *H. pylori* urease subunits were constitutively expressed.[66] The plasmid was maintained both *in vitro* or *in vivo*. Mice were inoculated with a single oral dose of the recombinant *S. typhimurium* 3261. Immunized mice developed serum and intestinal antibody responses and were protected from challenge with *H. pylori* as determined by failure of gastric antral biopsies to generate any urease activity *in vitro*. Sham immunized mice generated a significant degree of urease activity due to the presence of *H. pylori* following challenge. The success of this immunization with only one dose of bacteria contrasts significantly to the four or more doses of antigen typically required to induce protective immunity in mice when using bacterial toxin adjuvants to achieve similar levels of protection.

The authors also used a streptomycin-resistant strain of mouse-adapted *H. pylori* to challenge a separate group of immunized mice to facilitate the recovery of *H. pylori* from gastric biopsies. The bacterial load correlated well with the presence or absence of urease activity. Although *H. pylori* could be cultured from some mice immunized with urease-expressing *S. typhimurium*, the overall bacterial load for this group was only 63 colony forming unit (CFU.)/gastric biopsy compared to almost 3000 CFU. in sham immunized mice. Thus, mice could be protected, or the amount of *H. pylori* significantly decreased by immunization with recombinant attenuated *S. typhimurium*. Again, these mice were protected with only one dose of recombinant bacteria. If such an observation were consistently obtained, the problem of host immunity to the delivery vehicle, which might preclude subsequent use for booster immunizations, could be avoided.

Another group used the attenuated *S. typhimurium phoP^c* strain for expression of the *H. pylori* urease subunits.[63] The urease genes were carried on one of two plasmid systems. One system was designed for high levels of constitutive protein expression, while the other system was designed for phase variation of protein expression where only a subset of the *S. typhimurium* would be expressing the urease subunits at any given time. Both strains of recombinant *S. typhimurium phoP^c* were used to immunize BALB/c mice by two intranasal inoculations given at two-week intervals. Although the system designed for constitutive expression of urease failed to elicit protective immunity, this was probably due to loss of the plasmid. However, mice immunized with *S. typhimurium phoP^c* expressing urease under phase variation control responded with urease-specific serum antibody and $CD4^+$ T cell responses as measured by proliferation and cytokine production. This strain maintained the plasmid and almost two thirds of these mice were protected from challenge with *H. pylori*. Both the gastric biopsy urease test and direct enumeration of bacteria on histologic sections confirmed either the complete, or near absence of bacteria.

The use of Salmonella vectors for *H. pylori* vaccination is a recent development that needs further exploration in the murine model. It remains to be seen whether these bacterial vectors are as effective as CT or LT in stimulation long term immunity. This is a practical consideration since both adults and children are susceptible to infection. Additionally, the potential for use in therapeutically immunizing infected mice is of equal if not greater importance than prophylactic immunity given the high prevalence of people currently infected in developing nations. And, since a low inflammation strain of mice, Balb/c, was used, gastric disease could not be studied adequately in these experiments. Thus an evaluation as to the degree of post-immunization gastritis present following challenge needs to be performed. Proper characterization of this vaccine model will require histologic analysis although a separate group has now begun testing a Salmonella strain for use in humans (see above[37,38]).

8. MINING ALTERNATIVE ROUTES OF VACCINE DELIVERY

The first published study investigating the efficacy of immunization against *H. pylori* infection was performed in the piglet model.[34] In that study, no protective immunity was achieved through immunization by either the oral or parental route. The failure of the oral immunization protocol might be explained by the lack of use a mucosal adjuvant. Failure by parental immunization is consistent with what immunologists have believed about mucosal pathogens for decades, that protection of mucosal surfaces requires local (mucosal) induction of immunity. However, recent experiments suggest that other routes of immunization, including systemic, may prove to be more practical and effective at protecting the stomach from *H. pylori* infection than oral immunizaton. A recent comparative study of routes for mucosal delivery of a *H. pylori* urease vaccine in mice demonstrated that optimum immunity was elicited by rectal and intranasal delivery of the vaccine.[67] Currently, several laboratories including the laboratories of each of the authors have successfully employed intranasal immunization to protect and/or cure mice from *H. pylori* infection.[63,67] Although these immunizations still require the use of a mucosal adjuvant, toxicity is typically not at issue by this route. And as described above, an attenuated *S. typhimurium* recombinant vaccine expressing *H. pylori* urease A and B subunits has also been applied by intranasal inoculation with good efficacy. These uniform results are encouraging and suggest a means of vaccinating humans against *H. pylori* without the problems of traversing the harsh gastric environment or inducing diarrhea.

Delivery of a vaccine by an alternative route could have other benefits as well. It has now been amply demonstrated in both the *H. felis* and *H. pylori* mouse models, that challenge of immunized animals with infectious Helicobacter results in post-immunization gastritis, even when protection is demonstrated. The inflammation can be ameliorated by subsequent administration of antibiotic treatment, suggesting incomplete protection by immunization.[25,26] Additionally, most mouse immunizations for *H. pylori*, and the human clinical trial described above, have failed to completely protect against challenge. And in the human study two thirds of the subjects tested developed diarrhea due to the LT adjuvant.[36] And it bears remembering that prophylactic immunization has only been reasonably successful in the murine Helicobacter models but not for the larger models of Helicobacter infection. Finally, several nontoxic bacterial endotoxin adjuvants retain adjuvanticity by other routes but not necessarily the stomach, and smaller doses of both antigen and adjuvant could be administered by alternative routes.

Helicobacter vaccine research has challenged our fundamental understanding of how the immune system operates in mucosal tissues. In one of the first reports of successful immunization against *H. felis* in the mouse model, the efficacy of both parenteral and oral immunization were compared.[16] Despite the induction of systemic antibody by intravenous immunization, no protection was achieved by this route. However, intraperitoneal immunization resulted in protection of 55% of the challenged mice. Unfortunately, a combination of the success of their oral immunization, combined with a similar report by Czinn *et al.*, demonstrating success by the oral route,[15] and the earlier observation that systemic immunization was nonprotective in the *H. pylori*/pig model[34] caused most laboratories to focus almost exclusively on oral immunization.

The approach to *H. pylori* immunization has broadened significantly following initial reports that systemic immunization can induce protective immunity in mice.[68] Guy *et al.* have demonstrated that subcutaneous immunization of mice significantly reduces *H. pylori* numbers following challenge. This study has been followed by a more detailed analysis documenting that the tissue used for immunization can be critical in predicting the efficacy of the vaccination.[69] Although novel adjuvants were employed in that study our own experiments have indicated that intraperitoneal or subcutaneous injection of antigen with aluminim hydroxide, complete Freund's adjuvant (CFA), and incomplete Freund's adjuvant (IFA) are capable of inducing protective immunity against *H. felis* and *H. pylori* infection in mice.[51] Additionally, we have shown that both intraperitoneal and subcutaneous injection of *H. pylori* antigens with adjuvants such as aluminum hydroxide, CFA or IFA can induce protective immunity when administered to neonatal mice.[54] The use of systemic immunization has only just begun to be explored and will require extensive further investigation to determine its effectiveness in therapeutic immunization, length of protective immunity induced, effect on post immunization gastritis, and application to larger animals and humans.

REFERENCES

1. Warren, J. R., and Marshall, B. J., 1983, Unidentified curved bacilli on gastric epithelium in active chronic gastritis. *Lancet.* **i**:1273–1275.
2. Marshall, B. J., and Warren, J. R., 1984, Unidentified curved bacilli in the stomach of patients with gastritis and peptic ulceration. *Lancet.* **1**:1311–1315.
3. N.I.H., 1994, Consensus Conference, *Helicobacter pylori* in peptic ulcer disease. *J. Am. Med. Assoc.* **272**:65–69.
4. Graham, D. Y., 2000, Therapy of *Helicobacter pylori*: Current status and issues. *Gastroenterol* **118**:S2–S8.
5. Langenberg, W., Rauws, E. A. J., Oudbier, J. H., and Tytgat, G. N. J., 1990, Patient-to-patient transmission of *Campylobacter pylori* infection by fiberoptic gastroduodenoscopy and biopsy. *J. Infect. Dis* **161**:507–511.
6. Batchelder, M., *et al.*, 1996, Natural and experimental *Helicobacter mustelae* reinfection following successful antimicrobial eradication in ferrets. *Helicobacter* **1**:34–42.
7. Czinn, S. J., Bierman, J. C., Diters, R. W., Blanchard, T. J., and Leunk, R. D., 1996, Characterization and therapy for experimental infection by *Helicobacter mustelae* in ferrets. *Helicobacter* **1**:43–51.
8. Forman, D., Webb, P., and Parsonnet, J., 1994, *H. pylori* and gastric cancer. *Lancet.* **343**:243–244.
9. World Health Organization. in *Schistosomes, Liver Flukes and Helicobacter pylori* 177–241 (International Agency for Research on Cancer, Lyon, 1994).
10. Rupnow, M. F. T., Owens, D. K., Shachter, R., and Parsonnet, J., 1999, *Helicobacter pylori* vaccine development and use: A cost-effectiveness analysis using the Institute of Medicine methodology. *Helicobacter* **4**:272–280.

11. Fendrick, A. M., *et al.*, 1999, Clinical and economic effects of population-based *Helicobacter pylori* screening to prevent gastric cancer. *Arch. Int. Med.* **159**:142–148.
12. Nedrud, J., 1999, Animal Models for Gastric Helicobacter Immunology and Vaccine Studies. *FEMS Immunology and Medical Microbiology.*
13. Lee, A., Fox, J. G., Otto, G., and Murphy, J., 1990, A small animal model of human *Helicobacter pylori* active chronic gastritis. *Gastroenterol* **99**:1315–1323.
14. Czinn, S. J., and Nedrud, J. G., 1991, Oral immunization against *Helicobacter pylori. Infection Immun.* **59**:2359–2363.
15. Czinn, S. J., Cai, A., and Nedrud, J. G., 1993, Protection of germ-free mice from infection by *Helicobacter felis* after active oral or passive IgA immunization. *Vaccine* **11**:637–642.
16. Chen, M., Lee, A., Hazell, S., Hu, P., and Li, Y., 1993, Immunisation against gastric infection with *Helicobacter* species: first step in the prophylaxis of gastric cancer? *Zentralblatt für Bakteriolgie* **280**:155–165.
17. Radcliff, F. J., Chen, M., and Lee, A., 1996, Protective immunization against Helicobacter stimulates long-term immunity. *Vaccine* **14**:780–784.
18. Michetti, P., *et al.*, 1994, Immunization of Balb/c mice against *Helicobacter felis* infection with *Helicobacter pylori* urease. *Gastroenterol* **107**:1002–1011.
19. Ferrero, R. L., Thiberge, J.-M., Huerre, M., and Labigne, A., 1994, Recombinant antigens prepared from the urease subunits of *Helicobacter* spp.: Evidence of protection in a mouse model of gastric infection. *Infect. Immun.* **62**:4981–4989.
20. Ferrero, R. L., *et al.*, 1995, The *groES* homolog of *Helicobacter pylori* confers protective immunity against mucosal infection in mice. *Proc. Natl. Acad. of Sci., U. S. A.* **92**:6499–6503.
21. Corthesy-Theulaz, I. *et al.*, 1994, *H. pylori* urease B subunit as a therapeutic vaccine against *H., felis* infection (Abstract). *Gastroenterol* **106**:A668.
22. Doidge, C., *et al.*, 1994, Therapeutic immunization against Helicobacter infection (Letter). *Lancet.* **343**:913–914.
23. Cuenca, R., *et al.*, 1996, Therapeutic immunization against *Helicobacter mustelae* infection in naturally infected ferrets. *Gastroenterol* **110**:1770–1775.
24. Pappo, J., *et al.*, 1995, Effect of oral immunization with recombinant urease on murine *Helicobacter felis* gastritis. *Infect. Immun.* **63**:1246–1252.
25. Ermak, T. H., *et al.*, 1997, Gastritis in urease-immunized mice after *Helicobacter felis* challenge may be due to residual bacteria. *Gastroenterol* **113**:1118–1128.
26. Blanchard, T. G., Nedrud, J. G., Zagorski, B. M., and Czinn, S. J., 1997, Antimicrobial therapy as an adjunct to oral immunization significantly enhances the resolution of gastritis. *Gut* **41**:A63.
27. Radcliff, F. J., Hazell, S. L., Kolesnikow, T., Doidge, C., and Lee, A., 1997, Catalase, a novel antigen for *Helicobacter pylori* vaccination. *Infect. Immun.* **65**:4668–4674.
28. Marchetti, M. *et al.*, 1998, Protection against *Helicobacter pylori* infection in mice by intragastric vaccination with *H. pylori* antigens is achieved using a non-toxic mutant of *E. coli* heat-labile enterotoxin (LT) as adjuvant. *Vaccine* **16**:33–37.
29. Ghiara, P., *et al.*, 1997, Therapeutic intragastric vaccination against *Helicobacter pylori* in mice eradicates an otherwise chronic infection and confers protection against reinfection. *Infect. Immun.* **65**:4996–5002.
30. Fox, J. G., *et al.*, 1995, *Helicobacter pylori*-induced gastritis in the domestic cat. *Infect. Immun.* **63**:2674–2681.
31. Handt, L. K., *et al.*, 1994, *Helicobacter pylori* isolated from the domestic cat: Public health implications. *Infect. Immun.* **62**:2367–2374.
32. Perkins, S. E., *et al.*, 1998, Experimental infection in cats with a cagA+ human isolate of *Helicobacter pylori. Helicobacter* **3**:225–235.
33. Rossi, G., *et al.*, 2000, Immunohistochemical study of lymphocyte populations infiltrating the gastric mucosa of beagle dogs experimentally infected with *helicobacter pylori. Infect. Immun.* **68**:4769–4772.

34. Eaton, K. A., and Krakowka, S., 1992, Chronic active gastritis due to *Helicobacter pylori* in immunized Gnotobiotic piglets. *Gastroenterol* **103**:1580–1586.
35. Eaton, K. A., Ringler, S. S., and Krakowka, S., 1998, Vaccination of gnotobiotic piglets against *Helicobacter pylori*. *J. Infect. Dis.* **178**:1399–1405.
36. Michetti, P., *et al.*, 1999, Oral immunization with urease and *Escherihia coli* heat-labile enterotoxin is safe and immunogenic in *Helicobacter pylori*-infected adults. *Gastroenterol* **116**:804–812.
37. DiPetrillo, M. D., Tibbetts, T., Kleanthous, H., Killeen, K. P., and Hohmann, E. L., 2000, Safety and immunogenicity of *phoP/phoQ*-deleted *Salmonella typhi* expressing *Helicobacter pylori* urease in adult volunteers. *Vaccine* **18**:449–459.
38. Andelakopoulos, H., and Hohmann, E., 2000, Pilot study of *phoP/phoQ*-deleted *Salmonella enterica* serovar typhimurium expressing *Helicobacter pylori* urease in adult volunteers. *Infect. Immun.* **68**:2135–2141.
39. Blanchard, T. G., *et al.*, 1999, Antibody-independent protective mucosal immunity to gastric Helicobacter infection in mice. *Cell Immunol* **191**:74–80.
40. Ermak, T. H., *et al.*, 1998, Immunization of mice with urease vaccine affords protection against *Helicobacter pylori* infection in the absence of antibodies and is mediated by MHC class II-restricted responses. *J. Exp. Med.* **188**:2277–2288.
41. Blanchard, T. G., Czinn, S. J., Nedrud, J. G., and Redline, R. W., 1995, Helicobacter-associated gastritis in SCID mice. *Infect. Immun.* **63**:1113–1115.
42. Roth, K. A., Kapadia, S. B., Martin, S. M., and Lorenz, R. G., 1999, Cellular immune responses are essential for the development of *Helicobacter felis*-associated gastric pathology. *J. Immunol* **163**:1490–1497.
43. D'Elios, M. M., *et al.*, 1997, T helper 1 effector cells specific for *Helicobacter pylori* in the gastric antrum of patients with peptic ulcer disease. *J. Immunol* **158**:962–967.
44. Fan, X. J., Chua, A., O'Connell, M. A., Kelleher, D., and Keeling, P. W. N., 1993, Interferon-gamma and tumour necrosis factor production in patients with Helicobacter pylori infection. *Irish J. Medl. Sci.* **162**:408–411.
45. Fan, X. J., *et al.*, 1994, Gastric T lymphocyte responses to *Helicobacter pylori* colonisation. *Gut.* **35**:1379–1384.
46. Karttunen, R. A., *et al.*, 1997, Expression of mRNA for interferon-gamma, interleukin-10, and interleukin-12 (p40) in normal gastric mucosa and in mucosa infected with *Helicobacter pylori*. *Scand J. Gastroenterol* **32**:22–27.
47. Karttunen, R., Karttunen, T., Ekre, H.-P. T., and MacDonald, T. T., 1995, Interferon gamma and interleukin 4 secreting cells in the gastric antrum in *Helicobacter pylori* positive and negative gastritis. *Gut.* **36**:341–345.
48. Karttunen, R., *et al.*, 1990, *Helicobacter pylori* induces lymphocyte activation in peripheral blood cultures. *Clin. Exp. Immunol.* **82**:485–488.
49. Bamford, K. B., *et al.*, 1998, Lymphocytes in the human gastric mucosa during *Helicobacter pylori* have a T helper cell 1 phenotype. *Gastroenterol* **114**:482–492.
50. Pappo, J., *et al.*, 1999, Helicobacter pylori Infection in Immunized Mice Lacking Major Histocompatibility Complex Class I and Class II Functions. *Infect. Immun.* **67**:337–341.
51. Blanchard, T. G., *et al.*, 1999, Systemic vaccination inducing either Th1 or Th2 immunity protects mice from challenge with *H. pylori*. *Gastroenterol* **116**:A695.
52. Mohammadi, M., Nedrud, J., Redline, R., Lycke, N., and Czinn, S., 1997, Murine CD4 T cell responses to Helicobacter infection: TH1 cells enhance gastritis and TH2 cells reduce bacterial load. *Gastroenterol* **113**:1848–1857.
53. Radcliff, F. J., Ramsay, A. J., and Lee, A., 1996, Failure of immunisation against Helicobacter infection in IL-4 deficient mice: evidence for a TH2 immune response as the basis for protective immunity. *Gastroenterol* **110**:A997.
54. Eisenberg, J. C., *et al.*, 2000, Immunization of neonatal mice induces protective immunity against *Helicobacter pylori*. *Gastroenterol* **118**:2653.

55. Hu, L.-T., and Mobley, L. T., 1990, Purification and N-terminal analysis of urease from Helicobacter pylori. *Infect. Immun.* **58**:992–998.
56. Lee, C. K., *et al.*, 1995, Oral Immunization with recombinant *Helicobacter pylori* urease induces secretory IgA antibodies and protects mice from challenge with *Helicobacter felis*. *J. Infect. Dis.* **172**:161–172.
57. Holmgren, J., Lycke, N., and Czerkinsky, C., 1993, Cholera toxin and cholera B subunit as oral-mucosal adjuvant and antigen vector systems. *Vaccine* **11**:1179–1184.
58. Blanchard, T. G., Lycke, N., Czinn, S. J., and Nedrud, J. G., 1998, Recombinant cholera toxin B subunit is not an effective mucosal adjuvant for oral immunization of mice against *H. felis*. *Immunol* **94**:22–27.
59. Lee, A., and Chen, M., 1994, Successful immunization against gastric infection with *Helicobacter* species: Use of a cholera toxin B-subunit-whole-cell vaccine. *Infect. Immun.* **62**:3594–3597.
60. Weltzin, R., Guy, B., Thomas, W. D., Jr., Giannasca, P. J., and Monath, T. P., 2000, Parental adjuvant activities of *Escherichia coli* heat-labile toxin and its B subunti for immunization of mice against gastric *Helicobacter pylori* infection. *Infect. Immun.* **68**:2775–2782.
61. Weltzin, R., Kleanthous, H., Guirdkhoo, F., Monath, T. P., and Lee, C. K., 1997, Novel intranasal immunization techniques for antibody induction and protection of mice against gastric *Helicobacter felis* infection. *Vaccine* **15**:370–376.
62. Kleanthous, H., *et al.*, 1997, Effect of route of mucosal immunization with recombinat urease on gastric immune responses and protection against *H. pylori* infection (Abstract). *Immunol Cell Biol* 75 suppl **1**:A93.
63. Corthesy-Theulaz, I. E., *et al.*, 1998, Mice are protected from *Helicobacter pylori* infection by nasal immunization with attenuated *Salmonella typhimurium phoP^c* expressing urease A and B subunits. *Infect. Immun.* **66**:581–586.
64. Whary, M. T., *et al.*, 1997, Promotion of ulcerative duodenitis in young ferrets by oral immunization with Helicobacter mustelae and muramyl dipeptide. *Helicobacter* **2**:65–77.
65. Kim, S. Y., *et al.*, 1999, Induction of mucosal and systemic immune response by oral immunization with H. pylori lysates encapsulated in poly(D,L-lactide-co-glycolide microparticles. *Vaccine* **17**:607–616.
66. Gomez-Duarte, O. G., *et al.*, 1998, Protection of mice against gastric colonization by Helicobacter pylori by single oral dose immunization with attenuated *Salmonella typhimurium* producing urease subunits A and B. *Vaccine* **16**:460–471.
67. Kleanthous, H., *et al.*, 1998, Rectal and intranasal immunizations with recombinant urease induce distinct local and serum immune responses in mice and protect against *Helicobacter pylori* infection. *Infect. Immun.* **66**:2879–2886.
68. Guy, B., *et al.*, 1998, Systemic immunization with urease protects mice against *Helicobacter pylori* infection. *Vaccine* **16**:850–856.
69. Guy, B., Hessler, C., Fourage, S., Rokbi, B., and Quentin Millet, M.-J., 1999, Comparison between targeted and untargeted systemic immunizations with adjuvanted urease to cure *Helicobacter pylori* infection in mice. *Vaccine* **17**:1130–1135.

Index

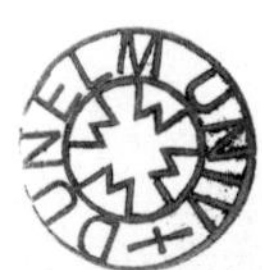